Genetic Theory
and
Abnormal Behavior

David Rosenthal, Ph.D.

Chief, Laboratory of Psychology
National Institute of Mental Health

McGraw-Hill Book Company

New York St. Louis San Francisco Düsseldorf London Mexico Panama Sydney Toronto

This book was set in Caledonia by The Maple
Press Company, and printed on permanent
paper and bound by The Maple Press Com-
pany. The designer was Merrill Haber; the
drawings were done by John Cordes, J. & R.
Technical Services, Inc. The editors were
Walter Maytham and Laura Warner. Paul B.
Poss supervised the production.

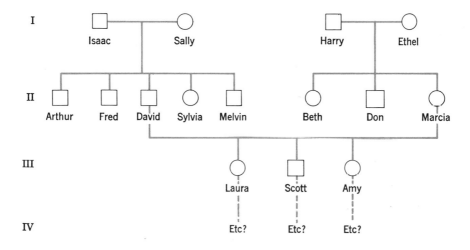

Preface

At the request of Dr. Norman Garmezy, I have taken time and energy from my research activities and other duties to write this textbook. At times during the course of writing, I have felt that I might be like the proverbial bellringer, sounding the knoll to an unhearing congregation. But reflection warrants that the time for such a book is now.

Although the book is intended for students of abnormal psychology, those who may have the greatest want of it are the potential teachers themselves. For many years, I have been continually surprised to learn how little most mental health devotees know about the possible hereditary contributions to the phenomena they are studying and teaching. Moreover, many do not want to know. These include not only most clinical psychologists, but psychiatrists, psychiatric social workers, nurses, social scientists, counselors, physicians, and others who must deal with mentally disturbed persons.

This avoidance behavior occurs especially among those with a psychodynamic bent, and among those who advocate a strict, behavioristic learning approach to all psychological phenomena. Yet B. F. Skinner

Note: The opinions expressed herein are those of the author and do not necessarily express the position of the National Institute of Mental Health.

has compared abnormal behavior to the patterns that occur on a tele-
vision screen when something goes wrong with the set, and Sigmund
Freud stated that: "It does not imply a mystical overvaluation of heredity
if we think it credible that, even before the ego exists, its subsequent
lines of development, tendencies and reactions are already determined."

One can readily find reasons to explain why the possible hereditary
aspects of abnormal behavior have been ignored so long by so many.

1 It seemed desirable to develop a homogeneous set of constructs
from a single domain to account for behavioral phenomena. Thus,
psychoanalysts concentrated on unconscious processes, ego defense
mechanisms, and related psychological and metapsychological concepts, all more or less systematized at a single integrative level.
Learning behaviorists concentrated on objectively perceived and
manipulatable stimulus-response contingencies and on reinforce-
ment schedules. To bring in variables from another domain, for
example, genetic or metabolic factors, would impose a strain on
the theoretical systems and complicate them terribly.

2 Many scientists concerned with social behavior and human values
had been unalterably shocked and revolted by the horror and
degradation stemming from racist interpretations and "applications" of genetic theory. The Nazi holocaust lingers vividly in
memory as the lowest, most evil point in man's history.

3 Most of the early literature on psychiatric genetics was written in
German, by Germans. Even those who were conversant with the
language avoided the literature and distrusted it. Moreover,
English presentations of that literature were sketchy at best, and
were often communicated in a high-handed, almost antagonistic
fashion that tended to alienate far more readers than it won over.

4 Psychiatric geneticists, though paying lip service to environmental
factors, evinced an almost total disregard of them in their theorizing, seemingly negating the possibility of a common meeting
ground for genetic and environmental variables. The conceptualization of how hereditary and environmental factors combine
to influence human behavior is a difficult enterprise at best.
Avoiding the issue was much easier than coming to grips with it.

Nevertheless, during the past decade, there developed among some
workers in the mental health professions a heightened awareness that
much of the variation observed in their patients could not be explained
solely in terms of the conceptual framework they were employing. The
exciting developments in molecular genetics and biology stimulated
interest in how the new-found knowledge in these fields might bear on

abnormal behavior.   New insights into the old literature on psychiatric genetics and new research on genetics of the behavioral disorders demanded attention.   Gradually, more psychologists and psychiatrists began to cast about for a better understanding of this area of study, not only to inform themselves but to carry out their teaching functions in as rounded and conscientious a manner as possible.   Unfortunately, they found the relevant literature to be fragmented, scattered, and somewhat confusing, in the main.   This book may help to make their task easier.

From an opposite point of view, the lack of hard, integrated knowledge in this field did much to encourage many teachers and practitioners to take strong "theoretical" positions, which more often represented preferred beliefs than systematically formulated interpretations of data. It also encouraged such eminent scientists as Julian Huxley and Linus Pauling, to name only two, to speculate about the nature of the metabolic dysfunction that causes schizophrenia.   Surely they would be appalled if laymen, however brilliant, but with only a smattering of information, made analogous speculations in their own fields.   However, Huxley and Pauling are representative of all men in that they cannot resist the irrepressible fascination with abnormal behavior that everyone feels and desires to express in some constructive way.

I have not found the writing of the book easy, since it must provide instruction for potential teachers as well as for students.   The reader may not find many hard, neatly drawn conclusions in the book, but he should find much information that had escaped him before.   In this sense, the book may inform more than it enlightens.

I have wished to do more than present a body of facts and research findings.   Rather, my intention has been to reason about the data where possible so that the reader may reason along with me in a step-by-step fashion.   In this way, he may get a feeling about some of the thinking that underlies research and theory in this field, and at the same time develop his own views in which he may disagree with my own reasoning and improve upon it.   My primary goal is to get students to see the great, untapped potential in this immature field and to stimulate a few to take an active interest in advancing it further.

Chapter 6 is the heart of the book, in part because schizophrenia is the prototypical mental illness, and in part because there is a more vast literature on schizophrenia, with respect to both research and theory, than all other behavioral disorders combined.   The first five chapters are primarily propaedeutic to it.   Chapter 2 presents only as much information about genetic principles that a reader needs to know to understand the subsequent chapters and to read the relevant literature with fair appreciation.   It cannot substitute for a course in genetics.   Interested readers who have no background in genetics may become intrigued enough to study the subject further.   Anyone who has had a course in genetics should simply skip this chapter.

Three acknowledgments are in order.   First, to Barbara McCandlish, my erstwhile assistant during the past year, who helped me in the translation of many of the German articles, and who was of tremendous value in the library research.   Second, to Dr. Gordon Allen, who kindly read a preliminary draft of the book and made many helpful suggestions.   Any errors that remain in the book are mine and not his.   And third, to my wife, Marcia, who bore the arduous task of typing the manuscript in its entirety, and who often helped in making decisions about other practical matters regarding preparation of the book.

DAVID ROSENTHAL

Contents

Chapter Six
Genetic Studies of Schizophrenia (Dementia Praecox)   92

Chapter Seven
Genetic Studies of Manic-depressive Psychosis   201

Chapter Eight
Genetic Studies of Psychopathy and Criminality   222

Chapter Nine
Genetic Studies of Psychoneurosis, Homosexuality, and Alcoholism   240

Chapter Ten
Some Methodological and Theoretical Considerations for Future Studies   264

Glossary of Genetic Terms   279

Name Index   301

Subject Index   309

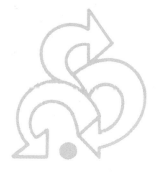

Chapter One

Evolution and Abnormal Behavior

Of all the facts of life, the most important is evolution. If psychology is to take its legitimate place within the family of life sciences, it must eventually integrate its basic theories and facts with those of evolution. If we are to understand abnormal behavior, we must do so in the context of a psychology so conceived and so formulated. These three simple statements constitute the conceptual framework that hopefully will lend vitality and a sense of orientation to the chapters that follow.

EVOLUTION AND NATURAL SELECTION

What is evolution? It is the history of all life on Earth (there may be other forms and histories of life elsewhere in the universe). It is the description of how life first began, of the first organisms, of the physical changes that occurred in these organisms, and of how these changes increased gradually and steadily and innumerably so that new forms or species of living things were constantly appearing and disappearing. We have all heard of viruses and one-celled organisms; of algae; of myriads of grasses, flowers, shrubs, and trees; of insects, birds, fishes,

1

amphibians, reptiles, and mammals. And we are ourselves in the family of man. This whole constellation of life makes one impressive kindred. It is important that we see ourselves as part of that kindred if we are to understand our behavior, and our misbehavior.

Why should species be forever changing? If we think of change as a necessary precursor to variety, and if we realize that variety increases the chances of at least some members of a species surviving in the face of a complex or changing world, then we can appreciate the advantages of change. It is this constant interplay between each organism and the world around it that results in what Charles Darwin called *natural selection*. More specifically, natural selection refers to the processes whereby some organisms perpetuate their kind by reproducing themselves while others fail to do so.

Darwin became aware early in his career that the characteristics of organisms that tended to be perpetuated were useful. The concept of usefulness, along with the concept of variation, was always of primary importance in his thinking. He was impressed, too, by the convergence of usefulness and variation in the domestication and breeding of animals. In such instances, man was carrying out an unconscious or a deliberate process of selection with regard to different characteristics. Darwin knew that man did not *cause* the variation that occurred with selective breeding. Also, he argued against the views of naturalists who "continually refer to external conditions, such as climate, food, etc., as the only possible cause of variation." In 1838, he "happened to read for amusement Malthus on *Population,* and being well prepared to appreciate the struggle for existence which everywhere goes on from long-continued observation of the habits of animals and plants, it at once struck me that under these circumstances favourable variations would tend to be preserved, and unfavourable ones to be destroyed. The result of this would be the formation of new species." It was of course the problem of species formation that had been Darwin's central scientific concern. In Malthus, he discovered the underlying principle for his theory of natural selection.

With respect to abnormal behavior, we ought to remind ourselves to ask whether, since it persists and seems to be perpetuated, it serves any useful purpose at all. We shall grapple with this question later.

At the heart of natural selection are two basic concepts: *survival* and *reproduction.* The phrase *survival of the fittest* is one that Darwin borrowed from Herbert Spencer to describe the *principle of preservation.*[1] It is often thought to epitomize evolution. Strictly speaking,

---

[1] Interestingly, Darwin thought of *survival of the fittest* as a "more accurate" term than *natural selection,* but he used the latter term "to mark its relation

it is a tautology, since, *by definition,* the fittest organisms are conceived as those who survive. In this sense, the phrase is better worded as *survival is the fittest.* But survival is not enough for evolutionary significance. The individual must also reproduce. If he fails to do so, he will not be "selected."

In reproduction, the units of heredity that are passed on from parent to offspring are called genes. When an individual's life ends, he is said to suffer death. If he fails to reproduce, he is said to suffer "genetic death." In the main, his death is a matter of consequence to himself alone. But his genetic death is a matter of consequence to his whole species, for the genes that he could have contributed to the common pool are forever lost.

The process of evolution has been going on for many hundreds of millions of years. During that great span of time, all organisms that did not have the genetic equipment that made for survival or for success in reproduction suffered genetic death. All our forebears, at whatever stage of evolution they appeared, built and locked into a gene pool, more and more with each passing generation, those genes that impelled toward survival and toward successful reproduction. As human beings, we feel and experience these impulsions deeply and profoundly. We call them *instincts* or *drives,* and we have labeled them self-preservation and sex, respectively. To a great extent, they govern and guide our behavior. When they fail us or we fail them, we are likely to suffer physical death or genetic death, and we are likely to experience difficulties in relation to other members of our species and to our own selves.

We share the genetic impulsions toward survival and reproduction with all forms of life that reproduce sexually, but of course we experience them differently and organize and modify them in accord with the physical features of our own species and the cultural characteristics of the group in which we live. But we can be sure that these impulsions will be strong forces in our behavior, and that they will both affect and be affected by all factors that might provoke abnormal behavior. When the impulsion toward self-preservation is affected, in any way for whatever reason, we can expect to find self-destructive or frankly suicidal behavior. When an individual becomes "mentally ill," we can also expect to find profound disturbances in his sexual life and behavior. In fact, self-destructive thoughts and behavior and sexual disturbance of varying degree and kind run rampant through *all* forms of mental illness.

---

to man's power of selection." Historically, Darwin's own term is the one that has survived and become common parlance among biological scientists.

SEX AND
EVOLUTION

The great evolutionary value of sexual reproduction is that, in comparison with asexual reproduction, it increases dramatically the probability of obtaining great variation among the members of a species. The greater variation, in turn, ensures a higher probability that the species will survive and that it will improve its chances of being able to cope successfully with the complex world around it and with possible sudden changes in that world. In this sense, then, sexual reproduction provides a mechanism that facilitates the process whereby the species tends constantly to improve itself.

All sexual reproduction involves two—and only two—sexes. Nevertheless, the specific roles of the two sexes in reproduction differ markedly across the phylogenetic scale. We are concerned here primarily with man. Our species has evolved sexually in accord with a few basic principles which probably hold true for all mammals. There have developed more or less marked differences between the sexes in overt physical characteristics and appearance which make it easier for the sexes to discriminate one another, thereby facilitating the mating process. This fact is readily apparent in man and the higher primates. The male tends to be larger, is generally capable of greater feats of strength than the female, and tends to be dominant. The evolution of these traits probably occurred in part because they were more likely to ensure that a male could protect himself and his social group or family and fend off other males. In man, where the female does not have a clearly demarcated estrus pattern, these traits allow successful mating with females who might not be entirely receptive otherwise. In mammals, too, the female ovulates, bears her young, and nurses and protects the young until they are able to fend for themselves. A mother who does not provide these services maximizes the probability that her young will not survive and that her own genes will thereby be eliminated from the common pool.

THE COURSE
OF EVOLUTION

By and large, evolutionary change is gradual. Many genes subserve the functions necessary for life in particular species. Such genes involve the impulsions to obtain nourishment, for example. Or they involve the mechanisms of digestion, absorption, and the distribution of nutritive elements through the body in the form of available energy;

of transfers of energy as in respiration; of elimination of wastes; of sensitivity or receptivity to the physical energies of the world (for example, light, sound, solidity), and the capacity to respond advantageously to those energies; and others too numerous to list. These become interrelated and interdependent so that the successful functioning of one depends on the successful functioning of another. Although the separate genes underlying these functions may be changeable and variable, the entire system to which they give rise must be somewhat stabilized, and the final, integrated mechanisms they subserve will ensure conservation with regard to the rate of evolutionary change.

For these reasons, although evolution depends on the principle of variation and change, it also involves a principle of *stability*. The principle of variation is best observed in the broad sweep of evolutionary development. The principle of stability is best seen in the predictability of species sameness from one generation to the next. Darwin and animal breeders of his time knew that "like produces like." Some species exist today that have hardly changed at all over hundreds of millions of years.

When sudden changes do occur in the evolutionary process, they are called *mutations*. Mutation means that a particular gene has suddenly changed and given rise to a new, different characteristic or set of characteristics. For example, among fruit flies with red eyes, a fruit fly with white eyes may suddenly appear. If for some reason the new characteristic increases the organism's chances of surviving and reproducing, the new gene is likely to be infused into the common gene pool, and its occurrence will tend to increase. If the new characteristic involves a marked change in a vital function, the individual is likely to die. We say that such a gene is *lethal*. If the new characteristic involves a marked difference or limitation in behavior, so that the individual harboring the gene behaves in ways that are incompatible with the species behavioral and reproductive patterns, the probability of his mating successfully is markedly reduced. We call such a gene *abnormal*.

Mutations occur constantly throughout the phylogenetic scale, but their rate of occurrence is low. Although they often give rise to genes that are lethal or abnormal, they are also often responsible for producing advantageous traits. Usually, mutations do not occur with sufficient frequency to infringe seriously on the principle of stability, so that species change tends to be gradual. Occasionally, a nonrecurring mutation may become incorporated into the evolutionary progression, but its chances of survival decrease with each passing generation unless it has an evolutionary advantage. Most useful mutations may start out as neutral or slightly harmful, but are retained as part of the species reserve of genetic variability, and may later serve a new need or fit into a new constellation of genes.

By and large, the evidence for evolution has been based on the long chain of small changes that have been found between different forms of life, from the smallest organisms to the largest. The progression and linking of species is most readily demonstrated by actual measurements of different physical characteristics and by revealing their similarities, and we therefore tend to think of evolution in terms of physical changes. In museums, we can see the evolutionary development in the size of the horse (from *Eohippus* to current breeds) and understand why his increased size and speed afoot helped him to survive.[2]

In any species we can see physical and behavioral characteristics that are especially suited to obtaining food, escaping danger, or winning a mate. Such observations serve to remind us that the physical characteristics that develop in evolution are relevant primarily to the kinds of behavior they subserve. In and of themselves, they are of little consequence. Evolution is, in fact, concerned above all with the *behaviors* of organisms, especially as these involve survival and reproduction, and we must constantly remind ourselves of this fact.

GENETIC VARIATION
AND BEHAVIOR

Genetic variation is well illustrated in man. We have only to think of the Watusi, who commonly grow to a height of 7 feet, as compared with the 4½-foot-tall pygmies; the different colors of skin—black, white, brown, yellow, and coppery red; the different types of hair—kinky, curly, wavy, or straight; different noses—sharp, long, protruding, flat, snub, or bulbous, with nostrils broad or fine; hair that is blonde, red, orange, sandy, brown, or black; bones that are large and thick or fine and small; and so on. Except for the relatively uncommon instances that occur sometimes in multiple births, no two human beings are genetically alike. For our purposes, it is important to understand the implications of this pervasive fact. Since genes influence so dramatically one's physical characteristics, they are likely to influence one's behavior and mental state as well. We know that newborn babies already vary markedly in their behavior. In fact, it is likely that any broad theory of psychology will have to take into account those genetic effects with which

[2] The course of evolution does not always follow such a direct process of gradual transformation. The development of the horse prior to *Eohippus* was a tortuous process. Periods of rapid transition were common in many species.

people begin life that are manifested as primary individual differences in constitutional makeup and behavior. Just as evolution finds a way to accommodate a principle of stability and a principle of variation at the same time, so must psychology find a way to accommodate principles of behavior that have sweeping generality as well as those that allow for the ever-recurring genetic-behavioral variations among all people.

If it is true that genes influence behavior (in the sense that they are the instrumentalities that lead to differences in the organization, structure, and chemistry of all systems in the body that mediate behavior), it is equally likely that they influence much behavior that we call abnormal. But what is abnormal behavior? The fact is that it is not always easy to define. In a statistical sense, we may try to measure the general behavior of a population quantitatively and say that anyone who deviates markedly from our observed behavioral pattern is abnormal. This view would regard such "abnormal" behavior as normal if it occurred in another population where it was considered acceptable. If we prefer a view that is absolutist rather than relativist, we may try to define abnormal behavior according to clear, strict criteria. For example, if an individual is unable to speak or walk or solve simple problems or keep from having convulsions or say things sensibly, we may say that he is behaving abnormally. Often, however, it is difficult to establish workable criteria for an absolutist view of abnormality.

The absolutist and relativist views of abnormality often become fused (really confused) or blurred. A genetic-evolutionary point of view can be more simply applied to an absolutist than to a relativist conception of abnormal behavior, but it can in fact embody both conceptions.

THE BRAIN AND EVOLUTION

For our purposes, the system in the body that is of primary consequence for behavior, and thus for abnormal behavior, is the nervous system, especially the brain. Man stands highest in the evolutionary scale in that his brain is relatively larger and more differentiated than that of any other species. But newly developed species and organs always reflect their evolutionary heritage; in a related sense, we often hear the phrase—*ontogeny recapitulates phylogeny*. It may help us in thinking about abnormal behavior to know at least a little bit about how man's brain is evolutionarily linked to different aspects of his behavior.

Man retains three types of brain which, in phylogenetically ascend-

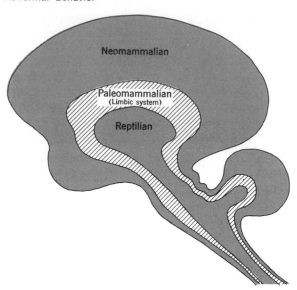

Figure 1-1. The three basic types of brains which in
the evolution of the mammalian forebrain became part
of man's inheritance. The paleomammalian brain,
corresponding to the so-called limbic system or
"visceral" brain, is an inheritance from lower mammals and has been shown to play an important role in
emotional behavior. (From P. D. MacLean, The brain
in relation to empathy and medical education, *J.
Nervous Mental Disease,* 1967, **144**(5). Reprinted
with permission of P. D. MacLean and The Williams &
Wilkins Company, Baltimore.)

ing order, have been called *reptilian, paleomammalian,* and *neomammalian* (see Figure 1-1). The oldest, or reptilian, brain includes structures that subserve primarily simple, automatically triggered types of
behavior. It is responsible for mediating sleep and wakefulness, alert-
ness or arousal, respiration and circulation, and reflexive types of response. It is basic for life, of course, but less interesting to us than
the others.

The paleomammalian brain sits astride the reptilian brain. It is
our heritage from the lower mammals. Together with a few other brain
structures that developed later, it comprises what has been called the
limbic system (see Figure 1-2). It is this system that essentially mediates the impulses to survival and reproduction. It is concerned with
oral functions—chewing, salivation, retching—and with behavior involved in the struggle to obtain food—searching, fighting, self-defense.
Thus the mechanisms for eating and assimilating food are intimately

linked with those required for hunting, that is, the angry attack, defense, or escape that may be called for in the search for food.   In man, this portion of the brain is particularly vulnerable to birth injury, head trauma, and infections.   It mediates, too, feelings associated with threats to survival: terror, fear, foreboding, and sensations of choking or a racing heart; it sometimes mediates anger and possibly strangeness, unreality, wanting to be alone, and feelings of persecution.   One can readily see the relevance of such mechanisms to the development of certain psychiatric conditions.

The limbic system also subserves expressive and feeling states conducive to sociability and other preliminaries of copulation.   Experiments show that stimulation of some parts of this system produces in male cats behavior indicating enhanced pleasure, grooming reactions, and sometimes penile erections, behaviors that are reminiscent of actions observable during feline courtship.   Comparable results are found in monkeys, and this indicates that the great evolutionary enlargement of some regions in the limbic system is associated in part with a shift from olfactory to visual influences in the guidance of sociosexual behavior.   Stimulation of these enlarged parts of the system in the squirrel

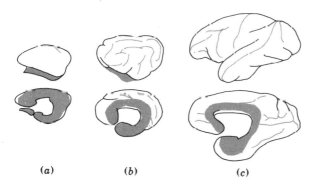

(a)   (b)   (c)

Figure 1-2.   The cortex of the paleomammalian brain (limbic system) is contained in the great limbic lobe surrounding the brain stem.   Shown in black is the location and relative size of the limbic lobe in the brains of (a) the rabbit, (b) the cat, and (c) the monkey.   The ring of limbic cortex is found as a common denominator in the brains of all mammals. The surrounding cortex of the neomammalian brain which undergoes a rapid expansion in evolution is shown in white.   (From P. D. MacLean, The brain in relation to empathy and medical education, *J. Nervous Mental Disease*, 1967, **144**(5).   Reprinted with permission of P. D. MacLean and The Williams & Wilkins Company, Baltimore.)

monkey results in penile erection and display. Such display to another male provides a means of exerting dominance, but to a female it is part of courtship. Of special interest, too, is the fact that the various parts of the limbic system have a close neural relationship, so that electrical stimulation of one part readily spills over into another. If stimulation of the part that induces chewing and salivation is prolonged, these behaviors may be followed by penile erection. In addition, the neural pathways for oral and genital responses converge in that region of the system that is central for the expression of angry, combative, and fearful behavior. In many psychiatric conditions, these functions become entangled and confused.

Man's third brain, the neomammalian, which is also called the *neocortex,* is his distinction and pride. It lies at the top of the other brain structures and envelops them. It appears late in evolution and is common to all primates, but is most extraordinarily developed in man. To this day, it is probably evolving more rapidly than any other bodily organ. The neocortex is responsible for man's vastly superior intellect and his indispensable capacity for language. It enables him to generate and manipulate symbols, to think logically, to conceptualize, to pose and solve complex problems, to recognize choices, and to render decisions. Such behaviors permit us a remarkable degree of flexibility and, therefore, versatility and variety in our behavior. Thus, the neocortex frees us from the more or less limited and constricted range of activities that characterizes all other species. But such behaviors are also vulnerable to psychiatric disturbances of various kinds. Beneath the neocortex, the older parts of the brain and their genetic impulses to carry out evolutionarily desirable behaviors often impinge on the possibilities of plasticity in our behavior. One pervasive attribute of all psychiatric disorders is that our prized plasticity suffers and diminishes. We usually, but not always wittingly, judge the severity of a psychiatric disorder by the extent to which this kind of diminution occurs. It is reasonable to believe that because the neocortex is still evolving relatively rapidly, more genetic "errors"[3] are being committed here than elsewhere in the body and that a number of behavioral disorders due to such errors are probably still occurring.

CULTURE AND EVOLUTION

The ability to survive and reproduce in a complex or changing world is known as *adaptation.* Each species becomes formed in ways that

---

[3] The term *genetic error* is used here to refer to mutating genes that lead to disadvantageous characteristics.

optimize this ability to adapt, usually to a fairly circumscribed set of conditions. If the conditions are very limited, particulate, and unchanging, the mechanisms mediating adaptation tend to be limited, particulate, and unchanging. If the conditions range more broadly and variably, the adaptive mechanisms are likely to be less rigidly patterned and to permit more varied behavior. In this sense, we may say that the environment shapes the species. It determines which genes will be selected.

But the appearance of man's neomammalian brain resulted in an entirely new adaptive relationship between himself and his world. It enabled him to learn to shape his environment to suit himself, thereby reversing the old evolutionary mechanism. He developed a mastery of fire, so that those who required more warmth and who would have died of cold could survive. He domesticated animals and planted crops, so that those who required more nourishment and who would have died when the food supply dwindled did not die. He used animals for transportation and as beasts of burden, so that weaker men and women who could not have borne such hardships were able to live and reproduce. In these instances, and in many, many others, the pattern of natural selection in man changed drastically in ways that we have not yet been able to appreciate fully. This is as true of people suffering from mental illnesses as of man generally. Whereas most mentally ill people up until recent times were not able to breed, because of the disabling effects of their symptoms, advances in medicine and psychiatry, and a moral code which is based on the treatment and welfare of the individual patient, have now enabled many mentally ill persons to marry and to have children, and the number is increasing all the time. This suggests that future generations may include many more mentally ill persons, and those predisposed to mental illness, than exist today.

The total of all changes that man wreaks on his surroundings, his accumulated learning, and the prescriptions and proscriptions that he devises with regard to his own behavior pass on from one generation to another as our cultural heritage. This heritage, in turn, becomes a major evolutionary force in that it mediates for almost all of us those behaviors that individuals had previously had to engage in themselves to ensure their own survival: the production, gathering, and distribution of food; insulation against extremes of climate; and warning and protection against catastrophic natural states or events such as floods, tornados, hurricanes, and aridity. It also influences to a great extent the patterns of mate selection and of reproduction.

At the same time, since a culture takes on the characteristics of an individual to the extent that it subserves and prescribes the behavior required for survival and reproduction, it becomes itself subject to growth and change in an evolutionary sense. It commits itself to the laws of natural selection. Such selection is governed to a large extent by competition for resources. This competition holds true as much for cultures as it does for individuals, and either cultures or individuals who fail to compete successfully will be eliminated. A culture must also be adaptive. It must be geared to the physical and surrounding cultural climates in which it finds itself. If it breeds too many individuals who are weak, diseased, inflexible, retarded, or mentally ill, its ability to adapt will be severely impaired.

A culture also serves as a major environmental milieu that determines who within it will be selected and who will not. It may do this in many ways. It may banish or destroy individuals who hold beliefs deemed alien to it, for example, religious or political beliefs. It may prohibit reproduction by many individuals, for example, priests and nuns. It may imprison or institutionalize certain individuals—such as criminals, mental defectives, and mentally ill persons—for long periods of time, thereby limiting their opportunities to reproduce. It may restrict matings to only certain individuals, as in antimiscegenation laws. It may limit individuals' reproductivity by laws against plural marriage. And it may foster reproductivity, as by antisterilization laws, or fail to limit it, by prohibiting birth control or abortion. Sometimes the persons whose reproductivity is banned or curtailed may be the ones who should perhaps be encouraged to have children, and sometimes the ones who are reproducing may be the ones who should perhaps be discouraged from having children. Sometimes the kinds of matings that are prohibited may be the ones that, because they increase genetic variation, are most consonant with the development of maximal evolutionary potential.

But cultures do not as a rule develop mores because of evolutionary concerns, and it is difficult to sum up and evaluate the total impact of a given culture on evolutionary development. One noteworthy exception is the almost universal taboo against incest, a type of inbreeding pattern that tends to increase the probability that some types of genetic disorder will occur among offspring. The examples indicated, and others too numerous to mention, point up how a culture, perhaps more rapidly than any other environmental force, may shape the characteristics of the individuals who comprise it.

Culture also influences selection with respect to adaptation, and in this sense it is of even greater concern to us here. The meaning of the term adaptation, as it applies to culture, is not identical with the meaning of the term as it applies to evolution, but adaptation is of central importance in both applications and in most conceptions of mental illness as well. In evolution, adaptation means the capacity of a species to develop structures or mechanisms that are relevant to the world around it and enable it to survive and reproduce. With regard to culture, adaptation refers to the individual's or group's ability to accept, share, or participate consentiently in the preservation, modification, or development of cultural norms and prohibitions. Individuals who do not or cannot adapt in this sense may have their lives or reproductivity curtailed by the culture. For example, one type of man—that is, one who is big, strong, insistent upon gratifying his desires with minimal delay, fearless, successful in personal and physical combat, and attractive to women—may have been a great success in a primitive form of society, but in our culture he may be frequently in trouble with the law. He may spend most of his life in jail, and may never reproduce. Thus his failure to adapt to the culture may become consonant with his failure to adapt in an evolutionary sense.

The same is true of many people with psychiatric disorders. For various reasons, such people often do not fit in with other groups. They behave differently, have ideas that are strange or alien to people with whom they are in contact, take extreme or incomprehensible positions, are eccentric, peripheral, or marginal, flout group codes, and otherwise fail to adapt to their primary culture. Some authorities actually *define* mental illness as just this failure in adaptation. Because such persons are often rejected and excluded by their age group, they are often unable to find a spouse and do not reproduce, so that, like our combative male, their failure in cultural adaptation overlaps with their failure in evolutionary adaptation. Whether the culture induces the maladaptive behavior in mentally ill persons or whether the individual's maladaptive behavior stems from genes he harbors is a basic issue in the field of abnormal behavior. A major portion of this book will be devoted to that issue.

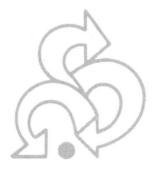

Chapter Two

Some Basic
Genetic
Concepts

Each of us began his behavioral career as a single cell. It is difficult to think of ourselves as a bit of matter of microscopic proportions, but between that cell and the complexly structured person who reads this sentence and comprehends its meaning there is an uninterrupted continuity and even a basic sameness. The genes in that cell recur in all the uncountable normal cells in the body that develops from it. They have never changed. If we are to achieve a fuller understanding of what we are and how we behave, we must eventually know more about these genes and what they do. In this chapter, we will review some of the basic concepts of genetics that we will eventually need to know to understand how knowledge about the genetics of abnormal behavior is achieved and what it tells us.

MITOSIS

Organisms are made of cells. A cell has two major parts: the nucleus and the surrounding cytoplasm. Somatic cells divide through a process known as *mitosis,* which is shown in Figure 2-1. Through mitosis, the original cell (Figure 2-1*a*) ends up as two duplicate daughter cells

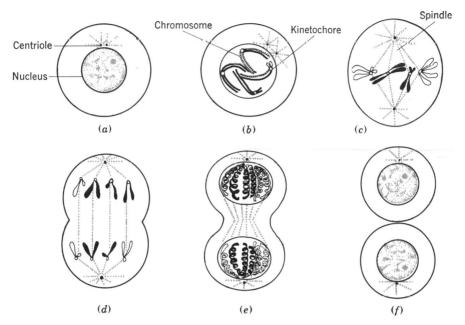

Figure 2-1. Diagram of cell division and mitosis. (Reprinted, with permission, from Curt Stern, *Principles of Human Genetics*, 2d ed., W. H. Freeman and Company, San Francisco, 1960.)

(Figure 2-1*f*), each of which will divide similarly. The chromosomes play the main role in this division. They reside in the nucleus and are the parts of the cell that concern us most. In the first stage, *interphase*, they are less distinctive, but in the next stage of cell division, *prophase*, they appear as elongated, double structures whose two identical parts lie nearly parallel to each other, attached at the kinetochore. Later, the centrioles move to opposite sides of the cell, and what looks like a spindle is formed (Figure 2-1*c*). At the same time, the chromosomes align themselves along the spindle's equatorial plane. This stage is known as *metaphase*. Each kinetochore divides, the sister kinetochores dragging the sister chromosomes toward the polarized centrioles in stages known as *anaphase* and *telophase* (Figure 2-1*d* and *e*). The chromosomes at one pole of the cell are identical with those at the other pole.

Different plants and animals have different numbers of chromosomes. Man has 46 chromosomes, or 23 pairs. Twenty-two pairs are called autosomes, but one pair is called the sex chromosomes, which are designated X and Y. The two chromosomes that make up a pair are said to be *homologous*. Genes occur contiguously in each chromo-

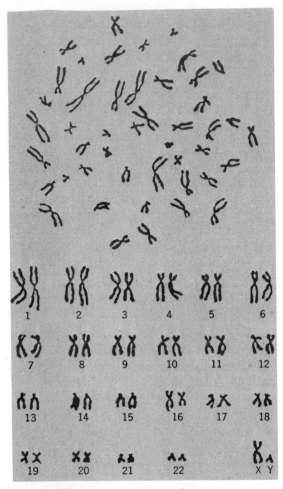

Figure 2-2. Chromosomes of normal human
male. (Reprinted, with permission, from L. S.
Penrose (ed.), *Recent Advances in Human Genetics*, J. and A. Churchill, London, 1961.)

some.   Figure 2-2 shows a photomicrograph or *karyotype* of the chromosomes of a normal male.   In the lower half of the figure, the chromosomes are arranged into appropriate pairs by size, shape, and structure, and numbered accordingly.   Each chromosome appears double because the preparation was made at a stage in which each chromosome had duplicated itself.   Note the great difference in size between the X and Y chromosomes.

MEIOSIS

In mitosis, the cells reproduce themselves. But the cells called the sex or germ cells can reproduce an entire organism. They have the ability to reduce the number of chromosomes to 23 by separating the pairs, so that only one of each pair of homologous chromosomes ends up in the resulting *gamete,* the sperm or the egg. The process of division leading to this reduction during gametogenesis is called *meiosis.* The sequence of events in meiosis is shown separately for males and females in Figure 2-3. Reduction is achieved because, while the cells are dividing twice, the chromosomes duplicate themselves only once.

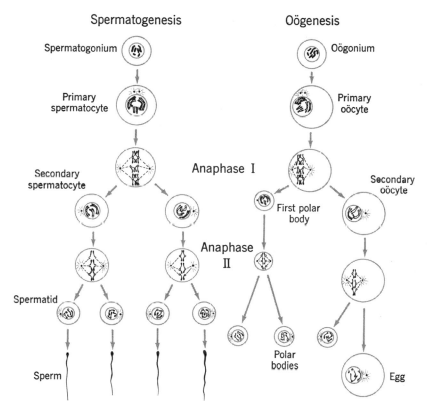

Figure 2-3. Diagram representing the meiotic sequence in the male and female animal: the process of spermatogenesis, resulting in the formation of four sperm; and oögenesis, resulting in the formation of one egg and three polar bodies. (Reprinted, with permission, from E. J. Gardner, *Principles of Genetics,* 2d ed., John Wiley & Sons, Inc., New York, 1960.)

The gametes are *haploid* or *monoploid,* whereas the somatic cells
of higher plants and animals are ordinarily *diploid;* that is, they have
two sets of chromosomes.   When a human sperm and an egg unite, the
resulting cell is diploid; it contains 46 chromosomes, 23 from each parental gamete.   The homologous chromosomes end up as pairs in the
fertilized cell.   It is important to remember, then, that half of a child's
inheritable characteristics come from his father and half from his
mother.   A human female has two X chromosomes, and a male has
one X and one Y.   A child must get one X chromosome from his mother,
but either an X or a Y from his father.   For the most part, it seems
to be a matter of chance whether the X- or the Y-carrying sperm from
the father fertilizes the egg.   Similarly, it is mostly a matter of chance
whether one or another of any homologous pair of autosomes is the
one that ends up in the fertilized cell.   A gene that causes an abnormality may be in a sex chromosome, in which case the disorder is said
to be *sex-linked,* or it may occur in any of the autosomes.

The place on a chromosome that a gene occupies is called its
locus.   Genes that occupy the same loci on homologous chromosomes
are called *alleles* of one another.   If an individual has the same gene
on a pair of homologous chromosomes, he is said to be *homozygous*
for that locus.   If the alleles in the homologous chromosomes differ,
he is said to be *heterozygous* for that locus.

TRAIT DOMINANCE

If a trait or characteristic is determined primarily by genes at a given
locus, one allele may be *dominant* over the other.   The second gene
is then said to be *recessive* to the first.   In genetics a capital letter
is usually used to designate the dominant gene, and a lowercase letter
the recessive gene.   For a given locus an individual may be:

> *AA*: homozygous for the dominant gene
> *aa*: homozygous for the recessive gene
> *Aa*: heterozygous

The designations *AA, aa,* and *Aa* are the kinds of symbols used
to identify *genotypes.*   The forms in which the genotypes are expressed
are called *phenotypes.*   Strictly speaking, dominance and recessiveness
refer to the phenotypes, not the genotypes, but usage and convenience
have led to these terms being applied to the genotypes as well.   Sometimes different genotypes may give rise to the same phenotype; for example, if *A* is completely dominant over *a,* the genotypes *AA* and *Aa*

Table 2-1

Mother

		A	a
	A	AA	Aa
Father			
	a	aA	aa

will give rise to phenotypes that are indistinguishable from one another. Conversely, a given trait such as deafness may derive from a dominant gene in some instances or from a recessive gene in others. There may in fact be several genes—and hence genotypes—that can cause deafness. Similarly, mental deficiency can be caused by more than one gene, and whether there is more than one major gene that can cause a severe psychosis like schizophrenia is not yet a settled question.

If there is a mating between two homozygous genotypes, AA and aa, each child must receive an A gene from one parent and an a gene from the other. That is, all children must be Aa. If both parents are heterozygous, or Aa, the possible genotypes of the children are as shown in Table 2-1.

A child may get one A from each parent and be AA, or one a from each parent and be aa. He may get an A from his father and an a from his mother, or an a from his father and an A from his mother. Both result in the child's being Aa, since Aa and aA are indistinguishable. If we have many matings of Aa parents, one-fourth of the children are likely to be AA, one-half are likely to be Aa, and one-fourth are likely to be aa. If A is completely dominant over a, three-fourths of the children will have one phenotype and one-fourth will have another.

If we have matings of AA × AA parents, all children must be AA, and aa × aa matings must result only in aa children.

With respect to a major psychosis like schizophrenia, some researchers believe that the illness is caused by a dominant gene, and others believe it is caused by a recessive gene. If the former were true, all schizophrenics, with a few rare exceptions, would be Ss; if the latter, all would be ss. We use the letter designations S and s arbitrarily to represent the hypothesized genes.

MENDELIAN RATIOS

Let us consider the genotypes that would occur in the children of different matings if schizophrenia is caused by a completely dominant gene.

A mating between two normal people will be $ss \times ss$. Since the recessive gene in this instance is designated normal, all children will be ss and normal. If a schizophrenic married a normal person, we would have $Ss \times ss$. (We temporarily exclude the possibility of a schizophrenic's being SS, since this genotype would be extremely rare.) Each child has an equal chance of getting the S or the s gene from his schizophrenic parent, in which case the child will be either Ss and schizophrenic or ss and normal. Among the offspring of many such marriages, we would expect half of the children to be schizophrenic. In the rare instances when two schizophrenics married, the parental genotypes would be $Ss \times Ss$. One-fourth of their children would be SS and schizophrenic, one-half would be Ss and schizophrenic, and one-fourth would be ss and normal. All together, three-fourths of the children would be schizophrenic.

Now let us consider what would occur in the children of different matings if schizophrenia were caused by a recessive gene. Most marriages between normal persons would be $SS \times SS$. (We now designate the dominant normal gene as S, the pathogenic recessive as s.) All their children would be SS and normal. Some marriages between normal persons would be $SS \times Ss$. Half their children would be SS and normal, and half would be Ss and also normal. A fewer number of marriages between normal persons would be $Ss \times Ss$. Among their children we would find one-fourth SS and normal, one-half Ss and normal, and one-fourth ss and schizophrenic. Marriages between a schizophrenic and a normal person would be of two types: (1) $ss \times SS$, in which case all children would be Ss and normal; and (2) $ss \times Ss$, in which case half the children would be Ss and normal and half would be ss and schizophrenic. Every marriage between two schizophrenics would be $ss \times ss$. All their children would also have to be ss and schizophrenic.

Some investigators have advocated two-gene theories of schizophrenia. They hold that two pairs of alleles are implicated in causing the illness, not just one pair. Some have thought both were recessive, some have thought both were dominant, and a recent investigator has maintained that one is dominant and the other recessive. To illustrate the types of predictions made by such theories, we will deal with the case where both genes are recessive. Let us designate the two pairs of alleles Ss and Zz. A given parent may pass on to his child SZ, Sz, sZ, or sz. The genotypes of the children from different combinations of transmitted parental genotypes are shown in Table 2-2.

The 16 matings produce 9 genotypes. Only 1 of the children ($sszz$) would be schizophrenic, and only 1 (SSZZ) would not be a carrier of any of the pathogenic recessive genes; 8 would carry one s gene

Table 2-2

	SZ	Sz	sZ	sz
SZ	SZ SZ	SZ Sz	SZ sZ	SZ sz
Sz	Sz SZ	Sz Sz	Sz sZ	Sz sz
sZ	sZ SZ	sZ Sz	sZ sZ	sZ sz
sz	sz SZ	sz Sz	sz sZ	sz sz

Genotype	Frequency
$SSZZ$	1
$SSZz$	2
$SSzz$	1
$SsZZ$	2
$SsZz$	4
$Sszz$	2
$ssZZ$	1
$ssZz$	2
$sszz$	1

and 8 would carry one z gene.   Aside from the schizophrenic genotype, 3 genotypes would be homozygous for the s gene and 3 would be homozygous for the z gene.   According to a strict recessive theory, 15 of the 16 children would be normal.

Let us now consider an alternative hypothesis for the genotypes in Table 2-2, namely, that the two pairs of alleles are independent of each other with regard to phenotypic expression.   Let us also make the assumption that the Ss alleles affect interest in socialization, so that the normal dominant S leads to gregariousness whereas the recessive s leads to social withdrawal.   Let us suppose too that the Zz alleles influence thought patterns, so that the normal dominant Z leads to well-organized, coherent thinking, whereas the recessive z leads to a loosening of the thought associations.

With these assumptions in mind, let us consider the relation between genotypes and phenotypes in Table 2-2.   There are four possible phenotypes: (1) sociable, coherent thinking; (2) sociable, loose associations; (3) asocial, coherent thinking; and (4) asocial, loose associations. The genotypes that lead to sociable, coherent thinking are SSZZ, SSZz, SsZZ, and SsZz. Counting the frequencies of these genotypes, we find 9 in all. The genotypes that lead to sociable, loose associations are SSzz and Sszz. There are 3 such children. The genotypes that lead to asocial, coherent thinking are ssZZ and ssZz. Again, there are 3 such children. The genotype that leads to asocial, loose associations is sszz. Only 1 child has it.

The ratio 9:3:3:1 for two such independently assorting genes was one of the classical discoveries of Gregor Mendel, who also demonstrated the 3:1 phenotype ratio for a pair of alleles with complete dominance. These ratios are often referred to as *Mendelian heredity*. Mendel recognized that the ratio 9:3:3:1 was a multiple of 3:1, that is, $(a + b)^n$. The 3:1 ratio for a single pair of alleles is a *monohybrid* ratio, and 9:3:3:1 is a *dihybrid* ratio. Applying the binomial expansion for three pairs of alleles, we find the trihybrid ratio to be 27:9:9:9:3:3:3:1. The paradigm can be extended to n pairs of alleles. This is clearly a powerful law in genetics.

GENES
AND DNA

As a matter of fact, complete dominance or recessiveness is much more the exception than the rule. Many factors influence phenotypic expression. In the schizophrenia illustration above, it is possible that some of the different genotypes that included the pathological alleles could have been associated with behavioral characteristics that might be considered abnormal but not frankly schizophrenic; other characteristics influenced by these alleles might even be considered desirable.

What are some of the factors involved in the relationship between genotype and phenotype that lead to abrogation of the Mendelian ratios? There are many. But before discussing them, we should know a little more about what genes do. First, we must recognize that a gene is essentially a chemical unit. Although any given gene probably has only a single primary action, each step of the biochemical processes in which it is involved may have many effects on the developing organism. Such multiple effects of a single gene are called *pleiotropic*. It is probable, then, that the effects of the action of one gene are likely to be influenced in turn by the actions of other genes, and there are probably few instances in which a single gene is solely responsible for the development of a given trait. Similarly, since each step in the chemical progression

influences what happens next, it is clear that any single gene may ultimately influence many characteristics rather than just one.

The chemical basis of genes is popularly called DNA (deoxyribonu-
clcic acid). It comprises about 40 percent of the chromosomes, and
is not found elsewhere in the cell. The now famous conceptualization
of DNA, the Watson-Crick model, is shown schematically in Figure
2-4. In the model, DNA is structured as a double helix. Each helix
is a sugar-phosphate chain. The helixes are joined by hydrogen bonds
which bind a purine and a pyrimidine. There are two purines—adenine
and guanine—and two pyrimidines—cytosine and thymine. The four
are called *nucleotides*. Adenine always pairs with thymine, guanine
with cytosine. Thcsc organic base pairs may occur in any order or
sequence. The sequence itself represents the way in which genetic
information is coded. When the helical strands separate, complementary
bases will be constituted and bonded at each purine or pyrimidine site

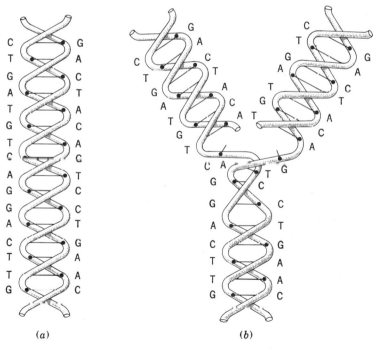

(a)   (b)

Figure 2-4. The double-helix model of (*a*) the gene and chromosome
structure and (*b*) its replication, suggested by the Watson-Crick hypothesis. The genetic "alphabet" of four nucleotides: A = adenine,
C = cytosine, G = guanine, and T = thymine. (Reprinted, with permission, from T. Dobzhansky, *Mankind Evolving*, Yale University Press,
New Haven, Conn., 1967.)

on the chain. In this way, each strand serves as a template from which the original double helix is replicated. This process is the key to reproduction in all living things.

Although DNA provides the information code for the building of proteins, or enzymes, it requires the help of RNA (ribonucleic acid) to get the job done. RNA is found both in cytoplasmic structures and elsewhere in the cell. It transmits the information provided by DNA. Its molecular structure is similar to that of DNA, but instead of thymine, it contains another pyrimidine, uracil. The concentration of DNA in the cell is much more uniform and constant than that of RNA, which changes with the metabolic activity of the cells.

Some leading contemporary geneticists are now classifying genes into four main categories according to the role they play in building a protein. These include (1) *structural genes,* which determine the particular structure or type of protein; (2) *regulatory genes,* which specify the nature of the control systems to which the protein responds in its normal functioning in the cell; (3) *architectural genes,* which are concerned with the integration of a protein into the structure of cells; and (4) *temporal genes,* which control the time at which the other types of genes are activated, and which program the sequence of events in cell differentiation. Such a classification suggests that we must be wary of any oversimplification in our thinking about the relations between genes and traits.

FACTORS ASSOCIATED WITH NON-MENDELIAN RATIOS

Sometimes, instead of dominance, we find what is called *intermediate inheritance.* In such cases, when both parents are homozygous for different alleles, the heterozygous progeny resemble neither. For example, in snapdragons, one parent may be red (RR) and the other white ($R'R'$). The filial generation will all be pink (RR'). Neither the R nor R' genes achieves complete dominance over the other. We also find various *degrees* of incomplete dominance with respect to many genes.

Some genes change, reduce, or amplify the visible effects of other genes; these are *modifiers.* Although a few modifying genes have been identified, it has generally been impossible to locate or identify them or even to analyze critically their individual effects. Often, it is not possible to tell whether certain characteristics are caused by modifiers or by environmental factors. Nevertheless, in genetic studies of mental disorders, modifying genes have often been proposed to explain findings that are not compatible with simple Mendelian ratios.

Sometimes a gene which is not an allele of another gene will mask the expression of the nonallelic gene. This phenomenon is *epistasis.* Dominance involves only genes that are alleles of one another.

Certain events occurring in the chromosomes themselves may also lead to non-Mendelian ratios. One has to do with genetic *linkage,* in which genes located close to one another on a given chromosome tend to segregate together and cause deviations from the expected 9:3:3:1 ratio. *Crossing over,* a very common phenomenon, is an interchange of chromosomal material between the maternal and paternal chromosomes. For example, if *A* and *B* are on the maternal chromosomes, and *a* and *b* on the paternal chromosome, through crossing over *A* and *b* could end up on one chromosome, and *a* and *B* on the other. An illlustration of how this process occurs is provided in Figure 2-5. We can readily see that crossing over is a mechanism that increases many times the possibilities of genetic variation and recombination.

Translocation is the exchange of chromosomal segments between nonhomologous chromosomes. Such exchanges are not normal, and may cause serious disorders such as mongolism. *Inversion* is rearrangement of a group of genes on a chromosome so that their position order is reversed. When a difference in phenotypes occurs because of differ-

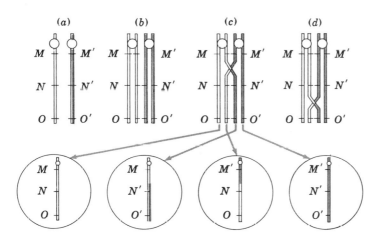

Figure 2-5. Crossing over. (*a*) A pair of homologous chromosomes heterozygous for three pairs of loci *M*, *M'*; *N*, *N'*; and *O*, *O'*. (*b*) Four-strand stage. (*c*) Crossing over between two of the four strands in the region between *M,M'* and *N,N'*. (*d*) Same in the region between *N,N'* and *O,O'*. In the lower row are the four types of reduced chromosome constitutions of the gametes resulting from crossing over in (*c*). (Reprinted, with permission, from Curt Stern, *Principles of Human Genetics,* 2d ed., W. H. Freeman and Company, San Francisco, 1960.)

ences in the positions of genes relative to other genes, it is called a *position effect*.

Deviations from Mendelian ratios may also be caused by *lethal* genes, which render the fertilized cell unable to develop. The "creeper" chicken, a freak with short, crooked legs, is caused by a dominant *C* gene. Matings of two creepers yield two creepers to one normal chick, instead of the expected 3:1 ratio. The *CC* chicks do not appear because all embryos with this genotype die on about the fourth day of incubation.

Mutation

Sometimes the chemical structure of genes changes spontaneously, possibly because of an error or misfit in the duplication of DNA. This phenomenon is known as *mutation*. Mutated genes reproduce themselves in the same way that unmutated genes do. Some genes are more mutable, others much less so. Although mutations are generally recognized by the unexpected, sudden appearance of a characteristic which is not normal to that species, it is probable that most genetic mutations occur without being detected, at least not immediately. The increase in phenotypic species variation to which they give rise may be very slight or may involve minor decrements in fertility or viability, thereby influencing natural selection in less obvious but in definite ways. Further, many—probably most—mutations are recessive, and mutations of recessive genes may remain undetected for a long time.

A mutation may occur in a somatic cell or in a germ cell. Most mutations with large effects are likely not to be useful. Occasionally, a mutation may become useful in a changing environment and facilitate adaptation. Mutations may also be induced, most notably by radiation. Many human abnormal conditions have been associated with mutated genes. A number of investigators have included schizophrenia in this mutation-caused group of disorders and some have even estimated the rate at which they believe the mutations to occur. It now seems likely that such calculations are based on insufficient evidence.

Phenocopies

Sometimes phenotypes resembling others that are genetically caused occur for different reasons. They are known as *phenocopies*. It is believed that, in such instances, environmental agents induce chemical changes similar to those occurring as the result of mutation. Phenocopies have been found in insects, birds, and mammals. They have been produced in the laboratory by high temperatures, by mechanical shaking of eggs at a critical period in their development, and by chemicals. In humans, certain diseases are induced by both the environment and heredity, as heart disease or high blood pressure. Some eye defects following measles cannot be distinguished from certain hereditary diseases. Deafness due to maternal rubella may simulate hereditary deafness. The infamous drug, thalidomide, produces fetal deformities resembling some genetic abnormalities. In psychiatric genetics, many investigators have assumed that some clinical conditions resembling various schizophrenic types of disorder are really phenocopies. However, since the specific nature of the contribution of heredity to schizophrenic disorders is still not clear, the inference of phenocopies seems premature and is as yet very difficult to test.

Sex linkage

Sex-linked traits seem superficially to flout Mendelian laws, but really conform very nicely. These are traits that are determined by genes on the sex chromosomes, and the gene is almost always on the X chromosome. In the rare Y-chromosome linkage, the gene is passed on directly from father to son. In typical sex linkage (X-chromosomal), the male of one generation exhibits a trait that does not occur in any of his children, and the trait turns up again in the male grandchildren. This skipping of a generation was noted by the ancient Greek philosophers, and has stimulated a not-uncommon belief that children get some of their heredity directly from their grandparents. Of course, children inherit all their genes from their parents, but in a loose sense the *trait* has been inherited from the grandfather.

Red-green color blindness is a sex-linked trait. It is caused by a relatively common recessive gene on the X chromosome. The Y chromosome has no allele for this gene, so that when a man has the gene on his X chromosome, the recessive gene acts like a dominant and the trait is expressed. If a woman has the gene on one X chromosome, she is very likely to have the normal dominant allele on the other X chromosome, and she will not manifest the trait. Because of some sex differences regarding the occurrence of mental illness in families, some investigators in the past considered the possibility of sex linkage in such disorders, but, with respect to schizophrenia, no such theory claims our attention today.

Rare recessive genes

Sometimes a trait pops up suddenly in a family that is not caused by a mutation but by a relatively rare recessive gene which both parents happen to have. Recessive genes are difficult to trace, but the probabilities of their occurrence can be calculated in relatives of individuals who show the trait caused by the gene. To aid the calculations, it is common to show the family relationships in pedigrees. Let us consider again a theory that was once widely held, that is, that schizophrenia is caused by a recessive gene. Now let us construct a made-up pedigree which could apply to many hospitalized schizophrenics today. Such a pedigree is shown as Figure 2-6.

In Figure 2-6, the Roman numerals represent the three generations shown. The Arabic numerals represent the descendants in each generation in the order of their birth for each marriage. A circle indicates a female, a square a male. A darkened square or circle indicates that this individual has the trait (in this case, schizophrenia). Others are unaffected.

We know first of all that II-2 has the trait caused by the recessive gene. Therefore, she has the gene in double dose, that is, on both homologous chromosomes. We know too, then, that she must have gotten one gene from each parent, and that each parent is a carrier, that is, has the gene in single dose. Thus each parent is Ss, and II-2 is ss. We know that II-1 and II-3 are not ss, since they are not schizophrenic. They must be SS or Ss. Since the parent mating is $Ss \times Ss$, the probability is $\frac{1}{3}$ that a normal child will be SS and $\frac{2}{3}$ that a normal child will be Ss. The probability that II-1 and II-3 are carriers is $\frac{2}{3}$ for each of them. Since a carrier has a 50:50 chance of passing the suspected s gene on to his children, the probability that the children III-1,2,3,6,7, or 8 are carriers is $\frac{2}{3} \times \frac{1}{2} = \frac{1}{3}$, for each. The children of II-2 *must* get the s gene from her. Therefore the probability that they are carriers is unity. In these calculations, we are assuming that the marital partners in generation II have a probability of zero of being carriers, on the ground that the gene occurs with low frequency in the population at large.

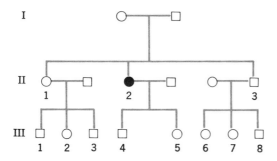

Figure 2-6.

Now let us assume that the first cousins III-1 and III-5 marry. What are their chances of having a schizophrenic child? The probability that III-1 has the s gene is $\frac{2}{3} \times \frac{1}{2}$ or $\frac{1}{3}$. The probability that III-5 has it is 1. If III-1 is in fact Ss, the mating $Ss \times Ss$ will result in one-fourth of their children being ss. We can now calculate the probability of a schizophrenic child resulting from the marriage. It is the product of all the separate probabilities, that is, $\frac{2}{3} \times \frac{1}{2} \times 1 \times \frac{1}{4} = \frac{1}{12}$. If one child should indeed turn out to be schizophrenic, we would then know that III-1 really is a carrier, that the mating is in fact $Ss \times Ss$, and that the probability of any additional child being ss is $\frac{1}{4}$.

Thus, in comparison with the general population, we expect a marked increase in a trait from cousin marriages if the trait is recessive and if the gene is relatively rare. Conversely, when such an increase occurs, it is taken as evidence that the trait is in fact caused by a recessive gene. It is not surprising then that research on psychiatric disorders has included studies of the offspring of consanguineous marriages. Later, we will try to evaluate these studies.

Penetrance

It is known that not every individual who carries a dominant gene or both recessive alleles will manifest the trait. The suppression of the phenotype could be caused by interaction with other genes or by environmental factors. If 80 percent of all individuals who have a dominant gene manifest the trait, the gene is said to have a *penetrance* of 80 percent. The *expressivity* of the gene is the degree to which it manifests itself in different affected individuals. The concept of penetrance has been used widely and freely in the genetics of psychiatric disorders to "explain" deviations from predicted Mendelian ratios. Although the concept could and perhaps should be useful in such studies, many geneticists feel that it is too often used to make ignorance respectable, and that in human genetics, it has been abused to the extent that it is in danger of falling into disrepute.

Multiple-factor inheritance

Of all the influences that blur Mendelian ratios, the most important is probably *multiple-factor inheritance*. When Mendel crossed tall and dwarf varieties of sweet peas, all the filial-generation plants (F_1) were tall ($AA \times aa = Aa + Aa$). When the tall F_1 plants were fertilized by their own pollen, two distinct types of plants appeared again in the second generation (F_2), tall ($\frac{3}{4}$) and short ($\frac{1}{4}$). If, however, tall and dwarf varieties of the tobacco plant (*Nicotiana*) are crossed, the

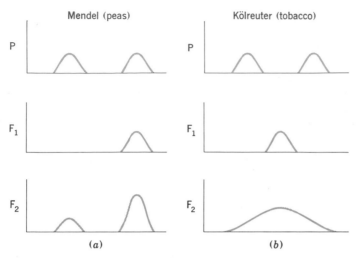

Figure 2-7. Curves representing the results of Mendel's experiments compared with those of Kölreuter. (*a*) P, F₁, and F₂ from Mendel's crosses with garden peas; (*b*) P, F₁, and F₂ from Kölreuter's crosses on tobacco plants. The ordinate represents the number of plants and the abscissa the range in size. (Reprinted, with permission, from E. J. Gardner, *Principles of Genetics,* John Wiley & Sons, Inc., New York, 1960.)

F_1 generation is intermediate in size between the two parent groups. If the F_1 progeny are crossed, the F_2 generation consists of plants that are continuously distributed in size, the distribution forming a normal (bell-shaped) curve whose average height is intermediate between the original parent groups. The contrast between the two types of inheritance is shown in Figure 2-7.

What happens in the tobacco plant is that many genes are acting on size in a cumulative way. The separate genes still segregate independently, in accord with Mendel's law, but it is not possible to detect the action of any single pair of alleles. Sometimes, when the number of allele pairs is small—for example, two or three—and when the phenotype can be classified according to degrees of the phenotype, the correspondence with Mendelian ratios can be demonstrated, these ratios permitting the determination of the number of genes involved.

Genes that act concertedly to produce a cumulative effect on the same character or phenotype are *polygenes*. Polygenic inheritance is characterized by the continuous phenotypical variation noted in *Nicotiana,* in contrast with the segregation of specific and distinctive phenotypes found in the sweet pea. Contributing to the distributions found are dominance, epistasis, cytoplasmic influences, gene interactions, and environmental factors. Many species characteristics, such as height, weight, skin color in humans, and numerous others, derive from polygenic inheritance. Most such traits involve so many genes, and the phenotypes are so continuously graded, that the classical methods of genetic analysis can no longer be applied. Instead, statistical methods have been devised to deal with this type of genetic variation. The field of investigation dealing with polygenic inheritance is known as *quantitative genetics*. It has been estimated that of all practical genetic experiments going on today, between 80 and 90 percent involve quantitative inheritance. With respect to schizophrenia, the view that this disorder has a polygenic basis has been gathering considerable support in the last few years.

THE HARDY-WEINBERG LAW

Although the genes of every individual have implications for the population to which he belongs, evolution is concerned primarily with the genes of entire populations and how the gene frequencies change. What happens to a pair of alleles in the course of generations? Will one allele, for example, a dominant gene, tend to increase in frequency as compared with the other? It should be clear that if one group of AA parents marries a group of aa parents, all their children will be Aa, so that in the offspring generation the dominant and recessive alleles will occur with equal frequency, just as in the parent generation. Now let us take the case where both parents are heterozygous (Aa). Let p stand for the proportion of A, and q for the proportion of a in the parent population, so that $p + q = 1$. The father and mother matings are shown in Table 2-3.

Among the total offspring population, which equals unity, the distribution of alleles is: $p^2(AA) + 2pq(Aa) + q^2(aa) = 1$. Neither allele has gained any advantage in frequency as compared with the other. If,

Table 2-3

Fathers

		$(p)A$	$(q)a$
Mothers	$(p)A$	$(p^2)AA$	$(pq)Aa$
	$(q)a$	$(pq)Aa$	$(q^2)aa$

in fact, in a very large population neither allele mutates more often, and neither allele has any advantage over the other in natural selection, and if marriages occur randomly with respect to the two alleles, not only the relative frequency of the genes, but the proportions of the allelic genotypes, will remain in equilibrium generation after generation. This important fact is known as the Hardy-Weinberg law. It is a central concept in the field of *population genetics.*

To illustrate how this law may be used, let us assume once again that schizophrenia is caused by a recessive gene. Let us assume too that we examine everyone in a population of 1,000 persons and find that 10 of them are schizophrenic (ss). The rest are not schizophrenic, but they could be SS or Ss. We want to know what is the frequency of the s gene in this population. The 10 ss individuals represent q^2 or 0.01 ($\frac{10}{1,000}$) of the population, and $q = \sqrt{0.01} = 0.1$. By definition, $p = 1 - q$ (since $p + q = 1$), or $p = 0.9$, and $p^2 = 0.81$; $pq = 0.1 \times 0.9$ or 0.09. Thus, in the entire population we have the following proportions:

$$p^2(SS) = 0.81$$
$$2pq(Ss) = 0.18$$
$$q^2(ss) = 0.01$$

Since, in fact, it is generally accepted that approximately 1 percent of the population is or becomes schizophrenic, we now can say that if the illness is caused by a recessive gene, then approximately 18 percent of the population are carriers of this gene.

The Hardy-Weinberg law illustrates the stability of the gene pool. It does not apply, however, when a genotype renders individuals more or less fit for a given environment than its counterpart genotype. It does not apply either when matings are not random with respect to the alleles involved. When people with a given genotype tend to marry others with the same genotype, the matings are no longer random, and are called *assortative matings.* It may be that schizophrenics marry other schizophrenics more often than would be expected by chance. If so, this would be an example of assortative mating. Assortative mating, like inbreeding in plants and animals, tends to reduce the proportion of heterozygotes in the population.

BALANCED POLYMORPHISM

Sometimes the heterozygote may have a selective advantage over a normal homozygote. With respect to the locus implicated in sickle-cell anemia, the individuals afflicted with this fatal disease are homozygous with respect to the recessive abnormal allele. Individuals who are heterozygotes, that is, who have the abnormal gene on one chromosome and the normal dominant gene on the other, are especially resistant to malaria and do not have sickle-cell anemia. Those who are homozygous with respect to the normal gene are more likely to contract malaria than are the heterozygotes. Thus the gene that can cause sickle-cell anemia, which in turn would ordinarily cause the gene to be eliminated, also protects against malaria, a fact which tends to favor its selection. The homozygous normal genotype and the heterozygotes eventually reach a point of equilibrium with respect to one another. This equal weighting of positive and negative selection effects is *balanced polymorphism*. It may be that the genes that lead to schizophrenia have a selective advantage when they occur in certain combinations, or in combination with other genes. Later we shall look at the evidence that suggests this possibility.

TWINS

With respect to heredity in abnormal behavior, and in intelligence and personality as well, probably the most common research technique involves the study of twins. Twins originate in two ways:

1 The newly fertilized egg, or *zygote*, divides as expected, but the initially single embryonic structure separates and gives rise to two distinct, complete individuals instead of one. Since all the cells have the same complement of genes and chromosomes, the two individuals deriving from this division are genetically identical. Such twins are *monozygotic* because they originate from the same single zygote.

2 Two maternal eggs are fertilized respectively by two sperm cells, thus forming two distinct individuals. Such twins are commonly called fraternal, but technically they should be called *dizygotic* because they originate as two separate zygotes.

Since the identical or monozygotic twins have exactly the same genes and chromosomes, they must necessarily be of the same sex. Fraternal or dizygotic twins are really ordinary brothers and sisters who happen to be born at the same time. Like any pair of siblings, they may be of the same or opposite sex.

When twins—or individuals of any other relationship—have the same trait or phenotype, they are said to be *concordant* for that trait. If the twins differ with respect to the trait, they are said to be *discordant* with regard to it. Monozygotic twins must be concordant for all traits that are clearly genetically determined, such as eye or hair color, blood types (A, B, O, Rh, and so on), and most other physical characteristics. The concordance rate for dizygotic twins will vary, depending on the mode of inheritance with respect to the trait involved. It should be clear that monozygotic twins will nearly always bear a strong resemblance to one another—as alike as two peas in a pod—but dizygotic twins will resemble each other no more than ordinary siblings. Differences in appearance between monozygotic twins could arise from discrepant prenatal conditions, birth difficulties, illnesses, injuries, nutritional differences, and perhaps other factors, such as life experiences, as well.

If a pair of twins differs with respect to a genetic trait like eye color, we know that they must be dizygotic. However, even when a pair of twins shares all the genetic traits that we can ascertain, the possibility still exists that they may be dizygotic. The best we can do is to state numerically the probability that the twins are in fact monozygotic.

Research involving twins generally assumes that if monozygotic twins are significantly more concordant with respect to a trait than dizygotic twins, the trait itself is genetically caused or influenced. It also assumes that intrapair environmental differences are the same for the two types of twins. With respect to behavioral traits, which often involve learning or other environmental factors, the validity of these assumptions has been seriously questioned. For many years, the most salient evidence for a genetic theory of schizophrenia has been based on the findings of twin studies. Later we shall review this evidence.

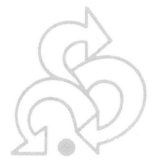

Chapter Three

Research
Strategies and
Methods

THE HEREDITY-ENVIRONMENT PROBLEM

When a trait or disorder follows a Mendelian pattern, we can be quite certain about the genetic basis of that disorder. If it does not, we must look for the factors that cause the deviation from Mendelian ratios and, in fact, question whether the disorder is genetically determined at all. Nongenetic factors are called *environmental*. Environmental factors can be cellular ones, such as cytoplasmic or other biological influences, or others perhaps less tangible or demonstrable.

When a trait or disorder is behavioral, that is, involves no known specific biological manifestation, we must be doubly careful to pay attention to the possible influence of environmental factors. This is true for two main reasons:

1 So much of behavior is learned, and so much behavior can be shaped or determined by external stimuli, that it is difficult to think of any behavior that may not be so influenced.

2 Behaviors are difficult to define or delimit; this is especially true of nonlaboratory human behaviors, which tend to shade off one

into another. To ascribe genetic bases to such behaviors, therefore, becomes a precarious enterprise, though not an impossible one.

In the strictest sense, there can be no genetic expression without environment. In turn, environment is meaningful only with regard to the particular organism whose form, structure, and capacity for behavioral response are programmed from conception by his specific complement of genes. From the moment of conception, and in the gamete stages as well, heredity (genes) and environment are always in interaction with one another, always influencing one another, in more or less degree. Ideally, of course, understanding these processes as fully as possible involves studying them as mutually dependent processes and recognizing their inevitable lifelong interaction. However, it helps us to do research on the problem if we simplify the actual state of affairs conceptually and think of the genes and environments separately and independently.

Research on the genetics of the behavioral disorders must take these principles into account. The approaches used in such investigations may be thought of as research strategies. There are a number of them that we can describe and evaluate with regard to the conclusiveness of the data derived by each. At this stage of our knowledge, we are not able to point to particular genes, chromosomes, or biochemical processes that cause the so-called functional behavioral disorders. We can only look at patterns of occurrence and statistical constellations and make inferences about hereditary influences from such information.

PEDIGREE ANALYSIS

In this method, the investigator first finds a case that is representative of the disorder he is studying. This individual is the *index case*. The investigator then examines each relative of the index case, both lineal (direct descent) and collateral (siblings, aunts, uncles, nephews, and so on). Ideally, he should see and examine each relative personally. Practically, this is often impossible. Many relatives may have died or migrated. Some may refuse to be seen. The investigator may in such instances have to rely on the verbal reports of relatives or friends, or if the relative has had contact with a physician, psychiatrist, clinic, or hospital, their reports may be available to the investigator. He should include every family member. Information about the number and sex of the relatives usually has to be obtained from the relatives themselves, but sometimes birth records can provide precise information. When all relatives are identified, the investigator plots the relationships in a manner similar to that shown in Figure 2-6.   Standard notational systems are available which facilitate communication about the individuals in the pedigree.   At least two generations are necessary for the analysis to be meaningful, but it is preferable to include more.   A similar pedigree must be compiled for each new index case, and the pedigrees then compared to see if they are consistent with a given Mendelian pattern.   Sometimes, for a given trait, a researcher may find pedigrees indicating both dominance and recessiveness.   This is the case in human albinism: both a dominant and a recessive gene can cause the condition.

CONSANGUINITY STUDIES

Most—but not all—investigators have given up hope of finding pedigree patterns that might throw light on the nature of genetic transmission in most of the functional behavioral disorders, that is, on whether the gene or genes involved are dominant or recessive.   Instead they may hold that if the incidence of a disorder among the relatives of patients with the same disorder is higher than the incidence in the general population, the disorder is genetic or at least genetically influenced.   Moreover, if a higher incidence among first-degree relatives (parents, sibs, children) than among second-degree relatives (aunts, nephews, grandparents) or relatives further removed can be demonstrated, we can infer a genetic basis for the disorder.   Such studies therefore depend on the strength of the association between incidence and degree of consanguinity, or blood relationship.

Although such studies are well worth undertaking for their own sake, the inference of a genetic basis must be held in abeyance until it can be shown that the association between incidence and consanguinity cannot be explained on some other basis.   We might conceivably find a similar association with respect to some infectious diseases or with respect to a trait like poverty, where environmental factors may be of overriding importance.   As a matter of fact, just such an association would be predicted by many clinical psychologists and psychiatrists who hold that the occurrence of functional behavioral disorders results from peculiar or unusual behavior that takes place in certain families.

Determination of incidence in the general population

Consanguinity studies depend first of all on knowing what the incidence of the disorder in the population is.   It is important to make a distinction between *incidence* and *prevalence*.   If we were to collect data on a certain day regarding all persons with schizophrenia, we would have an example of the prevalence of schizophrenia in the population, that is, how many cases exist at a certain time. To know the incidence, however, we must also know who, in the same population, has been schizophrenic at some time in the past and who will develop the illness in the future. Clearly, it is more difficult to obtain reliable incidence figures.

Four of the most common sampling methods used to determine incidence involve the following sources of subjects:

1 *Normal probands.* The investigator begins with a randomly selected sample of *unaffected* subjects and determines the incidence of the disorder among their relatives.

2 *Past birth registers.* The investigator obtains a random sample or a consecutive series of names from a birth register that may date back 50 or 60 years, and he traces each one's psychiatric history.

3 *Total census.* For practical reasons, the investigator limits his sample to a defined geographical area in which he examines and diagnoses every person in the specified part of the population.

4 A fourth, less widely used, method is based on all new cases that occur in a given period of time, for example, one year.

Each method has its own problems, and the reader can probably think of many of them. None is easy to carry out. One could readily think of another method, at least as desirable as the others, in which the investigation begins with a large, randomly selected group (or *cohort*) of babies and follows them through the period of life in which they would be expected to show the disorder, if they are going to show it at all. This period is called the *age of risk.* Of course, this method poses problems that may be even greater than those in the four methods cited.

Incidence in relatives

To determine the incidence of a disorder among relatives, the investigator must begin with a series of cases who have the disorder. As noted earlier, the pivotal subjects with whom the study starts are known as the index cases (or *probands* or *propositi*). How one collects his index cases is critical, since biases may crop up readily in such work. For example, in the pedigree method, an investigator may have been particularly impressed by a pedigree with a large number of afflicted individuals. If he publishes this pedigree alone as representative of the genetics of the disorder, he may well be overlooking other pedigrees where the number and distribution of affected family members differ markedly. As we saw in the previous chapter, in genetics we always deal with probabilities, since for each locus either one of two alleles may be passed on by each parent to each child. With each conception, the same chances of particular combinations of alleles occurring repeat themselves anew. By chance alone, unusual frequencies of one particular combination can be expected to occur sometimes in families.

It is common knowledge too that our attention tends to be drawn to the unusual or the unexpected, or to those events that fit in with our particular frame of reference or system of beliefs. Therefore, if we rely only on reports by individuals—whether lay or professional—to find our index cases, we have an excellent chance of introducing bias into our sample. Ways of obtaining systematic samples of index cases exist and should of course be used.

Let us assume now that we have collected such an unbiased, systematic sample. How do we determine the incidence of the disorder among the involved relatives? For genetic analysis, we are not interested in a simple count alone; we want to know how consistent the figures are with a particular mode of genetic transmission. To illustrate a method used commonly, the Weinberg proband method, let us postulate a disorder that is caused by a recessive gene, and let us consider 16 couples with both partners heterozygotes, each couple having two children. Among the 32 offspring, we expect one-fourth, or 8, of the children to be affected. The most likely distribution of affected cases among the families is shown in Table 3-1.

Now let us assume that an investigator embarks on a study of this disorder. He begins by searching systematically for index cases, and indeed he finds all the affected children in Table 3-1. There are 8

Table 3-1
Most Likely Distribution of Affected Cases among Families When the Gene Is Recessive

Families	Families	Families	Families
1 $AA*$	5 AN	9 NN	13 NN
2 AN	6 AN	10 NN	14 NN
3 AN	7 AN	11 NN	15 NN
4 AN	8 NN	12 NN	16 NN

$* A$ = affected; N = nonaffected.

such children represented in 7 families. If he wished to calculate the
incidence of the the disorder among the siblings, he could include the
index cases, which means he finds 8 of 14 children affected, or 57.1
percent, or he could exclude the index cases and count only the sibs
who were not index cases, or zero percent. Clearly, both procedures
would be genetically misleading. It is important to observe that 9 of
the families who could have contributed index cases, but by chance
did not, remain completely unknown to the investigator, who must then
make some allowance for the lost families. The Weinberg proband
method makes this correction.

In this method, the family is counted once for each instance of
the disorder it contains, but the proband is rejected as well. The probability p that a child of heterozygous parents will be affected is calculated
by the formula:

$$p = \frac{\Sigma[x(x-1)]}{\Sigma[x(s-1)]}$$

where

x = number of affected children in family, including the proband
s = total number of children in family
n = number of families with respect to different values of x

The calculations for the data given in Table 3-1 are set forth in
Table 3-2.

Of course, we are interested not only in incidences that occur in
families where both parents are heterozygous or in other instances where
neither parent is affected. Sometimes marriages occur between an
affected and a nonaffected person and, more rarely, between two affected
persons. We will not present here the different methods that have been
devised for these respective marital situations. The problem from the
geneticist's point of view is already demonstrated by the above illustration of the Weinberg proband method. Later, we will discuss the strategic value of studies involving marriages between two affected persons.

Table 3-2

Method of Calculation Used in the Weinberg Proband Method

n	x	$\Sigma[x(x-1)]$	s	$x(s-1)$	$\Sigma[x(s-1)]$
1	2	$\Sigma(2) = 2$	2	$2(2-1) = 2$	$\Sigma(2) = 2$
6	1	$\Sigma(0) = 0$	2	$1(2-1) = 1$	$\Sigma(1) = 6$
		Total = 2			Total = 8
$p = \frac{2}{8} = 0.25$					

However, another common methodological problem should be discussed at this point. An investigator is likely to find that a sizable number of relatives of his index cases are of variable ages and that some others have died or disappeared from view at different ages. Should they be counted or excluded? Should the well twenty-year-old brother of a schizophrenic be counted as nonaffected? How about a forty-year-old brother? May not either one yet develop the illness?

In a disorder like schizophrenia, the age of onset, as measured by age at first hospitalization, typically occurs some time after childhood. By the forties or fifties, new admissions for this disorder are infrequent, and sometimes the diagnosis at later ages is questionable. We can actually chart the age of first admissions for males and females in the entire population and apportion to each relative a remaining-risk value, depending on the point on the curve where his age places him. This method is rather tedious, especially for large samples, and some corrections need to be added as well. The aforementioned Weinberg proposed a shorter method which gives a fair approximation to the more laborious procedure.

In Weinberg's short method, the investigator decides on an age of risk that he thinks will provide the best approximation to the rate of affected cases that would eventuate if all relatives lived long lives and could be followed to their death. With regard to schizophrenia, the age of risk most commonly used is fifteen to forty-five. Every relative in this age range is counted as half a subject. Relatives younger than fifteen are not counted at all and those over forty-five are counted as full risk-completed subjects. The investigator does not arrive at a precise knowledge of the actual incidence in his sample, but makes what is known as a *morbidity-risk estimate*. This estimate could be made

Table 3-3
Illustration of the Weinberg Short Method to Calculate Morbidity Risk

Age	Affected Ss (z)	All Ss in Sample (n)	Risk Completed (r)	Corrected Sample Size (n × r)
0–14	0	100	0	0
15–45	10	200	0.5	100
46+	20	300	1.0	300
Total	30	600		400

Morbidity-risk estimate: $m = \dfrac{\Sigma(z)}{\Sigma(n \times r)} = \dfrac{30}{400} = 0.075$, or 7.5 percent to approach the actual incidence very closely by selecting the most suitable age of risk, but to do this we would first have to know what the actual incidence is, and of course this is what we are trying to find out.

The calculation of a morbidity-risk estimate by Weinberg's short method is given in the imaginary example of Table 3-3. The standard error of m can also be calculated:

$$\sigma_m = \sqrt{\frac{m(1 - m)}{N}}$$

where $N = \Sigma(n \times r)$. In the above illustration,

$$\sigma_m = \sqrt{\frac{0.075(1 - 0.075)}{400}}$$
$$= \pm 0.013$$

With this method, the investigator must be wary of two major sources of possible error. One has to do with the distribution of the age at onset in the general population and in the sample under study. If both distributions are normal, or if age at onset is evenly or similarly distributed in both, there is no problem. If not, then the estimate may be considerably biased. The second error involves a possible correlation in age at onset between relatives. If this is not taken into account, the estimate will be misleading. Compared with these possible sources of error, σ_m may be small or even negligible.

At this point, it is well worth reminding ourselves that family-incidence studies per se tell us nothing about the cause of the disorder. Neither do pedigree studies, unless the pedigrees or the family incidences show a clear Mendelian pattern. When the latter occurs, the inference of a genetic cause can be made with fair confidence, since it is hardly possible that any environmental factors could produce the disorders in the same ratios. In the functional behavioral disorders, however, clear Mendelian patterns do not occur. We are therefore still faced with the problem of devising research strategies that can provide definite evidence for a genetic cause or an environmental cause. If we find both, we must devise studies to determine what the specific genetic and environmental causes are and how they combine to produce the clinically observed disorder.

Consanguineous marriages

Recessive genes that cause severe disorders tend to occur with very low frequency in the general population. Therefore, the chance of a mating occurring between two persons who are both carriers of the gene will be extremely small indeed. If only 1 person in 100 carries the gene, the probability of a marriage between two carriers is 0.01×0.01, or 0.0001; and of their children, only 1 in 4 will be affected, that is, have the gene in double dose. If, however, one suspects that a disorder is caused by a recessive gene, one can expect to find an increased incidence of the disorder among the children of cousin marriages. This problem was discussed in Chapter 2 in connection with Figure 2-6.

The investigator employing this research strategy may follow either of two methods.

1 He may first try to find all cousin marriages that took place in stipulated years past, and then examine all their progeny to see if the incidence of the disorder among them is greater than that in the general population. This is clearly a forbidding task, since it is difficult, if not impossible, to learn which marriages of long ago involved cousins, and since the numbers required to obtain a sample size that would permit a reliable calculation of incidence would have to be fairly large.

2 He may obtain a cohort of subjects who have the disorder and find out what proportion of them came from cousin marriages. Since it is difficult to find the rate of cousin marriages in the population at large, he may select a group of control subjects and determine the proportion of cousin marriages among their parents. The rates of cousin marriages among parents of both groups may then be compared. A higher rate for the index group would be presumptive evidence of a recessive gene contributing to the cause of illness.

One difficulty of the latter method is that information about whether or not parental marriages are consanguineous has in most instances to be obtained from the subjects, parents, or relatives, who may not always be reliable. Another problem arises from the possibility that people who marry their first cousins may do so because of personality difficulties, and that the latter may be instrumental in inducing behavioral disorders in their children. Thus the inference of a causative recessive gene from such studies alone may be precarious.

Dual mating studies

Dual matings are so called because both marital partners have the trait or disorder under study. If the disorder is caused by a single gene, each parent will be a heterozygote if the gene is dominant (except in rare instances), and each will be a homozygote if the gene is recessive. In matings where one partner has the disorder and the other does not, we do not know if the nonaffected partner is a carrier or not. Hence, dual mating studies are particularly strategic. If the gene is dominant, matings will be of the $Aa \times Aa$ variety. The offspring will be one-fourth AA, one-half Aa, and one-fourth aa. Thus, 75 percent of the offspring should show the disorder. If the gene is recessive, matings will be $aa \times aa$. All children will also be aa and all should be affected. Deviations from such rates require the postulation of other factors, such as incomplete penetrance or genetic modifiers to account for the deviations, or abandonment of the single-gene hypothesis; or they may reflect the importance of nongenetic factors.

TWIN STUDIES

Before systematic studies of psychiatric disorders were done, many case reports of twins were published. They tended to be mostly cases of monozygotic (MZ) pairs who were concordant for the disorder. There was less interest in dizygotic (DZ) or in discordant pairs. Later, investigators realized that if they did not have strict control over their sampling of twins, they would be getting an excess of concordant MZ pairs. In the main, they have obtained their twin samples from resident hospital populations, from consecutive admissions to hospitals, or from twin registers.

In some instances, investigators have had to learn which patients were twins by asking the patients themselves or their relatives. It is possible that some twins are missed this way, especially if clerks who carry out the inquiry are not assiduous. Some twins might prefer not to admit their twinship. One way to avoid such possibilities is to check the name and birth date of each admitted patient against birth records that report twin births. This is a laborious task.

If one samples from resident hospital populations, one is likely to include a relative excess of chronic, severely ill cases. Those who had improved and were discharged are more likely to be missed. This could produce inflated concordance rates if chronicity or severity of illness is associated with concordance. When one samples from consecutive admissions, the subjects are likely to be young, and the cotwins may still have many years to live before completing the risk period. If one begins with a twins' register, in which the birth of all twins over a period of many years is recorded, one finds that many twins have died or emigrated or cannot be found, and among the rest only a small

fraction have the disorder.   This procedure is also arduous and time-
consuming.   Each method has its advantages and disadvantages.

When the investigator has collected his index twins, he must determine if each is an MZ or DZ twin.   Zygosity determination may pose
several problems.   Sometimes the cotwin is dead or not available.   The
investigator may discard the pair, which could introduce a bias, or he
may rely on the testimony of the index twin or relatives to decide about
the zygosity of the pair.   The testimony may not be reliable.   Sometimes photographs are available and helpful.   Similarity in appearance
is not always sufficient to make an accurate zygosity determination.   Obvious dissimilarities in certain traits, however, clearly label the twins
as DZ.   Birth information may be helpful.   If the twins developed in
one chorion (a fetal membrane), they must be MZ.   If there were two
chorions, the pair could be MZ or DZ.   The best assurance of accuracy
is provided by serological tests of blood characteristics known to be
caused by single, major genes.   The accuracy can be increased if the
same tests of the twins' parents are available.

A problem may arise if a given investigator determines both the
zygosity of the twins and the presence or absence of the trait or disorder
in the cotwin.   If the trait or symptoms in the cotwin are ambiguous,
knowledge of zygosity may influence the investigator to make a judgment
of concordance or discordance that he might not have made without
that knowledge.

If he finds even a single pair of MZ twins discordant for a given
disorder, does that not constitute proof that the disorder is not genetically caused since both twins have the same genes?   The answer is
no, since the responsible gene or genes may not show complete penetrance.   However, the discordance does show that other factors that
are nongenetic are influencing the phenotype, either by enhancing expression in the affected twin or by retarding it in the nonaffected twin.

Since concordance in the functional-behavioral disorders is based
on behavioral similarities, are there not many environmental factors that
induce MZ twins to behave like one another, in sickness as well as
in health?   Would not a higher concordance rate in MZ than DZ twins
simply be reflecting this fact?   Certainly the possibility exists, but it
must be proved.   Even today, parents tend to dress their MZ twins
alike and treat them similarly, and this behavior was even more prevalent
in times past.

The twins are often mistaken for one another by all sorts of people
of close or distant relationship.   The twins themselves perceive the identity between them and are influenced by this perception.   They often
become closely attached to one another and feel part of each other,
almost like Siamese twins, who are in fact MZ twins that are physically

attached together. They tend to share the same friends and experiences. If they behave alike in early infancy and childhood, they will tend to elicit similar responses from caretakers and in turn respond similarly to them. People often expect—almost require—MZ twins to be alike. Thus, they are subject to a number of pressures toward psychological similarity, both internal and external.

However, there are concomitant pressures toward dissimilarity in MZ twins as well. They are more likely to have been subject to prenatal circulatory influences which place one twin at a disadvantage, so that he will be born smaller, and perhaps always be smaller, less able physically and intellectually, and perhaps psychologically less competent generally than the more fortunate twin. Parents and other acquaintances may exaggerate minuscule differences between them to help in identifying each. Some parents, influenced by modern rearing views, prefer to deny that their twins are in fact identical and deliberately contrive to treat them differently. The twins themselves often develop complementary roles which tend to differentiate them behaviorally and psychologically. They are sometimes mirror images of one another, in which case one is right-handed and the other left-handed, and they perhaps exhibit differing psychological traits as well.

DZ twins, who are more likely to look and behave differently from birth, will tend to elicit more varied responses from caretakers and others all through life. They may experience some of the same external pressures toward similarity that MZ twins experience, but the greater inappropriateness of such pressures in the case of DZ twins may make for psychological problems of a different kind. This is especially true if the twins are of opposite sex.

The Weinberg difference method

It would be possible to obtain an estimate of the sampling bias in a series of twins if we knew the proportions of different kinds of twins in the general population. In the United States, approximately one-third of all twins are MZ, one-third same-sexed DZ, and one-third opposite-sexed DZ. However, these ratios may vary from one state or country to another, or from one race to another. This variation occurs mostly because of DZ births, the frequency of which is influenced by genetic factors, and others such as maternal age, average family size, or fertility drugs. MZ twinning does not seem to be affected by such factors. In Scandinavia and in American Negroes, twins occur about once in every 70 births, but in Japan they occur about once in 145 births. These differences primarily reflect variations in DZ births.

However, DZ births are like ordinary births in that each DZ twin has a separate complement of genes from each parent. The proportion of males (♂) and females (♀) among them will be the same as the proportion among all births. Each child has an equal chance of being ♂ or ♀, and each pair has an equal chance of being ♂ ♂, ♀ ♀, ♂ ♀, or ♀ ♂. Thus the number of opposite-sexed pairs should be equal to the number of same-sexed pairs. The Weinberg difference method takes advantage of this fact.

In this method, one simply counts the number of opposite-sexed twins in the sample. From among all same-sexed pairs, an equal number should be same-sexed DZ. The remaining pairs should be MZ. Thus, a quick and ready method is available to estimate the number of MZ pairs expected in the sample. If the actual count by zygosity diagnostic methods differs significantly from this estimate, the investigator can infer that some biasing factor has influenced his sample.

Concordance and heritability in twins

Investigators have calculated concordance as either a *pairwise* concordance rate or a *proband* concordance rate. The pairwise concordance rate is simply the proportion of affected twin pairs in which both members are affected, that is, $C/(C + D)$, where C and D = the number of pairs in a twin sample who are concordant and discordant for the trait, respectively. If the twin sample comprised all cases in a geographical or total population, the same formula would represent the concordance rate for that population. If it is not a total sample, it may be that the concordant pairs are overrepresented, since each such pair has a double chance of *ascertainment* (coming into the sample) as compared with the discordant pairs. To allow for this possibility, a corrected or transformed pairwise concordance rate may be calculated by the formula:

$$\frac{\frac{1}{2}(C + x)}{\frac{1}{2}(C + x) + D}$$

where C and D again equal the total number of concordant and discordant pairs, respectively, and x equals the number of concordant pairs in which each twin was independently found in the original sampling, and not found as a result of the fact that his cotwin was an index case.

The proband concordance rate is obtained by the application of Weinberg's proband method, which treats twin pairs as sibships of two. It answers the question: If one twin is affected, what is the probability that his cotwin will also be affected? It is calculated as

$$\frac{C + x}{C + x + D}$$

where C, x, and D have the same meanings as before.

Typically, the concordance rates are calculated for MZ and DZ pairs separately, and then compared. If the rate for MZ pairs is significantly greater, the investigator is inclined to infer that the trait is inherited. When he does, he is making the assumption that intrapair environmental differences are the same in MZ and DZ twins. As we saw, this assumption may or may not be tenable, depending on the trait or disorder in question, and the relevance of MZ-DZ psychological differences and of other environmental factors to that particular trait or disorder. Ideally, the tenability of the assumption should be assessed independently with respect to each trait or disorder studied.

The ratio between concordance rates in MZ and DZ twins is often used in the calculation of *heritability,* the degree to which the phenotype (trait or disorder) is caused by the genotype. In more technical, precise language, it is the genetic variance expressed as a proportion of the phenotypic variance, or

$$h^2 = \frac{\sigma_g^2}{\sigma_p^2} = \frac{\sigma_g^2}{\sigma_g^2 + \sigma_e^2}$$

where

h^2 = heritability
σ_g^2 = genetic variance
σ_e^2 = variance due to environment
σ_p^2 = phenotypic variance

Heritability is thus considered useful as an indicator of how much of the disorder is attributable to heredity and approximately how much to environment.

With respect to disorders whose presence or absence can be decided on a yes or no basis, heritability in twins has usually been calculated by the formula

$$H = \frac{CMZ - CDZ}{100 - CDZ}$$

where H = heritability, and CMZ and CDZ = the concordance rates for MZ and DZ twins, respectively. Often, only same-sexed pairs are included in the DZ group. When $CDZ \geq CMZ$, H = zero or is genetically noncontributory. A peculiar characteristic of this formula is that if CMZ = 100 percent and CDZ is any value less than that, that is, from zero to 99 percent, H = 1.00. Thus this can be a clumsy and perhaps misleading measure of heritability, especially when CMZ and CDZ are both large. The assumption that the relevant intrapair environmental differences are equal in MZ and DZ pairs must still be met.

Twins reared apart

Since MZ twins may exert a strong psychological influence on one another, and since they may be reared "alike" if they grow up in the same household, efforts have been made to find MZ twins who were separated at early ages and who grew up without knowing one another. Concordance rates among such twins can be compared with those of DZ twins reared apart and with MZ twins reared together. The first comparison would yield a better estimate of heritability in that the environmental factors are more likely to be randomized equally between MZ and DZ pairs. The comparison with MZ twins reared together could provide some evidence about the contribution to the concordance rates of environmental factors involved in common rearing.

Discordant MZ twins

Since MZ twins are genetically the same, differences between them must be the result of environmental factors. As noted before, such factors may involve prenatal influences, disease, nutrition, injury, rearing, life experiences of various kinds, and so on. One could possibly find out which of these environmental factors contributed to the differences if one studied intensively pairs of discordant MZ twins. The power of the method is increased if one can find discordant MZ triplets or quadruplets, since in such instances the genotypic template is repeated more than once and the range of environmental variations across them is increased. In the case of MZ quadruplets, for example, one can arrange them into six pairs in which each individual has the same genetic complement, and compare each pair with respect to any given environmental variable. Of course, such subjects are rare.

Discordant MZ twins may be used not only to learn about environmental contributions to a disorder, but to learn about the nature of the inherited factor as well. The rationale follows this line of thought. We assume first that there is some genetic involvement in the disorder. One MZ twin shows the expected phenotype; the second does not. It is the second twin that interests us. Since he has the implicated genotype but does not show the disorder, perhaps he reveals in his personality functioning those traits that reflect the inherited predisposition to the disorder. Knowledge about the inherited antecedents of a disorder could provide the understanding we need to learn how the disorder develops at all.

This thinking gives rise to the following research strategy. Assume that the disorder in question is schizophrenia. We first find a series of tests and measures that discriminate schizophrenics and normal controls generally. These tests and measures are administered to a series of discordant MZ twins. We are interested primarily in those measures on which *both* the schizophrenic and nonschizophrenic twin perform like schizophrenics generally. Such measures could be presumed to reflect the inherited predisposition, since both the schizophrenic and nonschizophrenic subjects with the implicated genotype perform similarly, whereas normal controls differ from both. Conversely, on those tests and measures where the schizophrenic twin performs like schizophrenics generally, whereas the nonschizophrenic cotwin performs like normal controls, we can then safely infer that the performances on such tasks reflect the effects of the clinical condition, rather than the predisposition to it.

QUANTITATIVE DISORDERS

Ordinarily, psychological studies of the severe behavioral disorders compare a group of index cases who have the disorder with a control group that does not. Similarly, in most genetic studies involving twins or other relatives of index cases, each relative is said to have or not to have the disorder. However, in many instances the relative may not have a clear case of the disorder but he may not be psychologically normal either. How should he be classified?

The question can be turned around. What if the disorder in question is not caused by a single major gene but is in fact polygenic? Then should not the disorder itself be graduated with respect to the severity and types of symptoms that fall within the framework of that disorder in a sizable population? Many people may not be frankly schizophrenic, but they may be "different," odd, eccentric, show unusual thought or speech patterns, daydream a lot, stay off by themselves, show little emotion, react too little or too much, and so forth. If such traits are observed in the cotwin of a schizophrenic index case, should the pair be counted as concordant or discordant? Perhaps it would be wiser to measure these characteristics and express the degree of similarity between relatives in quantitative terms rather than to say simply that both do or do not have the same disorder. We shall deal with this point again later.

For now, let us assume that the behavioral disorders lend themselves more appropriately to quantitative measurement than to dichotomous classification. We may wish to grade subjects with respect to their degree of "schizophrenicity" or neuroticism, or we may simply grade them with respect to specific traits, such as amount of daydreaming, degree of thought disturbance, anxiety, depressiveness, and so on. One could use tests or ratings to measure the traits. With such data, we would dispense with the concept of concordance and think in terms of the closeness of association between relatives regarding the trait measured. Are MZ twins, for example, more likely to have similar scores than DZ twins? The degree of association in each type of twins may be expressed by the intraclass correlation, which compares the variances between and within twin pairs, that is,

$$\frac{\sigma_b{}^2 - \sigma_w{}^2}{\sigma_b{}^2 + \sigma_w{}^2}$$

It is calculated as follows:

$$r_i = \frac{\Sigma(X_i - a)(Y_i - a)}{ns^2} = \frac{\Sigma(X_iY_i - na^2)}{ns^2}$$

where

a = mean of all measurements
X_iY_i = measurements on ith pair of twins
n = number of twin pairs
s^2 = variance of total sample about a

The intraclass correlation differs from the usual product-moment correlation in that the investigator has a clear basis for assigning subjects to one of two groups in the usual type of correlation, for example, father or son. In the case of twins, either one could be assigned to group A or group B. Therefore, in the intraclass correlation, the coefficient is derived from a mean and standard deviation based on *all* measurements, as shown in the formula for r_i above. It can be shown that r_i represents a linear function of the ratio of two variances, so that

$$1 - r_{MZ} = \frac{V_{MZ}}{V} \quad \text{and} \quad 1 - r_{DZ} = \frac{V_{DZ}}{V}$$

where V equals the total variance.

When the score for twin X equals the score for his cotwin Y in every pair, the correlation will be perfect, that is, 1.00. If the intrapair scores vary randomly, the correlation will be zero. Differences in r_i between MZ and DZ twins are taken as presumptive evidence of an inherited factor when the aforementioned assumptions about twins and additivity of genetic and environmental variances can be met.

It is also possible to obtain a measure of heritability when we have quantitative measures of twins. The one that is best known is Holzinger's heritability index:

$$H = \frac{r_{MZ} - r_{DZ}}{1 - r_{DZ}} = \frac{\sigma_{DZ}{}^2 - \sigma_{MZ}{}^2}{\sigma_{DZ}{}^2}$$

For various reasons, H is an unsatisfactory index of heritability. Let us recall that heritability represents the proportion of the phenotypic variance due to genetic variance, or

$$h^2 = \frac{\sigma_g^2}{\sigma_p^2}$$

Jensen (1967) derives a measure of what he calls the total true-score phenotypic variance, that is, total variance minus error variance, or

$$\sigma_p^2 = \sigma_g^2 + \sigma_E^2 + \sigma_e^2$$

where σ_E^2 = systematic environmental variance (between families) and σ_e^2 = unsystematic or random environmental variance (within families). If we divide this equation by σ_p^2, we obtain

$$1 = h^2 + E^2 + e^2$$

where $E^2 = \sigma_E^2/\sigma_p^2$ = proportion of total variance due to environmental differences between families, and $e^2 = \sigma_e^2/\sigma_p^2$ = proportion of within-family environmental variance.

Let us represent the correlation between two sets of individuals, A and B, on a given trait, where

ρg_{AB} = genetic correlation between A and B
ρE_{AB} = correlation between relevant environmental factors regarding A and B

Then,

$$r_{AB} = \rho g_{AB} h^2 + \rho E_{AB} E^2$$

Now, to determine heritability based on two groups of paired individuals AB and CD in which the genetic correlation in one group (ρg_{AB}) is greater than the genetic correlation in the other (ρg_{CD}), as in the case of MZ and DZ twins, the generalized formula becomes

$$h^2 = \frac{r_{AB} - r_{CD} - E^2(\rho E_{AB} - \rho E_{CD})}{\rho g_{AB} - \rho g_{CD}}$$

The problem remaining to the investigator is the determination of E^2 and e^2. With respect to psychological factors in the environment, a solution is not easy. One could assume that environmental factors for MZ twins reared together are perfectly correlated, $\rho E = 1$, and not at all correlated for MZ twins reared apart, $\rho E = 0$, but it is likely that one would fall into error on both counts. One could also assume that environmental factors are similarly correlated for both MZ and DZ twins, or $\rho E_{MZ} = \rho E_{DZ}$. This is the usual assumption that has been made in the past when heritability has been measured, but, at least with regard to many psychopathological conditions, the assumption is

probably not tenable. A more satisfactory procedure would be to estimate or to determine empirically the environmental (psychological or
otherwise) correlations regarding factors that may possibly be relevant
to the condition.

The attempt to describe a proper measure of heritability leads to a
troublesome point, namely, that it is the conceptualization of environment in genetic studies of behavioral disorders that most dismays psychologists. Rearing together and rearing apart hardly constitute functional independent variables. A serious behavioral scientist may want
to know how a specific organism (or genotype) responds to different
but specified stimuli of varying intensity programmed according to different schedules. Some aspects of the environment may be functional
with respect to a given response (i.e., elicit that response), whereas
others may not. In the behavioral disorders, we want to know the
specific stimuli (rearing conditions, maternal response patterns to the
child, experiences with peers, attitudes toward self, deprivations, frustra-
tions, conflicts, and so on) that provoke normal, neurotic, psychotic,
or other deviant behavior in different individuals, and what the genetic
characteristics are of those who respond to these external or internal
stimuli with similar kinds of pathological responses. Research toward
such ends can be designed, and much work along these lines has already
been done with animals. The science of human behavioral genetics
and behavioral pathology will come into its own when it is able to
generate and implement the designs needed to provide such knowledge.

Methods exist in quantitative genetics for evaluating heritability
in traits that are caused in good part by polygenes, even when the
traits are classified dichotomously. For example, some mice and rats
are adversely affected by high-pitched tones. Their responses can be
graded in severity, but investigators tend to classify their animals into
those who develop convulsions and those who do not. The convulsions
are classified as *threshold characters.* Similarly, human intelligence is
generally thought to be influenced polygenically, but individuals are
often classified simply as normal, borderline, or defective according to
predetermined cutoff scores on a test.

If the functional behavioral disorders are polygenically determined,
we can estimate their heritability from two sets of incidence figures:
those for relatives of index cases and those for the general population.
Since, as indicated earlier, it is difficult to obtain accurately the population incidence, investigators often substitute instead the incidence among
the relatives of normal controls.

This method, developed by Falconer, is too involved to be detailed
here. The measure it yields is called the heritability of *liability.* Liability includes both *susceptibility* (native tendencies to the disorder) and

the external circumstances that make it more or less likely that the
disorder will develop—or pass the threshold. The method assumes that
the measure of liability is normally distributed, and that the variance
of liability is the same for the groups compared. It also assumes that
there is no correlation within families with respect to environmental
factors relevant to the disease liability.

Falconer has prepared a graph that makes it extremely easy to
estimate the heritability of liability when an investigator has obtained
the two necessary incidences. It is reproduced here as Figure 3-1.

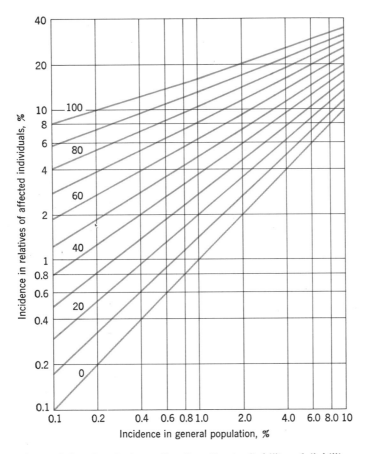

Figure 3-1. Graph for estimating the heritability of liability
from two observed incidences, when the relatives are sibs,
parents, or children. (From D. S. Falconer, The inheritance
of liability to certain diseases, estimated from the incidence
among relatives, *Ann. Human Genet.*, 1965, **29.** Reprinted
with permission of Cambridge University Press.)

The graph can be used only when the relatives are of first degree: parents, sibs, or children. The incidence among them is represented along the vertical axis. The population incidence can be represented by the relatives of the normal controls. It is plotted along the horizontal axis. Both the horizontal and vertical incidence scales are logarithmic. To estimate the heritability, one first reads along the horizontal axis to determine the point along it that represents the observed population incidence. Then one reads up vertically to the point that represents the observed familial incidence. The point where the two incidences intersect represents the heritability value. The sloping line to which it lies most closely tells the heritability value to the nearest 10 points. By interpolating, one can estimate the value obtained somewhat more accurately. When the two incidences are equal, heritability is zero.

Since most investigators concerned with familial psychiatric disorders collect data mainly on first-degree relatives, this graph can be widely useful. If one uses hospitalization as a threshold criterion, the heritability value may be too high in that if one member of a family is hospitalized, other members may be more likely to find their way to the hospital as well. Conversely, some families may tend to avoid hospitalization en bloc. Since index cases would be hospitalized and controls not, such tendencies, if they existed, could contribute to the observed incidences. The relatives of normal controls tend to have a slightly lower liability than the general population, and the incidence among them is not entirely suitable for evaluating the mean liability of the index cases and controls. This may introduce a slight error into the method, but not enough to cause concern. However, since intrafamilial correlations may well occur with respect to relevant environmental factors in many psychopathological conditions, Falconer's method provides primarily an index of the upper limit of their heritability.

ADOPTION STUDIES

In the usual family and twin studies of abnormal behavior, one of two possible causal factors tends to be emphasized: (1) heredity and (2) patterns of familial behavior that are noxious to the child. Regardless of which one holds the investigator's attention, the fact is that both may be operating at the same time. In truth, there is reason to believe that the two factors may be correlated, in the sense that the more the implicated abnormal genes occur in the parents, the more likely the parents are to pass on these genes to their children and the more likely they are to behave in abnormal ways with regard to their children. Although we have pointed up some research strategies that may help to provide information about the genetic contribution to these disorders despite the usual confounding of the two factors, the most direct strategy would be simply to separate the genetic and rearing variables entirely and to vary each one systematically with regard to the other. This goal can be achieved through adoption studies. There are several ways to carry out such studies, and we will describe a few, again using schizophrenia as the disorder in the proposed research models.

First, it should be pointed out that in Western cultures adoption ordinarily occurs as the result of some social, personal, or familial disruption. Conception out of wedlock is one common factor leading to adoption. Marital disharmony or loss of a spouse through death is another. Parental physical or mental illness, poverty, or indifference to the child are others. Social agencies exist to protect the child's interests and to provide him a good home. Most agencies are rightly wary of any interference with or disturbance of the adoption process that could cause anguish to the adoptee, the parents who place the child for adoption, or the adopting parents. Therefore, they may not at all welcome outside inquiries regarding any parties to the adoption, even if these inquiries come from sincere, judicious researchers with worthy medical, social, or scientific purposes. Different countries, states, and agencies work out their own policies regarding cooperation with such investigators.

Let us assume that we have in good faith obtained the necessary state and agency cooperation and that the following information is made available to us:

1 All nonfamilial adoptions during the past 50 years

2 The name(s), sex, date of birth, current address, and psychiatric history of each adoptee

3 The names, dates of birth, current addresses, children, and psychiatric histories of all biological parents and all adoptive parents of the adoptees.

We can now employ the following research models.

The adoptees' families method

We begin with adoptions that took place many years ago, for example, 30 to 50. These adoptees are now adults who have lived through enough of the risk period such that a number of them will now be schizophrenic. We find out who the schizophrenic adoptees are from their psychiatric histories and hospital records. These adoptees become our index cases. From among the remaining adoptees, we form a control group matched to the index cases with respect to age at transfer to the adoptive parents, age, sex, and social class of the adoptive parents. The control subjects, however, are free of any psychiatric history. We now determine the incidence of schizophrenic disorder among the biological and adoptive relatives of the index and control groups. The design is as follows:

Relatives
Biological   Adoptive

Reference   *Index*
Group

              Control

The entries in the four cells are the frequencies of the disorder among the corresponding type of relatives of the two groups. We may include only parents, sibs, and half-sibs of the adoptees, or we may extend the investigation to relatives of lesser degree. A higher incidence among the biological relatives of index cases than of controls indicates that heredity is contributing significantly to the disorder. A higher incidence among the adoptive relatives of index cases than of controls supports the view that rearing by, of, or with schizophrenics contributes to the development of the disorder.

The adoptees study method

In this research strategy, we begin with the biological parents of the adoptees. We search all their psychiatric histories and find those parents who have schizophrenic disorder. The children they gave up for adoption become the index cases. We then match to the index group adoptees of the same age at transfer for adoption, sex, age, and socioeconomic rearing status. The matched control group differs only in that the biological parents of these adoptees have no psychiatric history. We study the two groups of adoptees. A higher incidence of schizophrenic disorder in the index group indicates that heredity is contributing to the illness. The method assumes that the people who adopted the index and control groups of children are similar with respect to environmental factors that might give rise to the disorder.

The two groups of adoptees may also be studied intensively with respect to a wide variety of behaviors in controlled (test or laboratory) or natural situations. Differences between the two groups, apart from frank schizophrenic disorder, reflect the nature of the inherited factor insofar as that factor is manifested in personality functioning. By examining adoptees of different ages, it is theoretically possible to chart

the development of the inherited personality deviations from infancy
to adult schizophrenia.

The cross-fostering method

In genetic studies with animals, we might want to breed two strains
for a given dimension of behavior, for example, aggressiveness. Let
us say that in the first generation, we select those who are most and
least aggressive on a given test. We then breed the high aggressive
Ss with one another and the low aggressive Ss with one another. We
repeat the testing, selection, and inbreeding program until the nth generation, when we achieve maximal discrimination of the two groups.
We now need to know whether we have truly bred in genetic differences
with respect to the trait, or whether each succeeding generation became
more aggressive or more passive because it in turn had been reared
by a more aggressive or passive parent population. To answer this
question, we transpose the litters of the $n + 1$ generation so that the
offspring from the aggressive strain are fostered by passive dams, and
the passive strain litters by aggressive strain dams. This becomes the
test generation in which one can compare the relative contributions
of the genetic inbreeding and the type of rearing.

With this model in mind, we can now plan an analogous research
design in which the adoptees represent the $n + 1$ generation. We find
all adoptees who have a biological parent who is schizophrenic, but
whose adoptive parents are free of any psychiatric history. We also
find adoptees whose biological parents are both normal but who are
reared by an adoptive parent with schizophrenic disorder. The two
groups of adoptees are compared with respect to the incidence of schizophrenic disorder and other personality deviations.

Related methods

The bodies of information required for the research strategies just
presented are not often available. Lacking them, variations of the
adoptees' families method and the adoptees study method may still be
feasible.

Let us collect a series of schizophrenic subjects. We find out who
among them was adopted at an early age. This is the index group. We
match to them a series of schizophrenics who were reared by their
biological parents. The adoptive parents of the index group are compared with the biological parents of the matched group with respect
to the incidence of schizophrenic disorder and other psychopathology.
A higher incidence among the biological parents provides support for

the genetic hypothesis. This method does not have the refinements and controls of the others, but it has the advantage of not requiring the cooperation of adoption agencies or the ready availability of vast amounts of recorded information.

In a variation of the adoptees study method, we may begin with schizophrenic women who give birth at a mental hospital. Many of their children are placed in institutions or foster homes or given up for adoption. These children become the index cases. From lists provided by the cooperating social service and adoption agencies, babies similarly placed and matched to the index cases for sex and age are selected as controls. The two groups are compared as adults with respect to the incidence of schizophrenic disorder and other psychopathology. In this method, one must pay attention to the possibility that the mother's schizophrenic illness, or the medical treatment for it, could have had some noxious effect on the developing fetus and thereby contributed nongenetically to subsequent behavioral disorders among the index cases.

STUDIES OF HEREDITY-ENVIRONMENT INTERACTION

There is a severe illness called *favism* that is incurred by persons who have a certain sex-linked recessive gene and are on a diet that includes the fava bean. Both the gene frequency and the consumption of the fava bean vary considerably across populations. Some populations have a high incidence of favism because of the high frequency of the gene, others because of the high consumption of the bean. Susceptible groups who never eat the bean never have the disease. Is the disease genetically or environmentally determined?

The example actually illustrates a broad principle. Both genetic and environmental factors are always involved in the etiology of all disorders. Our task is to learn what the specific factors are and how they interact to produce the aberrant condition. Although we cannot know how they interact until we know precisely what they are, we are able to apportion in a statistical way the relative contributions to behavioral traits and disorders made by a given inferred genotype, a reasonably well-specified environment, and the interaction between them.

The research design enabling us to do this requires that we have at least two designated genotypes and two environments. To illustrate, let us begin with the cross-fostering research design described above. Let us assume that the results of such a study support the genetic hypothesis. We can then presume that among those adoptees who had a biological schizophrenic parent we have a representation of the genotype for schizophrenia. Among those adoptees with two normal biological parents, we expect normal genotypes. Similarly, we have two categories of environment: rearing by a schizophrenic parent and rearing by psychiatrically normal parents. We can add two groups to those used in the cross-fostering study: (1) a group with a biological schizophrenic parent, but also reared by a schizophrenic parent; (2) a group with both biological and rearing parents normal. The full design would look like this:

		Genotype	
		Schizophrenic	Normal
Rearing Environment	Schizophrenic		
	Normal		

The entries in the four cells could be either the frequency of schizophrenic disorder in the offspring or they could be measures of traits considered relevant to the study of schizophrenia. The n's in the cells should be sufficiently large to permit an analysis of variance in which we can apportion the contribution made by genotypes, by rearing, and by the interaction between them. In parallel studies, we could keep the same genotypes but vary the rearing or other environmental categories according to any theory of environmental etiology that seemed worth testing.

PREDICTION STUDIES

Prediction studies make no special effort in their design to separate out the genetic and environmental variables. Rather, they are concerned with being able to identify in young people (at any age from infancy to young adulthood) those traits or characteristics that are the psychophysiological or behavioral precursors of the subsequent disorder. The research designs are of two main types. Both begin with a cohort of subjects who have a "high risk" for developing the disorder.

The first is really postdictive in execution but predictive in intent. Here, the investigator begins with subjects who have shown evidence of psychological disturbance in childhood, that is, children who had been patients at a child guidance clinic but who are now adults. He conducts a search to find out who among them has developed the disorder, for example, schizophrenia. These become the index cases. From the clinic files, he matches to them subjects of the same sex, age, and social class who showed no psychiatric disorder in adulthood. The clinic records of the index and matched control groups are then compared with respect to symptom picture, rearing circumstances, family behavior patterns, and so on.   Found differences suggest the factors that are instrumental in leading to normality or to schizophrenia.

In the second type of study, the investigator typically begins with children of parents who have the disorder.   Usually, it is only one of the parents who has it, but if a sample can be collected in which both parents have the disorder, a much higher proportion of the children can be expected to develop it later.   As they grow up, the children are periodically studied intensively.   A matched group of children of the same sex, age, and class, but with both parents normal, serves as the control group.   Differences found between the two groups suggest those personality factors that are more likely to be implicated in the eventual development of the disorder.   The investigator has a postdictive option as well.   He can wait until a number of his subjects do develop the disorder, and then look back at his data to see which variables distinguished those index cases who developed the disorder from those who did not.   The method can be made more powerful in the latter type of analysis if the investigator begins his study by matching pairs of index cases, so that an index case who develops the disorder can be compared with his control index case who does not.

When the investigator identifies personality factors that discriminate index cases and controls, or index cases who develop the disorder as compared with those who do not, he is not likely to be in a position to judge the relative contributions of heredity and environment to the discriminating factors.   Nevertheless, aside from the high clinical value of such knowledge, the identification of the relevant factors serves to guide those interested in the genetics or environmental induction of the disorder by indicating which variable may be worth studying.

HEREDITY AS AN
INDEPENDENT VARIABLE

In many of the research designs and strategies described above, the research model departs radically from those traditionally employed by geneticists.   One reason for this is that in the functional behavioral disorders, we must still be concerned with the question of whether a genetic etiology is probable at all.   Geneticists working with plants or animals can answer this question easily by controlled breeding, as in the work of Mendel.   However, in human research, we have no control over breeding but must find where we can cases that represent the kind of breeding and rearing environment we would have deliberately planned if we wanted to study the genetics of a disorder in a controlled way. We may think of such groups of cases as *strategic populations* in that they have carried out their breeding and child rearing according to a research strategy we might have employed in the laboratory to probe the question of genetic etiology.

In the aforementioned designs, we were also concerned that environmental factors might be confounded with genetic factors. When we selected comparison groups of schizophrenic parents and of normal parents, we were testing experimentally whether the genes transmitted by the schizophrenic parents led to certain behavioral disorders in their children. In effect, we were treating these unknown, unobserved, hypothesized genes as if they comprised an independent variable. Conceptualized in this way, the research takes on the character and research methodology of any well-designed experiment on human behavior.

In studies employing discordant MZ twins, heredity is controlled, but it does not serve as an independent variable. Instead, the behavioral differences between the twins represent the dependent variable, and we embark on a search to find the explanation for the differences in the presumed independent variable which must be environmental. This is a sort of backward search carried out retrospectively, but it can be very useful. With respect to MZ twin research generally, we may use two kinds of postulates to guide us in the inferences we make regarding the explanations of differences or similarities between them.

DIFFERENCE POSTULATES.

1 Differences in outcome between the twins can be attributed to environmental factors.

2 If environmental factors A and B apply equally to both twins, differences in outcomes between them must be attributed to some other factor.

SIMILARITIES POSTULATES. When environmental factor A applies to twin X, but factor not-A or orthogonal factor B applies to twin Y, if both twins develop similar outcomes, we may consider two hypothetical relationships between factors and outcomes:

1 Factors A and B lead to the same outcome through independent pathways. The investigator must be prepared to accept and demonstrate two etiological factors instead of one. In the absence of such demonstration, this hypothesis is not parsimonious.

2 Neither A nor B can be considered to have a causal relationship to the particular outcome unless it can be shown that these factors are separately associated with a third factor C which in turn applies equally to both twins.

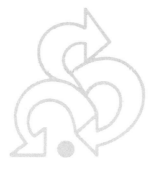

Chapter Four

Diagnosis and Unit Characters

We have been speaking blithely about the behavioral disorders as though we knew not only what they were, but also as if we knew that they were clear, distinctive, separate entities. This was necessary in order to demonstrate the genetic concepts and research strategies that are basic to this field. If we are to trace the transmission pattern of a gene, we must be able to associate it with a distinctive, single phenotypic entity. The entity may be simple, as the blood types A, B, AB, and O, which are specific characteristics, each deriving from the action of a single genotype at a single locus. The entity may also be a complex of phenotypic traits; for example, a single gene, *ch*, in the mouse causes death immediately after birth. Associated characteristics are: improper lung inflation, abnormal proportions of the skull, forehead, and face, abnormal sensory hairs of the face, skin covering only the forehead, and so on. Nevertheless, all together, the constellation of defects represents a single phenotypic entity. We may call it a disease or a syndrome, but the important thing is that it represents what geneticists call a *unit character*. We must be able to recognize or describe unit characters in the genetic study of behavioral disorders, or we may find ourselves in the position of a geneticist who might have looked for

a different gene to account for each of the phenotypic abnormalities
noted in the disease caused solely by the *ch* gene.

Probably the best way to present the scope and difficulty of the
problem of determining unit characters in the field of behavioral disorder
is to present a brief historical review of man's attempts to develop
diagnostic entities of mental illness.

First, we should recognize that mental disorders have long been
considered by physicians to lie within their sphere of competence. We
can trace this medical orientation in the Western world at least as far
back as Hippocrates. During the past two millennia, many brilliant
men have made attempts to classify mental disorders. They used a
wide variety of principles of classification, each reflecting the dominant
orientation and style of its time. Still current terms—*mania, melancholia, epilepsy,* and *hysteria*—as well as the now defunct *phrenitis* and
Scythian disease, were employed by Hippocrates himself. Celsus added
delirium (caused by fright), *cardiacum,* and *lethargus.* Arataeus coined
the terms *senile* and *secondary dementia.* Galen added the illnesses
anoia, moria, catalepsy, apoplexy, and others. Some of these terms have
remained in the medical literature to this day, but their definition and
description have been repeatedly revised. By and large, the historical
trend has been to increase the number of mental disease categories,
which in turn became increasingly differentiated.

But people who were not physicians also had some proprietary
interest in mental illnesses. Plato divided them into Natural Madness
(caused by physical diseases) and Divine Madness, which he classified
as Prophetic, Religious, Poetic, and Erotic, these being inspired respectively by Apollo, Dionysus, the Muses, and by Aphrodite and Eros.
Aristotle's conception of three souls—the vegetative, animal, and
rational—provided the basis for several classificatory schemes, including
one by Saint Thomas Aquinas, who believed that some conditions were
of supernatural origin and that hallucinations and insanity resulted from
the action of demons.

The Middle Ages demonstrate vividly that, although there always
existed a current of belief that mental illnesses stemmed from natural
or physical causes, they always were popularly classified and understood
in terms of a particular cultural context. At that time, religious beliefs
and practices dominated the minds and activities of men. A man's
life was an arena in which God and the devil contested for his soul.
Afflictions were sometimes thought to be a sign of God's grace, as in
the case of epileptic convulsions, but severe mental illness was almost
always taken as a sign that the victim was possessed by the devil. Because one's very soul was at stake, the sights and sounds of madness
must have inspired boundless awe and terror in the beholder, especially

in anyone who had the slightest doubt of his own mental stability, a doubt which always afflicts so many among us.

It is probable that in times long past, the ordinary man distinguished madness from mental deficiency. Mental deficiency could be recognized at an early age and could be presumed to have been present at birth. Madness, then as now, did not manifest itself until later, usually not before the victim had reached adulthood. When Jean Esquirol, a great French psychiatrist of the early nineteenth century, distinguished idiocy, which he considered to be a *congenital* defect, from dementia, which he described as an *acquired* defect, he was emphasizing these differences and minimizing the fact that *both* disorders tended to run in families. Esquirol's views were put forth at a time when the concept of *moral treatment* of insanity was at its height. The notion that madness was acquired, and could therefore be dispersed, fitted in very nicely with the philosophy of moral treatment and readily gained wide acceptance.

Nevertheless, the opposed view of biological transmission was not entirely submerged by Esquirol's theory. Another Frenchman, Benedict Morel, conceived of mental illness as constitutional, rather than accidental or acquired, and he added a new dimension to the concept, claiming that the illness became progressively degenerative as it passed down through successive generations. When the disease reached its severest point, usually in the fourth generation, the line died out. Morel's views were consonant with the excitement accompanying many new discoveries in the biological sciences and found a deeply responsive audience. Views analogous to his were put forth by an eminent English psychiatrist, Sir Frederick Mott, as late as the second decade of the present century.

German psychiatry, which dominated the last half of the nineteenth century, responded more to Morel than to Esquirol. It was a time of intellectual effervescence, with many great minds aspiring toward a resolution of the problem of mental illness.

Attempts were made to read order into the bewildering diversity and incomprehensibility of bizarre behaviors which constituted the only substance of this branch of medicine. Classification schemes multiplied profusely. Increased scientific sophistication led these new nosologists to propose classifications based on the onset, course, and outcome of the diverse clinical pictures seen. In their efforts to attain their objective, symptoms, or perhaps more properly, behaviors, were grouped, regrouped, and grouped again. Disease names such as *vesania* and *vecordia*, which were medical bywords 100 years ago, came and went, and only a tiny number of today's psychiatrists and psychologists even know that such designations once existed and were widely accepted.

At the very end of the nineteenth century, about the time when the work of Mendel was being rediscovered and the science of modern genetics really began, a German physician named Emil Kraepelin devised a classification scheme based on the principle of prognosis. He grouped together diseases known as *catatonia, hebephrenia,* and *paranoia,* which was very popular at the time, and from time to time added one or more others to this core group. He claimed that these entities were different manifestations of a single disease whose chief common feature was the more or less severe deterioration of mental functioning. He named the disease *dementia praecox,* a term which had been used by Morel about a half century earlier. Kraepelin also grouped together patients who had, among other things, periods of great excitement and depression, but who did *not* develop the picture of mental deterioration seen in dementia praecox. Such patients, he said, suffered from *manic-depressive insanity.* This reduction of the many earlier, more or less complicated classification schemes to two major diagnostic categories was hailed as a revolution in psychiatry.

In practice, the new scheme was not perfect. Patients who had the features of dementia praecox often recovered with minimal or no deteriorative signs, and patients with predominantly manic-depressive features often lapsed into a deteriorative state. Diagnoses had to be revised, sometimes years later, a procedure still not uncommon in Europe. More troublesome was the fact that (since the diagnosis was based on prognosis) it was often difficult to decide in new cases just what the prognosis should be.

Early in the twentieth century, a Swiss psychiatrist named Eugen Bleuler, who accepted Kraepelin's diagnostic scheme, decided to change the name of dementia praecox and to call the disorder *the group of schizophrenias.* One major reason for the change was that Bleuler found, as did everyone else, including Kraepelin, that not all cases that were clinically dementia praecox showed dementia, nor did they all have their onset at an early age or develop rapidly. Bleuler thought that the major feature of the disorder was the splitting of the psychic functions, not the apparent prognosis or subsequent dementia. Moreover, he was much impressed by the theories of Freud and Jung, and believed that many of the behaviors of his patients were meaningful in a psychoanalytic sense. In addition, Bleuler was not certain that the so-called group of schizophrenias really represented a single disease.

To this day, Kraepelin's basic view predominates in most of Europe and Japan, whereas Bleuler's view is prevalent in most of the United States and Switzerland. However, the term schizophrenia, used mostly in the singular, has now displaced the term dementia praecox throughout the world. Some psychiatrists do not believe in *any* psychiatric nosology, claiming that there is only mental illness of greater or lesser degree.

And some psychiatrists and many psychologists believe that such disorders should not be classified as illness at all, since they derive entirely from social and psychological influences.

Despite this lengthy history of various conflicting opinions based on observations that lacked hard, scientific support, research on heredity in mental disorder—a topic that had always provoked interest—began in earnest in the late nineteenth century, before Kraepelin's nosological revolution. Having neither modern genetical sophistication nor a modern nosology, the first investigators concerned themselves with a loose designation called *hereditary taint*. This could include not only the usual nervous, eccentric, or bizarre behaviors, but also other traits considered undesirable, such as left-handedness, stuttering, being hunchbacked, or using four-letter words to excess. The investigators started with a group of mental patients and a group of controls who might be friends and acquaintances of the investigator, and counted the number of relatives of each group who showed some hereditary taint. Typically, the findings revealed a high prevalence of taint in the families of both groups, from about 45 to 80 percent, with a somewhat higher rate for the relatives of the mental patients.

Modern psychiatric genetics began in the second decade of this century, and was guided by Ernst Rüdin in Munich, Germany. Among his colleagues we find most of the pioneers in this field. Rüdin, himself, took up the question of whether dementia praecox and manic-depressive psychosis were genetically distinct diseases, but he could find no simple answer to this question. These pioneers, who accepted the new nosology and the probability that they were dealing with genuine disease entities, applied the new methods of genetics with conviction and enthusiasm. They did family-prevalence studies of schizophrenia and evaluated its mode of genetic transmission; they calculated genetic penetrance, the proportion of homozygotes and heterozygotes in the population, and mutation rates of the culprit gene. They also began the first systematic twin studies regarding the two major psychoses.

Concurrent with this great outburst of activity in psychiatric genetics was another movement initiated by Freud and pursued avidly by his followers, some of whom engaged intensively in clinical studies of schizophrenic patients. Gradually, they came to the conclusion that the peculiar, noxious behavior of the patient's parents, particularly his mother, was a primary factor in the development of his psychosis. During this same period, the most influential psychiatrist in the United States, Adolf Meyer, developed the idea that schizophrenia was not a disease but a *psychobiological reaction* to a wide variety of stresses in the environment.

In fact, during the long history of developing and changing classification systems, voices were raised in protest against these nosologies, all of which were based on observations of essentially the same behaviors, which, however, were constantly regrouped according to different principles of classification. In ancient times, Asclepiades, a true monist, had said that all illness was based on patterns of tension and relaxation of body tissues (a principle that, in our own day, provides a basic rationale for personality diagnosis via handwriting analysis). At the beginning of the nineteenth century, Thomas Beddoes asked "whether it be not necessary either to confine insanity to one species, or to divide it into almost as many as there are cases." Later Heinrich Neumann stated: "There is only one kind of mental disorder; we call it insanity." Pierre Janet thought that psychiatric diagnosis referred more to the fortunes of the patient than to anything else. This view has found some support in modern investigations. As stated before, currently there are a number of prominent psychiatrists in the United States who are convinced that all psychiatric nosologies are meaningless, and that there is only a broad category of mental illness, whereas a few psychiatrists and many psychologists believe that the functional behavioral disorders should not be classified as illness at all.

Nevertheless, these objectors represent a minority. Psychiatric nosology and diagnosis persist, with new proposals of classification appearing regularly. Different countries often have their own diagnostic schemas. In the United States, the American Psychiatric Association has adopted or supported several such classifications. The current official one was published in 1952.[1] Many disorders are classified as *brain disorders* associated with clear tissue damage, circulatory disturbances, or toxicity. Some that are clearly hereditary, like Huntington's chorea, are referred to as "chronic brain syndrome associated with diseases of unknown or uncertain cause." *Mental deficiency* comprises another major diagnostic category.

The category of greatest concern to us is *psychotic disorders*. It has five subgroups. One is *involutional psychotic reaction,* which is presumed to be associated with metabolic or endocrine disturbance. The other four are referred to as "disorders of psychogenic origin or without clearly defined tangible cause or structural change." They include *affective reactions,* with three types of *manic-depressive reactions* and a *psychotic-depressive reaction; schizophrenic reactions,* with nine subtypes; *paranoid reactions,* with two subtypes; and a residual category simply called *psychotic reaction.*

In addition, there are *psychophysiologic autonomic and visceral disorders* "due to disturbance of innervation or of psychic control," ten subtypes; *psychoneurotic disorder* "of psychogenic origin or without

[1] Since this book was written, the American Psychiatric Association has proposed a new classification system.

clearly defined tangible cause or structural change," seven subtypes; *personality disorders,* also "of psychogenic origin," which are broken down into *personality pattern disturbance,* 4 subtypes, and a residual "other" subtype; and, last, *transient situational personality disorders,* with nine subtypes.

The geneticist who embarks on extensive investigations to study a unit character can be forgiven if, in the light of psychiatric nosology's history and current state, he approaches his task with misgivings or with frank pessimism. However, the fact is that many investigators have contributed important studies in this field. Later, we will review them. But the enticing possibility exists that genetic studies themselves may be the very ones that will eventually tell us what the unit characters are with respect to the behavioral disorders and what the principle of classification should be. At this time, at least, no other type of study holds out as much hope for a solution to the basic problems of psychiatric diagnosis and nosology.

In the meantime, problems of diagnosis confront the investigators and other scientists who wish to draw general conclusions from the many investigations done in so many countries. Studies have shown that the reliability of diagnosis is poor with respect to many disorders. Reliability tends to be higher, and substantial, with respect to a disorder like hospitalized, chronic schizophrenia; but when one studies relatives, most of whom are not hospitalized and sometimes not available for personal examination, then diagnostic reliability may be low indeed. The investigator needs to take various precautions in conducting and reporting his research, so that he can assure himself and critical readers that his diagnoses have not been influenced by his hypotheses and that consensus regarding the diagnoses can be obtained generally.

Ideally, the investigator should state precisely the criteria he uses for his diagnostic categories, and these should be published. Whenever possible, he should make the diagnosis on the basis of personal examination, and the nature and extent of the examination should be described. He should not know whether the subject he is examining is a relative of an index or control case or of an MZ or DZ twin. Ideally, he should not even know the diagnosis of the index group. If he is basing his diagnosis on hospital records or on the testimony of others, the persons who prepared the records or provided the testimony should not have known whether the subject was related to someone with a given diagnosis. And he should publish the case material and the examination report on which his diagnosis is based. Of course, it is seldom possible to achieve all these goals, but such precautions are the best insurance we have against the introduction of needless error. They should also expedite and illuminate the search for unit characters in the behavioral disorders.

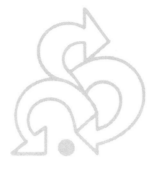

Chapter Five

Some Instructive Genetic Diseases

It is helpful to know something of the research history and accumulated knowledge about specific, relatively well-understood genetic diseases before attempting to evaluate the research findings on the functional-behavioral disorders themselves. We will review briefly several that are well known, that affect behavior in various ways, that represent different genetic mechanisms, and that illustrate some points that may have relevance to research in the functional-behavioral disorders.

PHENYLKETONURIA (PKU)

This disease has been traced to a single, recessive autosomal gene. Its most striking characteristic is moderate to severe mental deficiency, but not all affected children are quite so abnormal, and some may even pass for normal. The affected infant develops rather normally during the first few months, but then becomes dull and apathetic. Of untreated PKU patients, about 68 percent show microcephaly (small head), 25 percent have seizures, and 80 percent have an abnormal EEG (brain waves). The children tend to have fair hair, blue eyes, and lightly pigmented skin (about 60 percent) that may be eczematous in infancy (20 to 40 percent). They are smaller than normal children and have

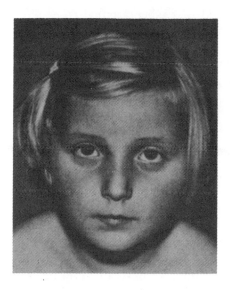 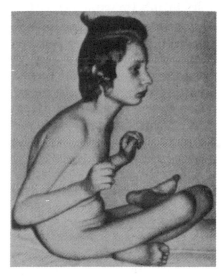

Figure 5-1. (*Left*) Engaging features and faraway look in a seven-year-old phenylpyruvic girl. (*Right*) Typical scissors posture in an eleven-year-old phenylpyruvic idiot. (Reprinted, with permission, from K. Lang, Die Phenylpyruvische, in Ergebnisse der inneren Medizin und Kinderheilkunde, vol. 6, Springer-Verlag OHG, Berlin-Göttingen-Heidelberg.)

an offensive body odor, due to the abnormal acid compound in the urine (see Figure 5-1).

Most have a stiff gait with short steps. About one-third are unable to walk, or have tremors. Over 60 percent are unable to talk. About 65 percent have an IQ less than 20; 20 percent between 21 and 50; and less than 2 percent above 60. Generally the PKU child is hyperactive, irritable, has an uncontrollable temper, shows hand play, abnormal postural attitudes, and agitated behavior. Ten percent show psychotic behavior, with destructiveness, self-injury, impulsiveness, and uncontrollable attacks of rage in the low-grade patient, and hallucinations, seclusiveness, and unpredictable behavior with episodes of excitement in the higher-grade patient.

Thus, there are a number of clear physical and behavioral characteristics that are common to the disorder, but these show considerable variation in range and degree (expressivity).

Incidence and distribution

Phenylketonuria was first described by Dr. Asbjörn Fölling in Norway in 1934. Jervis did the first large-scale genetic analysis of the disorder in the United States. He showed that when familial cases were found, they occurred largely among sibs, with both sexes equally represented, but very rarely in a parent or child of an index case. Such familial distributions are typical of severe recessive autosomal diseases.

When incidence of the disease was estimated from the number of institutionalized cases of north Europeans, it was found to be 1/25,000. In Oregon, through screening of infants, it was found to be 1/10,000. Thus the way in which one obtains one's sample influences the estimate. If $q^2 = 0.0001$, as in Oregon, $q = 0.01$, $p = 0.99$, and p^2, the proportion of people who are homozygous for the normal allele, $= 0.9801$. The proportion in the population who are carriers, $2pq$, equals 0.0198, or approximately 1 of every 50 individuals. The disease has been found in other parts of the world, for example, Japan, Czechoslovakia, and the Middle East, and appears, even more rarely, among Negroes and Jews. PKU represents only about 0.64 percent of institutionalized mental defectives.

Parents of PKU children have been found to have about 40 percent affected children, instead of the theoretically expected 25 percent. The excess was traced primarily to ascertainment bias. With proper corrections, the incidence was indeed found to be 25 percent.

Twin studies

Because of the rarity of the disease and the relatively low frequency of twin births, very few cases of affected twins have been found. Among six MZ pairs reported, concordance was 100 percent. Among five DZ or probably DZ pairs, both concordance and discordance was found, as expected, but the numbers are too small to calculate a concordance rate.

The nature of the disease

What is inherited is a disorder in the metabolism of phenylalanine, one of the basic amino acids involved in the building of body proteins. It is important to note that it is this *defect* that is inherited, not the disease. The latter is acquired in large part, and is influenced by normal diets which contain phenylalanine. Since tests are available to identify PKU in infants, when such children are found they are fed diets low in phenylalanine. With such treatment, the eczema usually clears, pigmentation increases, most of the neurologic signs are ameliorated, the patient becomes less restless and irritable, attention span increases, motor performance and difficulties improve, the EEG improves or is normalized, seizures lessen or are eliminated, and intellectual impairment is decreased and may be prevented in some cases. Once the impairment has occurred, however, it is irreversible.

It has often been assumed that if the behavioral disorders indeed had hereditary causes, the affected individuals were beyond hope and treatment. The PKU story indicates that such an attitude of therapeutic nihilism is not warranted.

One additional fact about PKU merits our attention. Although the pathological allele is completely recessive with respect to behavioral expression, it is not completely recessive with respect to metabolic expression. That is, heterozygous carriers of the allele show no higher incidence of mental defect, decreased intelligence, psychosis, or other behavioral disorders than do individuals homozygous for the normal allele. However, they do show a reduced capacity to metabolize phenylalanine after a tolerance test and under basal conditions. This reduction in capacity is not sufficient to generate the disease aspects of PKU. It does enable the carriers to be readily identified, which can be a great advantage, even though the chemical tests generate about 15 percent overlap between the heterozygotes and normal homozygotes.

HUNTINGTON'S CHOREA

This disease has been traced to an autosomal dominant gene. Huntington described the disease in an article entitled "On Chorea" in 1872. The name, chorea, comes from the Greek word meaning dance, and was used because the illness is characterized by spasmodic twitchings. The age of onset, as determined primarily by the appearance of such choreiform movements, has been reported anywhere from childhood to old age. The mean age of onset, however, has been estimated to be about thirty-five, and the average time between onset and death is almost 15 years. Since the disease is fatal, the age of onset is important in that most afflicted individuals have already reached the age when they can marry, have children, and transmit the pathological gene. The age of onset has several parallels with schizophrenia. In both, age of onset follows an approximately normal curve and may occur anywhere from childhood to advanced years, the mean time of onset occurs after reaching marriageable ages, and the earlier the onset the poorer the prognosis.

Emotional disturbance frequently precedes the onset of choreic movements, often appearing as neurosis or psychosis. Gradually, the chorea becomes more severe and intellectual deterioration and mental changes occur, often leading to insanity and a slowly progressing dementia. Psychoses often occur early in the disease, sometimes preceding the onset of chorea and dementia. Schizophrenia (paranoid and simplex), hypomania, and depressive psychoses are not uncommonly reported. About 7 percent of those affected but not institutionalized commit suicide. Typically, the EEG is flat, or shows an excess of theta and beta rhythms. Neurologically, one finds progressive abnormalities of speech and gait, and usually widespread cortical degeneration. Unlike PKU, however, the underlying biochemical abnormality in Huntington's chorea has not been found, even though the disease was described 62 years before PKU. Neither has an identified metabolic error been found in schizophrenia, despite many years of search.

Incidence and distribution

Since the dominant gene is passed on directly from parent to child, the disease clusters in families through lineal descent, and hence tends to concentrate regionally where these families live. Affected kindreds have been reported in most European countries, and in Japan and Australia. The incidences reported vary from 0.33 per 100,000 population in Japan to 6.5 per 100,000 in Northhamptonshire, England. As usual, the thoroughness of the sampling procedure influences the rate reported. A well-done Michigan study reporting an incidence of 1 case per 24,300 persons estimated that only about half the living affected persons were seen and examined. As in schizophrenia, the disease affects men and women equally. But we must point out that the incidence of both Huntington's chorea and PKU are much, much rarer than the incidence of schizophrenia, which is usually estimated to be about 1 per 100 population. This high frequency of schizophrenia, in contrast with the low rate found in other severe genetic diseases, has influenced many people's belief that this disorder has some other cause.

The gene that causes Huntington's chorea has been estimated to have a mutation rate of 5.4×10^{-6}. Supportive evidence for the low mutation rate is suggested by the rarity of unaffected parents when the latter have survived the generally accepted upper limit of age for manifestation of the disorder. As expected for a dominant trait, about half the children of affected individuals develop the illness, as shown in Figure 5-2.

Familial characteristics

Since the disease is dominant and appears in half the members of kindreds harboring the pathological gene, one would expect the nonaffected members of these kindreds to be as normal as the general population. But in fact, investigators have repeatedly found other disorders

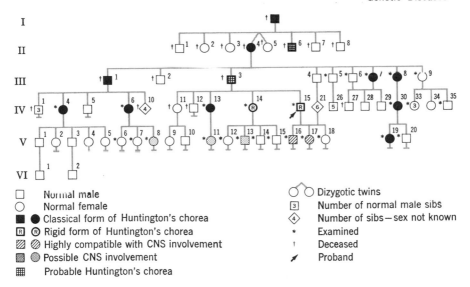

Figure 5-2. Pedigree of family with Huntington's chorea. (Reprinted, with permission, from R. M. Goodman et al., Huntington's chorea: A multidisciplinary study of affected parents and first generation offspring, *AMA Arch. Neurol. Psychiat.*, 1966, **15**.)

occurring commonly in these kindreds: mental deficiency, convulsive disorders, alcoholism, behavioral abnormalities, suicide, criminal tendencies, and insanity. The Michigan study also reported Parkinsonism, cerebellar syndromes, spastic quadriplegia, and dementia. It may be that the clearly neurological syndromes represent unusual manifestations of the gene for Huntington's chorea, or they may be chance associations. The same might be said for the behavioral disorders, but the latter could conceivably result as well from the psychological impact of being a member of a family that harbors the dread gene and not knowing if the disease will strike one next. It may be too that individuals in such families are limited in their marital opportunities and marry people with genetic proneness to other disorders.

Parallels may be found in schizophrenia. Investigators have repeatedly reported other mental disorders in the families of schizophrenics, including the ones found in Huntington families: mental deficiency, suicide, criminal tendencies, alcoholism, and so on. Could such behavioral anomalies be abetted by simply finding oneself in an affected family and feeling that one might be contaminated as well? Or are such behaviors simply incomplete manifestations of the suspected schizophrenic genotype? Do the spouses of schizophrenics contribute significantly to these disorders in their children? Later, we shall deal with the evidence bearing on these questions.

Detecting premorbid manifestations

Recently, investigators have begun to employ psychological testing in combination with intensive neurological examinations to see if they can discriminate the affected and the nonaffected young children of Huntington patients. In one study, 13 children, aged 3 to 20, were studied. Of these, 1 child (age 12) was diagnosed as Huntington's chorea, based on the neurological examination; 2 children, aged 13 and 14, were thought to have cerebral involvement, and 3 others, aged 6, $14\frac{1}{2}$, and 16, had possible cerebral involvement. The remaining 7 had no significant organic signs. On psychological tests, the offspring showed considerable variability. The 6 judged organic had a mean IQ of 86; the nonorganic, 108. With respect to personality, the organic children showed feelings of incompetence or task-related anxiety, sullen-depressiveness, and hostile resentment. They also tended to be dependent and immature and emotionally inhibited; interestingly, however, so did the children judged nonorganic. Of the total group, 4 were called maladjusted; 6, questionably maladjusted. Only 2 were adequately adjusted. Thus, even the probably nonaffected children tend to have psychological-behavioral disturbances.

This study follows the strategy of the prediction studies described in the previous chapter, and illustrates the potential fruitfulness of such studies. Later we shall review analogous studies with respect to schizophrenia. It is of interest to us, too, that in a 1925 study, an investigator, using cruder examination methods, could not distinguish potential choreic and nonchoreic siblings with respect to early temperamental traits and behavior, and concluded that there was no reliable indicator in early life of the later development of the disease. The modern study reveals the potential value of more precise examination methods, especially well-conceived psychological tests. However, the investigators would have to follow their cases for many years to have a complete, definitive study.

DOWN'S SYNDROME, OR MONGOLISM

This disorder has been traced not to a particular gene but to chromosomal abnormalities. It is detectable soon after birth because of the accompanying severe mental retardation. The children's facial characteristics reminded Langdon Down of mongoloid features, and prompted him in 1866 to call the disorder Mongolian idiocy. The children's physical growth is retarded, they have unusual *dermatoglyphic* (finger, palm, or footprint) patterns, short hands and small heads, and other somatic defects as well. About 75 percent show an abnormal EEG, and there are diffuse neuropathological changes, but no nerve lesions are visible and no constant biochemical abnormalities have as yet been found (see Figure 5-3).

Behavioral characteristics

Motorically, these children show poor muscle tone, incoordination, absence of the Moro reflex, and a tendency to sit in a squatting position and to keep their mouth open. Intellectually, their linguistic abilities are usually damaged and deviant. They tend to have higher intelligence test scores during their first five years of life. Their mean IQ has ranged from about 30 to 47 in different studies. Interestingly, they generally have a happy disposition and are highly responsive to their environments. They often have powers of mimicry and love of music and rhythm. Writing, drawing, and simple industrial tasks are within their scope, but not higher intellectual functions.

Incidence and distribution

The incidence among newborns has been calculated to be about 15 in 10,000 births. However, calculations based on studies of spontaneous abortion suggest that the incidence at conception may be about 1 in 200, which is more than three times higher than the birth incidence. The incidence among Negroes is thought to be much lower. Although the syndrome has been reported in nearly all non-European populations, reliable incidence figures among them are usually not available. There is little concentration of cases in families. There have been 13 known mongoloid women who had children, among whom 5 were mongoloid, 2 mentally retarded, 3 stillborn, and 4 normal.

Nonhereditary factors

For a long time, it was known that women who had Down's-syndrome children tended to be older than the average mother. Whereas the mean age of women in the general population giving birth is about 28.5, the mean age of mothers bearing mongoloid babies is 36.6. Although women over 40 produce only 4 percent of all babies, 40 percent

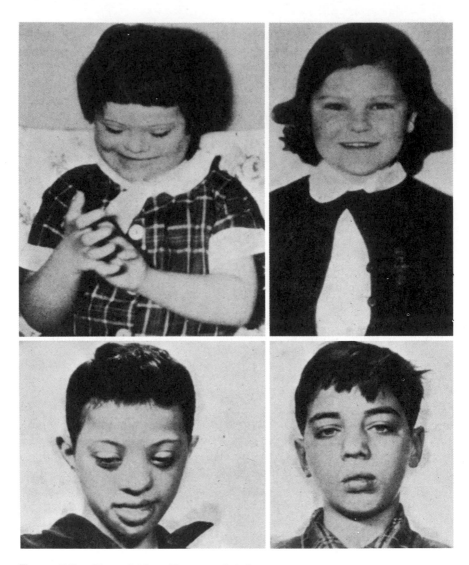

Figure 5-3. Mongoloids with normal twin partners proved dizygotic by skin grafts. (From G. Allen and G. S. Baroff, Mongoloid twins and their siblings, *Acta Genet.*, 1955, **5.** Reprinted with permission of S. Karger.)

of all mothers who bear Down's-syndrome babies are over 40. These figures indicated to investigators that a simple genetic explanation of the disorder was not likely, and some concluded that heredity might not even be an important factor, especially since there was hardly any clustering of cases in families at all.

Table 5-1
Concordance for Down's Syndrome by Twin Index Cases*

Zygosity	Concordant	Discordant	Total
MZ twins	6	0	6
DZ twins:			
Same sex	0	8	8
Opposite sexes	0	15	15
Unknown	6	3	9
Total	12	26	38

* Data from Allen and Baroff, 1955.

Twin studies

Case reports of Down's syndrome in twins had long indicated that MZ pairs were almost invariably concordant and DZ pairs almost always discordant. Table 5-1 shows the findings of a systematically collected sample. Without going into details about the distribution of MZ and DZ twins in the table, we may note the complete reversal of pairwise concordance rates in the two types of twins. This finding clearly supported the view that the disorder had no simple genetic explanation, but at the same time provided very strong evidence of an inherited basis for the syndrome. Similarly, in schizophrenia, twin studies for a long time provided the most salient evidence that heredity played an important role in that disorder, although findings in other types of studies were also consistent with that view.

Hereditary factors

The discovery that man had 46 chromosomes was first reported in 1956. Three years later, a report indicated that Down's children had 47 chromosomes. In 1960, a Down's child selected for study because of his mother's youthful age revealed a chromosomal translocation rather than an extra chromosome. And in 1961, a Down's child was found to have *mosaicism* (a condition in which part of the individual is made up of tissue genetically or chromosomally different from the remaining part). Thus, once a method for demonstrating human karyotypes was sufficiently perfected, the discoveries of chromosomal abnormalities followed quickly, and multiple but related causes for Down's syndrome were found.

However, most cases by far, 92 percent, have *trisomy* 21, or three chromosomes of the twenty-first type. The trisomy is traced to *nondisjunction*, that is, the failure of one pair of chromosomes to separate properly during meiosis, so that instead of each of the two pairs of #21 chromosomes ending up in each of two resulting gametes, one pair plus one chromosome ends up in one gamete, whereas the other gamete contains only the one remaining chromosome. The cells of older women are more likely to foster nondisjunction, which accounts for the higher incidence of Down's babies among them. It is the gamete containing the three chromosomes that is fertilized. If the gamete containing the one chromosome had been fertilized, the resulting zygote would not have developed or survived, since the complete complement of autosomes seems to be necessary for survival.

TURNER'S SYNDROME

In contrast with the case in which one of the autosomes is missing, individuals who are lacking one of the sex chromosomes may survive quite well, although they show a number of abnormalities. Such is the case in Turner's syndrome. Those lacking the sex chromosome are designated XO, the O representing the missing X or Y chromosome. No YO individual has been found. Individuals with Turner's syndrome are phenotypically female, but they lack ovarian tissue. They have short stature and infantile sex development. Usually, one also observes webbed neck, a shieldlike chest, cardiac defects, a deformity of the forearm, and polydactylism (too many fingers or toes) (see Figure 5-4). Although the abnormalities are present at birth, the clinical signs first appear with certainty in puberty, that is, with the failure to develop secondary sex characteristics. The subject on examination is found to have a high FSH (follicle-stimulating hormone) blood level without estrogen production. The buccal epithelial cells reveal an absence of the normal female chromatin mass. This mass is the *sex chromatin* or *Barr body*, a spot that lies against the nuclear membrane of resting female cells and does not occur in male cells.

Turner described the syndrome in 1938. In 1959, three of Turner's cases were shown to be XO, with only 45 chromosomes in their karyotype. However, subsequent reports indicated that XO cases accounted for only about one-half of all Turner's cases. Among other cases with this syndrome, some involve a chromosomal mosaicism and others a structural abnormality of one of the X chromosomes. Thus, three different kinds of chromosomal abnormalities have been subsumed in this syndrome. In some cases of Turner's syndrome, no chromosomal abnormality has been found at all.

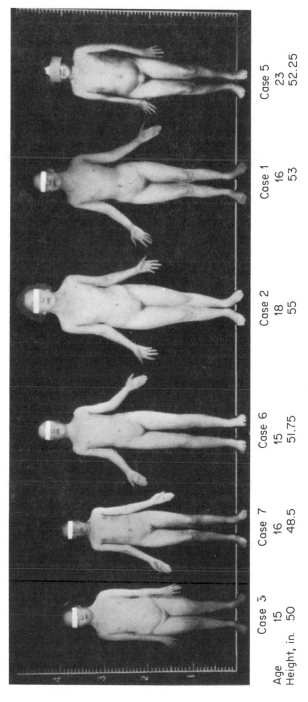

	Case 3	Case 7	Case 6	Case 2	Case 1	Case 5
Age	15	16	15	18	16	23
Height, in.	50	48.5	51.75	55	53	52.25

Figure 5-4. Patients with Turner's syndrome, illustrating infantilism, webbed neck, and cubitus valgus. (From J. J. Turner, A syndrome of infantilism, congenital webbed neck and cubitus valgus, *Endocrinology*, 1938, **23**. Reprinted with permission of J. B. Lippincott Co.)

Incidence and distribution

The incidence of XO monosomics at birth has been reported to be about 4/10,000. The total of all Turner's syndrome cases, including the mosaics and abnormal X-chromosome structures, may be assumed to be about one-third higher than that. However, the number of XO conceptions is much higher. It has been estimated that of about 14 such conceptions, only 1 survives. These XO births show no association with birth order or age of mother, but seem to be distributed proportionately among all births. Familial instances of the disorder are exceedingly rare. Parental consanguinity is also rare. The syndrome seems not to be associated with maternal illness or complications in pregnancy. Interestingly, it has been possible to determine in many XO cases whether it is the paternal or maternal sex chromosome that has been lost. The parents themselves have a normal karyotype. From a genetic point of view, it is clear that with only one X chromosome, the possibility of dominance of X alleles does not arise as in the normal female. In fact, the ordinarily recessive sex-linked phenotypes of a parent are manifested when the X chromosome is inherited from that parent. Another point of interest is that reports have indicated an association between Turner's syndrome and twinning in that a disproportionately large number of such cases have been found among MZ twins. The possibility of a parallel association between schizophrenia and twinship has also been raised.

Associated behavioral characteristics

Turner's-syndrome cases reveal no known neurological defect or any typical speech or motor defect. Their IQ distribution is like that of the normal population, but on the WAIS (Wechsler Adult Intelligence Scale) the verbal scale score tends to be higher than the performance scale. Factor analysis attributes this finding to a relatively high verbal-comprehension ability as against a deficit in perceptual organization. The latter finding was confirmed in studies using other tests. The Draw-a-Person test performance was characterized by a lack of feminine-looking figures and by general immaturity. Rorschach and TAT (Thematic Apperception Test) responses were characterized by an absence of the sexual and aggressive feelings that accompany the desire to be independent, mature females.

We must ask the question: If neurological and motor findings are essentially negative in such cases, and if the IQ distribution resembles that of the population at large, how shall we interpret the test findings reported? Two possibilities suggest themselves. The first is that the findings are direct reflections of the chromosomal abnormalities. The second is that the findings reflect the psychological impact of being so afflicted. In fact, some test findings may have one cause, some the other. For example, it may be that the deficit in perceptual organization stems directly from the chromosomal aberration. The absence of normal aggressive feelings may reflect a hormonal defect, a self-concept of unworthiness or self-abnegation, or other social-psychological factors such as a sense of being abnormal, a freak, or a misfit. Actually, chromosomal, hormonal, and psychological factors could conceivably act in concert to condition the kinds of test responses found. In the functional-behavioral disorders, for example, schizophrenia, test-response differences between index subjects and their controls could similarly reflect genetic factors, the clinical condition itself, or psychological factors associated with both of these and with life experiences as well. This problem currently occupies many investigators of schizophrenia.

KLINEFELTER'S SYNDROME

Individuals with Turner's syndrome may be thought of as incomplete females. They are classified clinically as cases of ovarian dysgenesis. Individuals with Klinefelter's syndrome are phenotypic males who may be thought of as incomplete males or male-female mixtures. Clinically, they represent a category of seminiferous tubule dysgenesis. Whereas Turner's cases lack a sex chromosome, Klinefelter's cases have one or more sex chromosomes too many. About 60 to 70 percent are XXY. Mosaicism is present in about 20 percent of the cases. Other variants include XXXY, XXXXY, XXYY, and XXXYY. The variants with two Y chromosomes are probably the least common. The more common mosaics tend to have some cells that are XXY and some that are XX in some cases, that is, XXY/XX, or XY in others, that is, XXY/XY.

Klinefelter and his colleagues described the disorder in 1942 as a clinical condition in male patients who suffered from increased development of the breasts (gynecomastia), lack of spermatogenesis, and increased excretion of FSH (follicle-stimulating hormone). Although the chromosomal abnormalities can be detected at birth by sex-chromatin studies, the syndrome itself first becomes clearly apparent at puberty. In addition to the symptoms mentioned, one also finds eunuchoid stature, the female escutcheon, and decreased body hair. Some may shave infrequently and some have no beard at all. Puberty is prolonged, as is growth (sometimes till age thirty) so that the average height of such individuals is about 6 feet. The penis may be small or average size, but the testes are invariably tiny, seldom exceeding 1.5 centimeters in

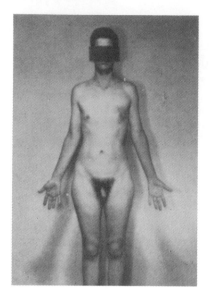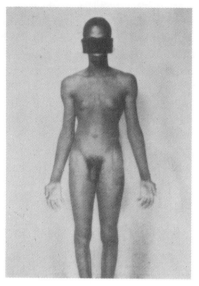

Figure 5-5. Major physical features in Klinefelter's syndrome. (*Left*)
Case D. H. 4; (*right*) case J. W. 3. Feminine habitus is frequently
marked as shown in D. H. 4. Paucity of body hair, abundant head hair,
lack of acne, eunuchoid stature, gynecomastia, small penis, and female
escutcheon are nearly always present. (Penis is normal size in J. W. 3.)
The testes are invariably tiny. (From R. A. Rohde, Chromatin-positive
Klinefelter's syndrome: Clinical and cytogenetic studies, *J. Chronic Diseases*, 1963, **16.** Reprinted with permission of Pergamon Press.)

length. The patients are almost always sterile. Skeletomuscular abnormalities are common, but there are no clearly associated neurological
abnormalities and no characteristic speech defect (see Figure 5-5).

Incidence and distribution

Using sex-chromatin studies at birth, investigators have reported
the incidence of the syndrome to be about 2/1,000 to 3/1,000. Among
male patients in mental institutions about 1 percent were found to be
positive for sex chromatin. The incidence of the disorder is much higher
than that of Turner's syndrome, in good part, probably, because mortality is much lower. In fact, despite the many disabilities, it has been
reported that there seems to be no major shortening of life-span in
Klinefelter's cases.

As in Down's syndrome, the average maternal age at birth is higher
for the mothers of Klinefelter's-syndrome children than for the average
mother in the population at large. Again, maternal nondisjunction seems

to be primarily involved. Red-green color blindness, which is an X-linked recessive trait, can be used to determine the relative frequency of maternal versus paternal nondisjunction. Because individuals with Klinefelter's syndrome have more than one X chromosome, these individuals have a very low frequency of red-green color blindness, as compared with normal males.

Some investigators have reported chromatin-negative cases of Klinefelter's syndrome, but doubts have been expressed regarding the frequency of this type, or whether such a homogeneous group indeed exists. In schizophrenia, similar problems arise regarding which cases should or should not be included in that syndrome. It is noteworthy, too, that primary hypogonadism due to radiation, orchitis, inflammation, or trauma (such as surgery) during childhood may produce a phenotype indistinguishable from Klinefelter's syndrome. In schizophrenia, the question has been debated whether some forms of the diagnostic group were primarily genetically caused whereas others were primarily due to environmental causes.

Associated behavioral characteristics

About 25 percent of Klinefelter's-syndrome cases have below normal intelligence. It is unfortunate that a larger number of systematically obtained samples have not been compiled in which the subjects are examined intensively by psychiatrists and psychologists. A provocative study is reported in which, during a one-year period, 12 males were referred to a cytogenetics laboratory for study of hypogonadism. Of the 12 cases, 8 had Klinefelter's syndrome. All 8 were sex-chromatin-positive. Of these, 2 had below normal intelligence; 4 had married, 1 of whom was now twice divorced. Of the 4 single subjects, 1 was age 17, another 27. The remaining 6 ranged in age from 44 to 74. The 2 single subjects who were older were admitted homosexuals. Another subject was considered to be probably homosexual on the grounds that he openly expressed a strong dislike for women and that he had a positive serological test for syphilis.

Two patients had had psychiatric care for psychoses which the author called schizophrenia. Two others had been under observation for suspected psychoses. The seventeen-year-old had been judged delinquent by the juvenile court and sentenced to a detention center. Another patient had had repeated lengthy prison terms, and had spent 34 years incarcerated. The two remaining patients were diagnosed "psychoneurotic with somatic complaints attributable to conversion hysteria."

Are these diverse behavioral disorders primary expressions of the chromosomal abnormalities, or are they secondary and reactive to their abnormal sexual status? The author, a cytogeneticist (Rohde, 1963) says of his patients:

> During puberty, the first stigmata may be tiny testes, excessively long legs, delayed onset of puberty, or gynecomastia. These patients are frequently harrassed by their schoolmates in locker and shower rooms, at boy's camps, and other places where their bodies are exposed revealing gynecomastia, small genitalia, tiny testes, lack of hair development, eunochoid stature, etc. During adulthood, additional peculiarities appear, such as decreased shaving frequency, feminine habitus, impotence, small ejaculate, muscular weakness, homosexuality, and psychiatric problems. Those who marry face concern with coital relationships and the invariable factor of sterility. Older patients are prone to premature Leydig cell failure which further accentuates their existing difficulties.

One patient had offered to wear a brassiere during high school gymnasium periods to cover his gynecomastia. Another said he "went to prison to have the breasts removed." Clearly, the psychological problems posed by the syndrome are pervasive and profound.

If in fact there is a higher incidence of severe psychiatric disturbance among Klinefelter's-syndrome cases than in Turner's-syndrome cases, the difference might reflect the possibility that males, whose masculinity is lowered or impugned for various reasons, may be subjected to greater psychological turmoil than females with parallel problems in sex identification. Of course, the difference could possibly be the result of the chromosomal and hormonal differences between the two disorders. Such questions are worth exploring, and they may indeed throw light on behavioral disorders generally. The fact that four of the eight subjects above were psychotic or possibly psychotic suggests that the pathways to psychoses like schizophrenia may be multiple and varied.

DIABETES MELLITUS

"Diabetes mellitus is in many respects a geneticist's nightmare. As a disease, it presents almost every impediment to a proper genetic study which can be recognized" (Neel et al., 1965). The genetic bases of the previous disorders described in this chapter have been discovered and their diagnosis—or unit character—has been rather clearly delineated. In schizophrenia and the other functional-behavioral disorders, we do not have matters so tidily packaged. The other disorders are relatively rare; schizophrenia is comparatively common. What problems and data do we encounter when we take a close look at a well-known disease that has no agreed-upon cause, that occurs rather commonly, and whose definition is not certain? Such a disease is diabetes mellitus. The quotation above is the lead paragraph of a fine article by some distinguished American scientists. Probably no other disease presents so many striking parallels to schizophrenia with regard to problems, findings, research strategies, and conceptual difficulties. By examining them, we should be better prepared to appreciate the body of knowledge accumulated in studies of schizophrenia.

What are the impediments that these authors mention?

1 The nature of the basic defect is unknown. Therefore, the disease may be heterogeneous (have different causes).

2 The frequency of the disorder in the general population is not well defined. It is therefore difficult to test hypotheses that draw on the concept of gene frequency.

3 It is not clear whether diabetes mellitus should be regarded as a distinct, qualitative departure from the norm (that is, from normal glucose metabolism) or as the tail of a continuous distribution in which some individuals have secondary complications that give the impression of a discrete disease.

4 The frequency with which the disease is diagnosed appears to be strongly influenced by environmental variables.

5 The disease may become apparent at any age from one to one-hundred. The geneticist may therefore be working with only a fraction of the possible cases.

6 Juvenile diabetics seldom reproduce.

7 There are well-known problems in the reproducibility of certain diagnostic procedures.

Each one of the above types of impediment applies to schizophrenia as well.

The familial nature of diabetes was reported as far back as 1696. In 1835, Ambrosiani discovered that diabetics had higher blood-sugar levels (hyperglycemia) than nondiabetics. To this day, hyperglycemia is the only essential sign of the disorder. In 1933 and 1934, several studies, using sound statistical methods, established that the prevalence of diabetes was higher among relatives of diabetics than of control subjects. Clinically, diabetes has been divided into two main types: (1) juvenile; and (2) adult-onset. Their characteristics are shown in Table 5-2.

Not only do the contrasts shown in the table occur between the

Table 5-2

Some Contrasting Characteristics of Juvenile and Adult-onset Diabetes

Juvenile Diabetes	*Adult-onset Diabetes*
Onset during growing period	Onset during adulthood
Severe ketoacidosis in insulin withdrawal	Absence of severe ketoacidosis
Normal, or hypersensitivity to insulin	Subnormal sensitivity to insulin
Severe weight loss	Obesity
Nonresponsive to hypoglycemic sulfonylureas	Responsive to hypoglycemic sulfonylureas
Decreased pancreatic and plasma insulin content	No such decrease

two types, but to make things worse, intermediate forms occur as well. Moreover, classification of diabetes mellitus based on carbohydrate metabolism differs from clinical classification. To complicate matters further, there are conditions called chemical or latent diabetes, which is asymptomatic diabetes, and "stress" hyperglycemia. The clinical course varies widely and many persons with the predisposition never have overt disease. Similarly, in schizophrenia, we do not know if prepubertal schizophrenic-type disorders belong with later cases, or whether late-onset cases should be included as well. Should cases diagnosed by tests, but clinically not symptomatic, be called schizophrenic? Some cases are called latent schizophrenia, and some "stress" reactions may be called schizophrenic. The clinical course varies widely, and many "predisposed" individuals do not show the disease clinically. Are all these part of one generic disorder?

Incidence and distribution

One finds a high level of incidence and prevalence of diabetes mellitus among all human races and societies. A slightly increased incidence has been reported among Jews. A United States National Health Survey made in 1960 estimated the frequency of recognized diabetes mellitus as shown in Table 5-3.

However, prevalence rates that have been reported increase with improved methods of detecting hyperglycemia or predisposition to the disease. Whereas studies of overt diabetics (with correction for age) give rates of about 3.5 percent, prevalence figures as high as 6.2 percent are obtained with a glucose-tolerance test (GTT). The ethnic variability regarding the clinical disease has not been successfully related to

Table 5-3

Prevalence of Recognized Diabetes Mellitus (Rates per 100 Persons)

Age	Males	Females
0–24	0.11	0.07
25–44	0.49	0.38
45–54	1.12	1.37
55–64	2.52	3.15
65–74	3.44	5.03
75+	3.15	3.88

environmental factors, which suggests that genetic heterogeneity may account for the differences.

Studies of the relatives of diabetics and control subjects yield the prevalence rates shown in Table 5-4. This table shows a clear difference between the relatives of index and control subjects and between the rates yielded by the clinical and GTT methods.

Twin studies

One study using the clinical method reported concordance rates of 48 and 2 percent for MZ and DZ twins, respectively. One study using the GTT method reported concordance rates of 65 and 22 percent for MZ and DZ twins, respectively. It is not clear why clinical concordance in MZ twins is so much lower than the expected 100 percent.

Table 5-4

Prevalence of Diabetes Mellitus among Relatives of Index Cases and Controls

Study	Relationship	Diagnostic Method	Percent Affected Index	Percent Affected Control
Pincus and White, 1933	Parents	Clinical	8.33	1.96
Pincus and White, 1933	Sibs	Clinical	5.85	0.62
Hanhart, 1953	Close relatives	Clinical	5.3	1.2
Conn and Fajans, 1961	Close relatives	Oral GTT	18.0	<1.0
Conn and Fajans, 1961	Close relatives	Cortisone GTT	26.0	4.0

Even with the GTT method, 35 percent are still discordant. In schizophrenia, comparable rates are reported in twins. The lower than expected rates have been attributed to incomplete penetrance (which has itself not been explained). Another proffered explanation, based on the assumed high frequency of the gene in the population, has led to the inference that diabetics are more fertile (some evidence suggests that diabetics have larger than average families) or that the gene favors some other survival characteristic. In schizophrenia, fertility is clearly *reduced,* but assumptions that the implicated gene(s) favors survival have been proposed.

Mode of inheritance

The authors of the first genetic study of diabetes mellitus concluded that the mechanism involved an autosomal recessive gene. The following year, another group of investigators attributed the disorder to a gene that showed irregular (or incomplete) dominance. Since then, both the recessive and dominance theories have had their advocates. One pair of authors suggested that the disorder might be sex-linked, but later withdrew this proposal. One author proposed that the juveniles who developed the more severe form of the illness were homozygotes, whereas those developing the milder adult forms were heterozygotes. Studies were made of the offspring of diabetic couples to see if such findings might help to decide which theory was correct, but they did not. Some authors recognized the possibility that their conjugal diabetics came from a hospital sample that might have been weighted for severity of diabetes, thereby yielding an excess of affected offspring beyond expectation. In the 1960s, the theory of polygenic or multifactorial inheritance began to win adherents. Newer findings have strengthened the case for this mode of inheritance. Attempts to pin down possible implicated environmental factors persist. This recital of theories and events could have been made verbatim for schizophrenia.

Different investigators have postulated different causes of diabetes mellitus, for example, an abnormal insulin molecule, an excess of insulin antagonists, an initial overproduction of insulin followed by excessive antagonist activity, or a too-high rate of release of fatty acids and ketone bodies for oxidation with an impaired sensitivity to insulin. It has also been proposed that the primary defect has nothing to do with insulin at all but results from an abnormality in the basement membrane of the small blood vessels. In schizophrenia, different investigators and theorists have at one time or another implicated almost every organ system in the body and innumerable metabolites or environmental agents as the source of the primary defect.

Associated behavioral characteristics

Diabetics show a normal IQ distribution, but diabetic children seem to be relatively superior in verbal expression and retarded in performance. Some studies purport to show an emotional basis for the onset of the disease, but other studies do not support this view. Some studies suggest that diabetics react physiologically when stressed, and that recurrent acidosis and diabetic regulation, in general, have an emotional basis. At least one study finds no evidence for this view. Some have claimed to find in diabetics a particular personality pattern that is distinctive. One author claims to identify a clear-cut clinical picture that he calls diabetic psychosis. Depression, anxiety, maladjustment, and psychopathic behavior have been found in diabetics. Some experimentors have raised the question whether the disease produces psychological problems that lead to abnormal behavior. Psychological tests are now being brought to bear on the study of these issues, but as yet no definite conclusions can be stated.

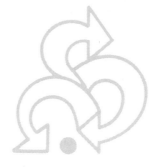

Chapter Six

Genetic Studies of
Schizophrenia
(Dementia Praecox)

To appreciate the nature of the disorders called schizophrenic, and the research findings and theories regarding them, the reader should have seen and interacted with at least one schizophrenic, but preferably many, because the clinical manifestations vary so widely. Since many readers, especially students, may not have had such an experience, or may not have appreciated the experiences they did have, it is desirable to present a brief, well-described case as an introduction to this chapter and as a concrete illustration of what is meant by schizophrenia. No case could serve this purpose better than one by the great clinical psychiatrist, Emile Kraepelin, who was a master of observation, descriptive recording, and systematization. These talents were sharpened during his early professional training when he spent several years in the laboratory of Wilhelm Wundt, the pioneering experimental psychologist. The following is part of an 1894 "Lecture on Dementia Praecox (Insanity of Adolescence)."[1]

> Gentlemen, You have before you today a strongly-built and well-nourished man, aged twenty-one, who entered the hospital a few weeks ago. He sits quietly looking in front of him, and does not raise his eyes when he is spoken to, but evidently understands all our questions

[1] Reprinted with permission of Philosophical Library, New York.

very well, for he answers quite relevantly, though slowly and often only after repeated questioning. From his brief remarks, made in a low tone, we gather that he thinks he is ill, without getting any more precise information about the nature of the illness and its symptoms. The patient attributes his malady to the onanism he has practised since he was ten years old. He thinks that he has thus incurred the guilt of a sin against the sixth commandment, has very much reduced his power of working, has made himself feel languid and miserable, and has become a hypochondriac. Thus, as the result of reading certain books, he imagined that he had a rupture and suffered from wasting of the spinal cord, neither of which was the case. He would not associate with his comrades any longer, because he thought they saw the result of his vice and made fun of him. The patient makes all these statements in an indifferent tone, without looking up or troubling about his surroundings. His expression betrays no emotion; he only laughs for a moment now and then. There is occasional wrinkling of the forehead or facial spasms. Round the mouth and nose a fine, changing twitching is constantly observed.

The patient gives us a correct account of his past experiences. His knowledge speaks for the high degree of his education: indeed, he was ready to enter the University a year ago. He also knows where he is and how long he has been here, but he is only very imperfectly acquainted with the names of the people round him, and says that he has never asked about them. He can only give a very meagre account of the general events of the last year. In answer to our questions, he declares that he is ready to remain in the hospital for the present. He would certainly prefer it if he could enter a profession, but he cannot say what he would like to take up. No physical disturbances can be definitely made out, except exaggerated knee-jerks.

At first sight, perhaps the patient reminds you of the states of depression which we have learned to recognise in former lectures. But on closer examination you will easily understand that, in spite of certain isolated points of resemblance, we have to deal with a disease having features of quite another kind. The patient makes his statements slowly and in monosyllables, not because his wish to answer meets with overpowering hindrances, but because he feels no desire to speak at all. He certainly hears and understands what is said to him very well, but he does not take the trouble to attend to it. He pays no heed, and answers whatever occurs to him without thinking. No visible effort of the will is to be noticed. All his movements are languid and expressionless, but are made without hindrance or trouble. There is no sign of emotional dejection, such as one would expect from the nature of his talk, and the patient remains quite dull throughout, experiencing neither fear nor hope nor desires. He is not at all deeply affected by what goes on before him, although he understands it without actual difficulty. It is all the same to him who appears or disappears where he is, or who talks to him and takes care of him, and he does not even once ask their names.

This peculiar and fundamental want of any *strong feeling of the impressions of life,* with unimpaired ability to understand and to remember, is really the diagnostic symptom of the disease we have before us. It becomes still plainer if we observe the patient for a time, and see that, in spite of his good education, he lies in bed for weeks and months, or sits about without feeling the slightest need of occupation. He broods, staring in front of him with expressionless features, over which a vacant smile occasionally plays, or at the best turns over the leaves of a book for a moment, apparently speechless, and not troubling about anything. Even when he has visitors, he sits without showing any interest, does not ask about what is happening at home, hardly even greets his parents, and goes back indifferently to the ward. He can hardly be induced to write a letter, and says that he has nothing to write about. But he occasionally composes a letter to the doctor, expressing all kinds of distorted, half-formed ideas, with a peculiar and silly play on words, in very fair style, but with little connection. He begs for "a little more *allegro* in the treatment," and "liberationary movement with a view to the widening of the horizon," will "*ergo* extort some wit in lectures," and "*nota bene* for God's sake only does not wish to be combined with the club of the harmless." "Professional work is the balm of life."

These scraps of writing, as well as his statements that he is pondering over the world, or putting himself together a moral philosophy, leave no doubt that, besides the emotional barrenness, there is also a high degree of *weakness* of *judgment* and *flightiness,* although the pure memory has suffered little, if at all. We have a *mental and emotional infirmity* to deal with, which reminds us only outwardly of the states of depression previously described. This infirmity is the incurable outcome of a very common history of disease, to which we will provisionally give the name of *Dementia Praecox.*

The development of the illness has been quite gradual. Our patient, whose parents suffered transitorily from "dejection," did not go to school till he was seven years old, as he was a delicate child and spoke badly, but when he did he learned quite well. He was considered to be a reserved and stubborn child. Having practised onanism at a very early age, he became more and more solitary in the last few years, and thought that he was laughed at by his brothers and sisters, and shut out from society because of his ugliness. For this reason he could not bear a looking-glass in his room. After passing the written examination on leaving school, a year ago, he gave up the *vivâ voce,* because he could not work any longer. He cried a great deal, masturbated much, ran about aimlessly, played in a senseless way on the piano, and began to write observations "'On the Nerve-play of Life,' which he cannot get on with." He was incapable of any kind of work, even physical, felt "done for," asked for a revolver, ate Swedish matches to destroy himself, and lost all affection for his family. From time to time he became excited and troublesome, and shouted out of the window at night. In the hospital, too, a state of excitement lasting for several days was observed, in which he chattered in a confused way, made faces, ran about at full speed, wrote disconnected scraps of composition, and crossed and recrossed them with flourishes and unmeaning combinations of letters. After this a state of tranquillity ensued, in which he could give absolutely no account of his extraordinary behaviour.

Besides the mental and emotional imbecility, we meet with other very significant features in the case before us. The first of these is the silly, vacant *laugh*, which is constantly observed in dementia praecox. There is no joyous humor corresponding to this laugh: indeed, some patients complain that they cannot help laughing, without feeling at all inclined to laugh. Other important symptoms are *making faces* or grimacing and the fine muscular twitching in the face which is also very characteristic of dementia praecox. Then we must notice the tendency to peculiar, distorted turns of speech—*senseless playing with syllables and words*—as it often assumes very extraordinary forms in this disease. Lastly, I may call your attention to the fact that, when you offer him your hand, the patient does not grasp it, but only *stretches his own hand out stiffly to meet it*. Here we have the first sign of a disturbance which is often developed in dementia praecox in the most astounding way.

DEFINITION OF THE DISORDER

Eugen Bleuler completed writing his classic work, *Dementia praecox, or The Group of Schizophrenias* in 1908. He said that he owed almost exclusively to Kraepelin the grouping and description of the separate symptoms. What then did Bleuler add to Kraepelin? It was largely an "attempt to advance and enlarge the concepts of psychopathology," an attempt that was "nothing less than the application of Freud's ideas to dementia praecox." In the process, the modern concept of schizophrenia was born. Bleuler protested that the term *dementia praecox* "only designates the disease, not the diseased." Also, the term had no adjectival form, thus making communication clumsy. Yet neither was Bleuler happy with the term *schizophrenia*, which means a splitting of the psychic functions, but he could think of nothing better. Moreover, he too was forced to compromise with language usage in a way that has been misleading, saying that "for the sake of convenience, I use the word in the singular although it is apparent that the group includes several diseases."

For Bleuler, the term designated "a group of psychoses whose course was at times chronic, at times marked by intermittent attacks." The disease process could "stop or retrograde at any stage," but a return to complete recovery never occurred. It was "characterized by a specific type of alteration of thinking, feeling, and relation to the external world which appears nowhere else in this particular fashion. . . . If the disease is marked, the personality loses its unity." Following Freud's student, Jung, Bleuler talked in terms of complexes. At times, one or another complex dominated the personality of affected persons, a complex that was not integrated with drives or ideas. Fragments of ideas were connected in illogical ways. Concepts lost their completeness. Thought associations were bizarre, unpredictable, disconnected, or suddenly blocked altogether. Emotions were lacking or incompatible with concomitant intellectual processes.

Accessory or secondary symptoms included hallucinations (especially hearing nonexistent voices); delusions (especially of persecution and grandiosity); confusion, stupor, excitatory or melancholic fluctuations of feelings; and peculiar motoric signs (called catatonic) such as fixity of posture or limb position or mutism, and repetitive, manneristic, stereotyped movements. Following Kraepelin in part, Bleuler accepted four major subtypes of schizophrenia:

1 *Paranoid.* Hallucinations or delusions continuously dominate the clinical picture.

2 *Catatonia.* Catatonic signs predominate.

3 *Hebephrenia.* Accessory symptoms appear, but are not dominant. Rather, this form has an acute beginning, usually at a young age, and often ends up in a state of psychic disorganization, or "dementia."

4 *Simple.* Accessory signs do not occur, but only the fundamental ones. A progression of affective and intellectual weakness occurs. Motivation and interests, including interest in one's self, diminish or disappear.

Bleuler also emphasized the fact that symptoms existed in "varying degrees and shadings on the entire scale from pathological to normal." Moreover, he pointed out that "milder cases, latent schizophrenics with far less manifest symptoms, are many times more common than the overt, manifest cases." This statement has important implications for genetic studies of schizophrenia, since these milder cases could be genetically linked to the more severe forms, yet they might be missed if not all family members are personally examined.

Bleuler's fundamental or primary symptoms of the illness are:

1 Thought associations lose their continuity.

2 Emotional deterioration is prominent.

3 Ambivalence, that is, having opposite or contrary feelings, desires, or thoughts at the same time.

4 Autism, or living in a world of one's own, detached from reality, absorbed in an inner life.

5 Deterioration of attention, or lack of active interests.

6 Abulia, or lack of will or initiative (but sometimes its opposite, hyperbulia).

7 The ego is never entirely intact.

8 A type of "dementia" characterized by many mistakes in thinking and acting, or by stupidity and foolishness, although the individual is capable of sound intellectual feats and, at times, normal behavior.

9 Inadequate adaptation to the environment: lack of a definite goal, disregard of reality, confusion, sudden fancies, or peculiarities.

By contrast, the simple functions of sensation, perception, orientation, memory, consciousness, and motility remain intact. No one has ever substantially improved on Kraepelin's and Bleuler's characterizations of schizophrenic illness.

From the point of view of genetic theory and study, we need to make the following points:

1 Investigators tend to employ criteria of schizophrenia that are either more like Kraepelin's (in which case they would include only hospitalized, deteriorated cases in their sample) or more like Bleuler's. In the latter case, subjects who show signs of the fundamental symptoms, even if only in mild form, might be diagnosed schizophrenic.

2 In selecting index cases, it is easy to choose cases that are clearly schizophrenic by either Kraepelinian or Bleulerian standards. But in diagnosing relatives of index cases, the decision whether a case should be called schizophrenic or not may differ, depending on whether Kraepelinian or Bleulerian criteria are used, and such decisions may appreciably affect the statistical picture.

3 One can study the genetics of the disorder itself or any of its aspects, such as subtypes or symptoms, considered separately. The latter could be a fruitless enterprise, but it could as well illuminate the nature of the disorder.

DISTRIBUTION OF
THE DISORDER

Geographical distribution, culture, and social class

As far as we can tell, schizophrenia occurs and has occurred in the past in all major areas of the world. Not so long ago, however, a number of investigators believed that the disorder did not occur in so-called primitive societies, or occurred there at a very low rate. They thought that schizophrenia was a disease of civilization: the more complex the society, the more prevalent the disorder. Subsequent investigators challenged this view. They pointed out that the earlier reports were made by anthropologists and sociologists who were not sufficiently conversant with mental disorders, that reports based only on hospital admissions simply reflected the scarcity of such facilities and the reluctance of natives to be admitted, and that many psychotic persons were simply harbored and maintained by the families and tribes, and had not been identified or recognized as ill by the investigators.

Modern investigations afford some support for the latter view. However, it is true that the character or expression of mental disorders may vary with different cultures, and at least in some cultures may be difficult to identify as schizophrenic or not. Authors in the field reflect this uncertainty, sometimes using terms like "ill-defined" or "primitive" psychoses to describe cases. Aborigines have their own terms for these disorders. In Malay, *latah* is a disorder in which a person echoes the words or actions of others, and *amok* refers to violent outbursts, often homicidal, often with ideas of persecution and possession. The *windigo* psychosis of the Ojibwa and Cree tribes in Canada combines homicidal with cannibalistic behavior. We find "frenzied anxiety" in Kenya and "running wild" among the Fuegian tribes. Eskimos manifest "Arctic hysteria," which may combine predominant echoing behavior with trances, convulsions, violence, or foul language. In the Greenland Eskimo disorder *piblokto*, the affected women run around naked. Differential diagnosis may often be difficult in such cases, but many of these observed disorders may well be some form of schizophrenia. Some may be called organic because of infections or infestations which are common in many of the populations in which they are observed.

Several studies suggest that cultural factors may play a suppressive, evocative, or an etiological role with respect to schizophrenia, although no study provides proof of this possibility. One was carried out by Lin (1953) in three areas of Taiwan. The population was young, but the rates for schizophrenia were low: 0.18, 0.25, and 0.21 percent for the three areas, respectively, and 0.21 percent for the groups combined. Using the Weinberg short method and an age of risk between 16 and 40, Lin found the corrected incidence to be 0.59 percent, about three times the empirically observed figure. Even 0.59 percent is in the lower range of estimates in the Western world, but perhaps in this instance the correction is too large as well.

In a study by Leighton et al. (1963) the authors compared two Yoruba populations in Western Nigeria with a rural Canadian province called Sterling County, using the same measures. The figures are shown in Table 6-1. The ratings represent a continuum of psychiatric casualty from A (definite) to D (symptom-free). Significant differences were found between the groups with respect to A and D ratings, but it is the *significantly impaired* group that most concerns us, since this would be the group that contained any schizophrenics. In this respect, Sterling County has a rate double that of the Yoruba villages ($p < 0.01$).

Additional studies reporting cultural differences in rates of schizophrenia have been reported, notably by Murphy (1968). He found relatively high rates among the Tamil-speaking people of South India and Ceylon, the people of northwestern Croatia, Irish Catholics, and the Roman Catholics in Canada. He compared three traditional French-Canadian communities with three whose culture was less traditional and found a much higher prevalence of schizophrenia among women living in the traditional culture (2:1), especially married women over thirty-five, all of whom had similar life histories and clinical pictures. Other studies reported elevated prevalence rates among minority groups living in other-ethnic neighborhoods.

The overall evidence is not strong, nor can we be sure that, even if the figures reported are valid, they reflect true differences in the rate

---

Table 6-1
Main Psychiatric Rating and Impairment in Survey Respondents*

Rating	Villages (n = 262), %	Abeokuta (n = 64), %	Sterling County (n = 1,010), %
A	21	31	31
B	19	14	26
C	35	30	26
D	25	25	17
Significantly impaired	15	19	33

* Data from Leighton et al., 1963.

of schizophrenia, or cultural rather than genetic differences. Some studies have suggested that cultural change—from simple indigenous to complex alien—increases the frequency of schizophrenic illness, but these studies are all fraught with methodological difficulties. New studies may not solve the problem, since very few of the earlier isolated societies are now free of the influences of our more complex societies. Comparisons of different subcultures within our more complex societies also face difficult problems in method. Consequently, the hypothesis of a cultural contribution to etiology remains refractory to test and awaits resolution.

Within Western society, a number of studies have reported a larger number of schizophrenic cases among populations in the lower socio-economic classes than in the higher classes. A representative and well-known study is one by Hollingshead and Redlich (1957), part of whose data is shown in Table 6-2.

So many studies have now reported higher concentrations of schizophrenics among lowest classes that the finding itself is no longer seriously questioned. What does it mean? Several explanations of it have been offered. The four most cogent ones are:

1 The finding indicates that conditions of poverty, inadequate education, low status relative to one's fellow men, and intrafamilial living and rearing patterns common to the lower classes can cause or evoke schizophrenia. One study found a correlation between such stresses and schizophrenia (Langner and Michael, 1963).

Table 6-2

Incidence, Reentry, Continuous, and Prevalence Rates per 100,000 for Schizophrenics, by Class (Age and Sex Adjusted)*

Class	Incidence Rate	Reentry Rate	Continuous Rate	Prevalence Rate
I–II(high)	6	14	97	111
III	8	20	148	168
IV	10	21	269	300
V(low)	20	46	729	895
Chi-square	8.50	13.46	355.62	452.68
Degrees of freedom	3	3	3	3
p	<0.05	<0.01	<0.001	<0.001

* Adapted by permission from A. B. Hollingshead and R. C. Redlich, *Social Class and Mental Illness*, Table 17, John Wiley & Sons, Inc., New York, 1957.

2 Schizophrenic and schizophrenia-prone individuals simply drift downward into the lower-class population, usually into the large cities where they may achieve a kind of anonymity and toleration by others.

3 Families carrying the genes for schizophrenia are less able to cope with social and economic problems, are less likely to be upwardly mobile in the socioeconomic sense, and tend to accumulate at the bottom rung of the social ladder.

4 Prenatal care is much poorer among lower classes and contributes to higher rates of schizophrenia among them.

Up till now, no study has been able to prove that one hypothesis holds true to the exclusion of the others.

Distribution by sex and age

Schizophrenia strikes both sexes about equally. Nevertheless, the age at first admission to a hospital differs somewhat between the sexes. To demonstrate this point, we have selected two sets of data obtained during the era between World Wars I and II, since primarily male admissions to military and veterans hospitals during and shortly after the wars made comparative data between the sexes more difficult to obtain with reliability. The data are shown as curves in Figures 6-1 and 6-2.

The data in Figures 6-1 and 6-2 represent all first admissions in New York State between 1929 and 1931, and in all the United States during 1933. The curves are very much alike. One can readily find similar admission curves in other Western countries. Their major features are that the male admission rate accelerates postpubertally and peaks in the early twenties, in accord with the original views of dementia praecox, whereas for females, the rate climbs more slowly, does not peak until the thirties, and continues to exceed those for males in later life. In these particular curves, the male admissions exceed the females (by as much as 9 percent in New York). Some have thought that this excess might have reflected the greater psychological impact on males of the great depression. Alternative explanations are also possible.

Although schizophrenia has traditionally been thought of as a disease that has its onset during puberty or later, investigators eventually described severe behavioral disorders without observable organic brain defect in young children, and called these cases childhood or preadolescent schizophrenia. In addition, Kanner (1943) described a behavioral

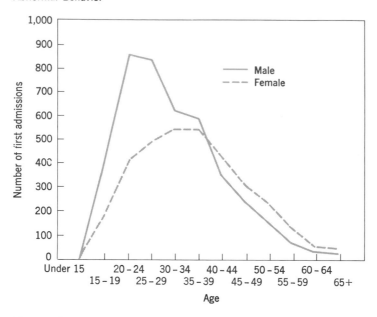

Figure 6-1. Number of first admissions for schizophrenia to state mental hospitals in New York, 1929 to 1931, by age and sex. (Based on data in B. Malzberg, A statistical study of age in relation to mental disease, *Mental Hygiene*, 1935, **19.**)

syndrome in infants and very young children which he called *early infantile autism.* Many investigators came to believe that this syndrome represented an unusually early form of schizophrenia, but others believed that neither it nor the preadolescent schizophrenias should be classified with the adult forms.

To see whether there might be some continuity among these possibly related disorders, we have done the following. Let us ignore for the moment the relative incidence of schizophrenia at any particular age. Instead, let us simply ask: What is the relative proportion of males and females among all new cases at each age? We can then plot the curves shown in Figure 6-3. In this figure, the data are plotted so that the combined male and female cases at any particular age sum to 100 percent. The age group up to four years is represented by the cases of early infantile autism reported by Kanner. The ages between five and fourteen are represented by the average of seven studies reporting numbers of cases by sex with respect to childhood or preadolescent schizophrenia. Ages fifteen and above are represented by the Malzberg data of Figure 6-1.

The continuity of the distributions by sex is rather striking, regardless of what interpretation we place upon it.   In Kanner's cases of early infantile autism, there are about four boys to every girl.   A somewhat lower ratio is reported by other investigators.   Among childhood cases called schizophrenic, the ratio of boys to girls is closer to 2.5:1.   In early adolescence, the ratio is about 2:1.   Thereafter, the gap narrows and reaches equality in the middle to late thirties.   By the late fifties, about two new female cases are admitted for every male.

If the three groups of disorders in fact have a common genetic basis, the curves suggest that the illness manifests itself earlier in males than females.   However, congenital factors that are not genetic could also account for the greater vulnerability in the infant or young male. As a matter of fact, a number of congenital infant disorders have comparable sex ratios, and Goldfarb (1968) reports finding signs of brain damage among his very young psychotic children.   Some investigators have suggested that the rates primarily reflect a greater parental anxiety about behavioral disorders in male children, and that males so afflicted

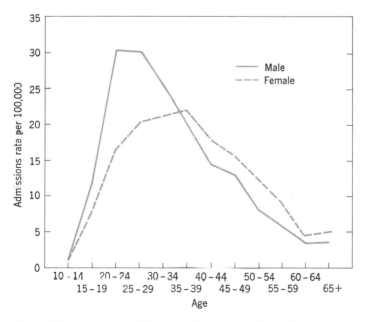

Figure 6-2. Number of first admissions for dementia praecox to state mental hospitals in the United States, 1933, by age and sex. (Based on data in C. Landis and J. D. Page, *Modern Society and Mental Disease,* Ferrar & Rinehart, Inc., New York, 1938.)

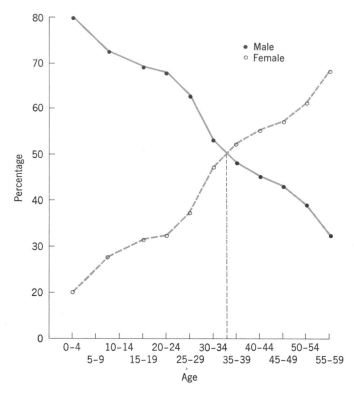

Figure 6-3. New admissions for schizophrenic type of psychoses at different ages.

are more combative, destructive, and less easy to manage, so that mothers are more prone to bring their boys for professional help than girls. Perhaps these possibilities will be better evaluated with further studies.

INCIDENCE AND PREVALENCE

Table 6-3 presents some major studies that have attempted to estimate the incidence of schizophrenia in different populations. They are grouped according to the method used. This table and a few others in this chapter are based in good part on summaries prepared by Zerbin-Rüdin (1967).

The studies cited are sufficient to make the following points. The median morbidity risk in Table 6-3 is about 0.8 percent, but we find considerable variation in the incidence rates reported, regardless of the method used. The largest rate is about four times the smallest for the normal proband method, twice as large for the birth-register method (with only three studies shown), and almost eight times as large for the census method. The smallest rate among all studies is about 3 cases per 1,000 population, the largest about 3 per 100, a difference that is about tenfold.

Such differences must be taken seriously. What do they mean? Can they be dismissed simply as errors of sampling? Possibly for the

Table 6-3
Incidence (Morbidity Risk) of Schizophrenia in Different Populations

Author	Risk Period	Location	Population Size (Weinberg Correction)	Morbidity Risk, %
Normal Proband Method				
Luxenburger, 1928	20–40	Munich	590.5	0.85 ± 0.37
Brugger, 1929	16–40	Basel	391	1.53 ± 0.62
Schulz, 1931	20–40	Munich	262.5	0.76 ± 0.54
M. Bleuler, 1932	17–40	Basel	508	0.98 ± 0.44
Panse, 1936	20–40	Berlin	287.5	0.35 ± 0.35
Birth-register Method				
Klemperer, 1933	16–40	Munich	349	1.40 ± 0.63
Fremming, 1951	15–45	Bornholm	3,777	0.90 ± 0.15
Helgason, 1964	15–49	Iceland	4,913.5	0.73 ± 0.12
Census Method				
Brugger, 1931	20–40	Thuringia	18,454	0.38 ± 0.05
Brugger, 1933	16–40	Allgäu	2,894	0.41 ± 0.12
Sjögren, 1935	15–40	Northern Sweden	4,390	0.68 ± 0.12
Strömgren, 1938	20–40	Bornholm	19,045	0.65 ± 0.05
Brugger, 1938	16–40	Rosenheim	1,643	0.36 + 0.15
Kaila, 1942	20–40	Finland	101,000	0.91 ± 0.02
Sjögren, 1948	20–40	Western Sweden	4,800	0.83 ± 0.13
Schade, 1950	15–45	Schwalm	1,929	0.52 ± 0.16
Böök, 1953	20–45	Northern Sweden	2,912	2.85 ± 0.31
Lin, 1953	16–40	Formosa	19,931 (uncorrected)	0.59
Essen-Möller, 1956	15–40	Southern Sweden	1,515	1.12 ± 0.27
Garrone, 1962	15–70	Geneva	67,662	2.4 ± 0.02

smaller studies, where a few cases might change the risk estimate appreciably, but probably not for the larger studies where big differences occur. Might they reflect real differences among the populations? Probably, at least in part. For example, it does appear that the rates are generally lower for Germany than Switzerland when one uses the normal proband method, and lower for Germany than Sweden or Switzerland when one uses the census method. The same investigator, Brugger, finds a much higher rate in Switzerland than in three German areas. It also appears possible that within Germany, the rate is higher for Munich than for the other areas studied.

From the genetic point of view, such differences, if they are real, suggest that the frequency of the implicated genotype varies from one population to another. Variations of gene frequencies across populations are common. From an environmentalist point of view, they suggest that it is the schizophrenia-inducing conditions that vary across populations. In different subpopulations in Japan, Kishimoto found uncorrected rates that varied from 0.31 to 3.35 percent, the highest rates occurring among isolated mountain villages. Similarly, the highest rate in Table 6-3, 2.85 percent, is found in a highly isolated population in northern Sweden (but the second highest rate occurs in an urban area). Such remarkably high rates could reflect the consequences of generations of inbreeding, or the possibility that small populations living in isolation in the same place thereby increase the risk of developing schizophrenic reactions.

Further variation in Table 6-3 could have arisen for many reasons.

1 The methods themselves differ.

2 The probands may differ (as in the normal proband method).

3 The birth registers include different years and may have different degrees of completeness and cases may be unequally difficult to track.

4 In the census method, investigators may vary in their diagnostic criteria, the proportion of the population they are able to examine personally, and the completeness of their examinations.

5 The extent of emigration.

6 The age of the population and the age of risk used.

Other factors probably contribute to the variations as well.

It is possible to group the studies in Table 6-3 in some way, for example, by country, and to obtain "average" rates for each country. Not surprisingly, these averages show less variation than the rates found in the separate studies, and tend therefore to be more alike. This averaging procedure has been carried out by various investigators who inferred that the rates for schizophrenia were much the same throughout the world because the "averages" of studies in different countries were of a similar order of magnitude. If the variation in Table 6-3 merely represents errors of some kind, the averaging may be justified. If, however, the variation represents real differences, the averaging can only help to obscure the differences and to put off attempts to explain them. Certainly, we cannot argue that the averaging itself, since it reduces variation, indicates that all the studies were random samples from a common population.

In the United States, 40 percent of all hospital beds are occupied by mental patients—about 750,000—and of these, over half are schizophrenic. Pugh and MacMahon, in a sophisticated analysis, concluded that there has been little change in rates of admission for the functional psychoses during this century, although rates of admission and prevalence rates rose for mental illness as a whole. However, Table 6-4 shows some of their data that suggest a possible relationship between wartime stress and admission rates for psychosis, that is, schizophrenic, manic-depressive, involutional, and paranoid psychoses combined.

Table 6-4 shows the admission rates for psychosis in the two age groups who were most affected by the war, that is, the men between twenty and thirty who were most draft-eligible and available for combat, and two older groups who were above draft age. The rates for the

Table 6-4
First Admissions to Mental Hospitals in the United States for Psychotic Disorders (Rates per 100,000 per Year)*

Sex	Age	1922	1939	1941	1942	1943	1944	1945
Male	20–24	50.2	46.3	47.0	51.8	65.0	85.3	88.3
	25–29	54.8	50.1	52.2	52.7	64.4	81.1	80.2
	45–49	36.6	38.9	36.9	35.9	32.0	32.2	33.2
	50–54	34.1	37.1	33.6	34.5	32.7	31.4	33.4
Total	15 70+	38.0	35.2	34.7	35.5	39.1	45.6	46.1
Female	20–24	29.6	34.6	38.3	37.6	34.5	40.0	41.5
	25–29	43.0	46.5	47.3	46.0	43.2	51.6	53.8
	45–49	62.3	58.7	61.3	58.6	55.9	58.3	62.8
	50–54	59.3	59.0	60.5	60.9	58.6	61.2	65.2
Total	15–70+	41.5	40.9	42.7	42.1	39.9	43.6	46.8

* Data from Pugh and MacMahon, 1962.

younger men rose strikingly, the increase ranging from about 60 to 90 percent.   The older men showed no increase at all.   The rates for the male population as a whole blur the increase among the younger men and suggest no appreciable change for males overall.   Among younger women, there was only a slight increase during the latter war years, perhaps reflecting their deprivation of or involvement with their men, but the increase was not very different from that of the older women, many of whom may have had sons in service.   The increases for the younger men would have had to be the result of increases in schizophrenia, since the other disorders subsumed under the category "psychosis" usually affect males much later in life.

It is also relevant that studies have indicated that the morbidity risk for American Negroes was about twice that of whites.   Although the possibility exists that the rates reflect genetic differences, studies of the African Negro do not lend strength to such a view.   Such data, and the Pugh-MacMahon data, if they do not reflect sampling artifacts, suggest that intense, prolonged stresses of certain kinds may indeed play some role in the etiology of schizophrenic disorders.   If this is true, genetic analysis must take such possibilities into account.

FAMILIAL
MORBIDITY RISK

The most reliable calculations of morbidity risk among relatives can be made among first-degree relatives, especially parents and sibs.   Usually, children of probands have not yet lived through a substantial part of the risk period, grandparents will have died or reached the age of senile disorders and become difficult to diagnose, and information regarding aunts, uncles, cousins, and other distant relations is likely to be less complete.   Morbidity-risk figures for parents and sibs in studies that have reported both are shown in Table 6-5.

In Table 6-5, and in the rest of this section, cases diagnosed as questionable, doubtful, or uncertain schizophrenia are not included because we know that the reliability of the diagnosis of certain schizophrenia is high whereas the diagnosis of the questionable cases is less reliable, and we wish to compare rates among relatives.   For other purposes, we might want to include such cases.   Where information about morbidity risk for the general population at the time of the study was reported, that information is included.

Since parents and sibs both share about half their genes with the schizophrenic index cases, we might expect the rates of illness to be the same for the two groups of relatives if the disorder has a genetic

Table 6-5

Morbidity-risk Estimates for Parents and Siblings of Schizophrenic Index Cases

Study	Age of Risk	Number of Probands	Parents	Sibs	Sibs-Parents Ratio	General Population
					Risk Estimates, %	
Brugger, 1928	15–40	85	4.3	10.3	2.4:1	1.53
Bleuler, 1930	20–40	100	2.0	4.9	2.5:1	
Schulz, 1932	15–40	660	2.6	6.7	2.6:1	0.76
Luxenburger, 1936	15–40	128	11.7	7.6	0.65:1	0.85
Smith, 1936	15–40	200	1.2	3.3	2.8:1	
Galatschjan, 1937	15–40	214	4.9	14.0	2.9:1	
Strömgren, 1938	20–40	195	0.7	6.7	9.6:1	0.48
Kallmann, 1938	15–45	1,047	2.7	7.5	2.8:1	0.35
Bleuler, 1941	15–40	100	5.6	10.4	1.9:1	1.53
Kallmann, 1946	15–45	691	9.2	14.3	1.6:1	
Böök, 1953	15–50	80	12.0	9.7	0.81:1	2.85
Slater, 1953	15–40	158	4.1	5.4	1.3:1	
Hallgren-Sjögren, 1959	20–40	247	0.2	5.7	28.5:1	0.83
Garrone, 1962	15–70	227	7.0	8.6	1.2:1	2.40

basis. However, we see that by and large, the rate for sibs is appreciably higher than that for parents. Exceptions occur only in the studies of Luxenburger and Böök. Two studies approach the expected equality—those of Garrone and Slater. In the 10 others, the rule of a higher rate for sibs than parents clearly applies.

The most likely explanation of this finding is that the parents of schizophrenics represent a select group, since schizophrenics are less likely than normals to marry and likely to have fewer children if they do marry. This is especially true for males. Therefore many potential schizophrenic parents are weeded out and do not find their way into the statistics of Table 6-5.

Multiple factors are likely to determine the selection or self-selection for parenthood of potential schizophrenics, and these could vary from place to place and from time to time. Such factors could involve the severity of prodromal disturbances, including the ability to work or assume marital responsibilities; psychological characteristics such as sexual drive and interest, sociability, and attitudes toward oneself; or sociological characteristics such as the cultural group's tolerance or acceptance of preschizophrenic personalities, especially as marriage partners. It may be this multiplicity of factors that makes for the extreme differences in rates reported for parents, from a low of 0.2 or 0.7 percent in the Hallgren-Sjögren and Strömgren studies to highs of 11.7 and 12.0 percent in the Luxenburger and Böök studies. The highest rate is 60 times greater than the lowest. The median rate for parents is about 4.2 percent.

By contrast, the rates for sibs, although they vary appreciably, are far more homogeneous, ranging from a low of 3.3 percent to a high of 14.3 percent, with a median value of about 7.5 percent. The considerable variation in the sib-parent risk ratio is contributed mostly by the variation among rates for parents. The median sib-parent risk ratio is about 2.5:1.

Nevertheless, the studies that report a higher risk for sibs tend to report a higher risk for parents as well. In fact, a rank difference or rho correlation between sibs and parents in Table 6-5 is about .78. This correlation is not associated with the size of the proband sample, since the correlations of sample size with rates for parents or for sibs are not significantly different from zero. However, we do find an association between rates for parents or for sibs and the general population, the rho correlations equaling .75 and .71, respectively. From the genetic point of view, these figures suggest that the frequency of the pathological gene(s) varies in different populations. However, such possible gene-frequency differences should not have a large effect on the rates that occur within families. The correlations may represent diagnostic preferences in different countries and investigators. Such findings would argue against averaging out the figures in Tables 6-3 and 6-5 to find a "representative" estimate of morbidity risk.

The environmentalist could argue similarly that nongenetic predisposing factors vary across populations, and that the varied incidences among relatives simply reflect this fact.

It is clear in any case that the expected rates of 25 or 50 percent for a recessive or dominant gene do not occur with respect to the sibs. The median expectancy is low indeed, although much higher than the rate for the general population. To attribute such large differences between observed and expected rates to reduced penetrance merely emphasizes our ignorance. It may be that rates based only on definite schizophrenia fail to provide all the information we need regarding mental illness in relatives. Later we shall examine this point more closely.

In Table 6-5, the morbidity-risk estimates for schizophrenia in sibs took no account of whether one of the parents of the index case was also schizophrenic. Does the risk estimate for sibs increase in such families or not? Table 6-6 shows six studies that provide information regarding this question. We can see that when at least one parent

Table 6-6

Morbidity Risk for Schizophrenia in Sibs of Schizophrenics When Neither Parent or at Least One Parent Is Schizophrenic

Study	Morbidity Risk, %		Increase, %
	Neither Parent Schizophrenic	At Least One Schizophrenic Parent	
Schulz, 1932	6.6	8.1	23
Luxenburger, 1936	6.7	12.2	82
Galatschjan, 1037	12.2	23.3	91
Kallmann, 1938	6.5	11.7	80
Böök, 1953	9.0	12.7	41
Garrone, 1962	5.5	33.7	513

is schizophrenic—as well as the index case—the morbidity risk for sibs increases strikingly. The smallest increase is 23 percent; the largest, more than fivefold. In half the studies the rate is almost doubled. The increased risk could reflect the fact that the schizophrenic parent is contributing the pathological gene(s) to many of his offspring. Such an increase would be expected whether one's genetic theory was recessive, dominant, or polygenic. An environmentalist, however, would also predict an increased rate among offspring who were reared by a schizophrenic parent.

What could the above data imply with respect to the possible mode of genetic transmission? From the viewpoint of dominance theory, how could we explain the finding in Table 6-6 that when neither parent was schizophrenic, the median risk among sibs of index cases was 6.65 percent? One might infer that in each couple, one parent—who had bred the schizophrenic index case as well—carried the pathological gene, but that he also carried other benign modifying genes that counteracted its effects. These modifying genes could have suppressed clinical manifestations both in the case of the gene-carrying parent—thereby enabling him to marry—and in his children, who show the illness much less often than a simple dominance theory would predict. The fact that this rate rises strikingly when one parent is clearly schizophrenic could be offered as support for this view, but we should then expect to find a risk frequency of 50 percent, whereas the median rate among the proband's sibs is only about 12.5 percent. Supporters of the dominance view could claim again that since this schizophrenic parent was able to marry and reproduce, he was not typical of schizophrenics, and that

he too carried some of the modifying genes that reduced clinical manifestation. They could also argue, more simply, that the pathological
gene shows only variable dominance with reduced penetrance, but we
are then left in the dark about why this may be so.

The argument for a polygenic theory runs much like that for the
single dominant plus multiple modifying genes, but it addresses itself
to the above data more easily, without having to account for deviations
from Mendelian ratios. It would hold that the nonschizophrenic parents
who produced the schizophrenic index cases were carriers of many of
the pathological genes, but not enough to be clinically schizophrenic
themselves. Chance combinations of these genes could make for variable frequencies of the illness among their children, and in Table 6-6,
the median risk for the probands' sibs happens to be 6.65 percent. A
schizophrenic parent carries more of these pathological genes, which are
then more likely to be passed on to the children, thereby leading to the
increased median rate which turns out to be an almost twofold increase.

A theory of recessiveness would express no surprise at finding couples in which neither spouse was schizophrenic but which bred schizophrenic children, although it too must account for the low rates among
probands' sibs, which are much less than the theoretical expectancy
of 25 percent. On the other hand, the discrepancy between the obtained
and expected rates is less for the recessivity than for the dominance
hypothesis. The discrepancy could again be accounted for by attribu-
tions of reduced penetrance and variable manifestation to the ss genotype, or by the postulation of modifying genes. When one parent is
definitely schizophrenic, his genotype is definitely ss instead of the more
likely Ss in the case of the nonschizophrenic parents (a few of whom
could possibly be ss). Since the schizophrenic parent passes on an
s gene all the time, whereas the nonschizophrenic parent passes on an
s gene about half the time, we might expect the rate for schizophrenia
in probands' sibs to be about twice as large when one parent is schizophrenic as it would be if neither parent were schizophrenic. This in
fact is the approximate ratio of the median rates given in Table 6-6.

We can examine the hypothesis of recessiveness further by seeing
whether consanguineous marriages may have been associated with
schizophrenia in their offspring (see Table 6-7). Of the eight studies
shown in Table 6-7 three report no increase of cousin marriages among the
parents of schizophrenics as compared with the rate of such marriages
in the general population. In a fourth study, Böök (1953), the author
expressed his belief that the difference between the two rates in his
study was not significant. In the Strömgren study, the difference between the two groups is less than three times the standard error of
the index group. In two additional studies, the frequency of cousin

Table 6-7

Frequency of Consanguineous Marriages

Author	Location	Frequency among Parents of Schizophrenics, %	Frequency in the General Population, %
Kallmann, 1938	Berlin	No elevated rate	
Strömgren, 1938	Bornholm	6.5 ± 2.2	1.3 ± 0.6
Weinberg and Lobstein, 1943	Amsterdam Jews	13.6	Not stated
Kallmann, 1946	New York	5.7	Not stated
Böök, 1953	Northern Sweden	6.8 ± 2.3	2.2 ± 0.4
Zerbin-Rüdin, 1960	Germany	1.2 ± 0.5	About the same
Garrone, 1962	Geneva	3.5	0.35
Hanhart, 1965	Switzerland	No elevated rate	

marriages in the general population was not known. In the Amsterdam study, the authors were dealing with a relatively small, self-isolating population in which one would expect the frequency of cousin marriages to be high generally. Thus, from these data alone, it is not possible to conclude that the incidence of cousin marriages is greater among the parents of schizophrenics than among those in the population at large. However, when the incidence of the disease is as high as the ones reported in Table 6-3, the probability of finding increased cousin marriages among probands' parents is low, since the postulated recessive gene responsible for the illness would occur with high frequency in the general population, and many marriages would occur between unrelated gene carriers. This method is most relevant to rare diseases. Thus, we find no clear support for the recessive hypothesis based on studies of consanguineous marriages, but neither can we rule it out on these grounds alone.

If we assume that a polygenic mode of inheritance is correct, we can calculate the heritability of liability to the disorder by using the studies in Table 6-5 that provide the necessary information. The calculations may be carried out easily with the use of Falconer's nomograph (Figure 3-2, page 54). The heritabilities are shown in Table 6-8.

It can be readily seen that the heritability estimates fluctuate with the variations in Table 6-5 with respect to observed incidences among parents and sibs. Among parents, heritabilities vary from zero to 85 percent, with a median value of 45 percent. Among sibs, the variation

Table 6-8

Estimations of the Heritability of Schizophrenia Based on an Assumed Quantitative Mode of Inheritance in First-degree Relatives

	Heritability Estimates, %*	
Study	Parents	Sibs
Brugger, 1928	34	73
Schulz, 1932	42	73
Luxenburger, 1936	85	69
Strömgren, 1938	7	73
Kallmann, 1938	52	83
Bleuler, 1941	47	73
Böök, 1953	61	51
Hallgren-Sjögren, 1959	0	60
Garrone, 1962	45	52

* Since within-family environmental correlations probably exist, the estimates are intended to represent upper limits rather than accurate estimates of heritability.

is much less, with a clear modal value of 73 percent. Thus, from a methodological standpoint, the estimates in Table 6-8 reflect an expected close link to and dependency upon the original data on which they are based. If the greater consistency of the figures regarding sibs derives from a closer and more consistent approximation of veridicality than do the figures regarding parents, then 73 percent may represent the best approximation we can make of an estimation of the upper limit of heritability of liability to schizophrenia under uncontrolled and unspecified life conditions.

Of five studies reporting the risk of schizophrenia among children of a schizophrenic parent, four are above the median risk value of 7.5 percent noted for sibs of a schizophrenic, although both children and sibs are first-degree relatives of a schizophrenic index case. The figures are shown in Table 6-9.

Whereas the median risk value for sibs was 7.5 percent, the median risk value for the children in Table 6-9 is 9.7 percent. The absolute difference between the two values is small and perhaps it should be ignored. However, if we had considered the possibility that schizophrenics who are able to marry and become parents have a more benign form of the illness, we might have expected that their children would be similarly protected and would therefore have a *lower* morbidity risk than sibs. Apparently, this is not the case. An environmentalist might be tempted to argue that the possibly increased risk for children as compared with sibs represents the additional hazard of being reared by a schizophrenic parent or in disturbed and broken homes.

The morbidity risk for second-degree relatives, who share approximately one-fourth their genes with a schizophrenic index case, is shown in Table 6-10. This table demonstrates that the morbidity risk is indeed lower among second-order relatives. The median risk value in the table is 2.1 percent. If we accepted the median risk value for sibs or children as the criterion value for first-degree relatives, we would expect the median value for second-degree relatives to be 3.75 or 4.85 percent. However, it is appreciably lower than that. Indeed, a few of the risk values found fall within the range of risk for the population at large. But again, the absolute differences are not large and may simply reflect sampling errors. For example, it may be that as the relationship moves beyond one of first degree, a number of cases are missed or lost. It is possible, too, that the further removed the relationship is from personal contact with and influence by the schizophrenic index case or the conditions that contributed to his becoming schizophrenic, the more sharply reduced is the likelihood that a relative will develop a frank schizophrenic illness.

Among six studies reporting the morbidity risk in third-degree relatives, who share about one-eighth their genes with the schizophrenic index case, the risk estimates are 0.5, 0.8, 1.4, 1.9, 2.8, and 5.5 percent, respectively. The median value is 1.65 percent, which is approximately one-fourth of the median risk value of 7.5 percent for sibs, and is therefore consistent with expectation based on that value. But this risk is only slightly larger than the risk for the population at large.

Table 6-9

Morbidity Risk for Schizophrenia in Children of a Schizophrenic Parent

Study	Number of Probands	Morbidity Risk, %
Hoffmann, 1921	51	7.0 ± 2.8
Oppler, 1932	109	9.7 ± 1.7
Gengnagel, 1933	44	8.3 ± 2.8
Kallmann, 1938	525	13.9 ± 1.3
Garrone, 1962	27	16.9 ± 4.3

What happens if, instead of reducing the probability of gene concentration in our sample by selecting increasingly more distant relatives, we try to *build up* the possible concentration of pathological genes? We can do this by examining the morbidity risk for children *both* of whose parents are schizophrenic. A summary of five studies using this strategy is shown in Table 6-11.

Unfortunately, Kallmann did not state the ages of his *Ss*, but he calculated the morbidity risk for certain schizophrenia in his sample to be 55.3 percent. Among the remaining four studies, we estimate the morbidity risk to be about 35 percent. Since an unqualified theory

Table 6-10

Morbidity Risk for Schizophrenia among Second-degree Relatives of a Schizophrenic Index Case

Study	Number of Probands	Morbidity Risk, %
Grandparents		
Bleuler, 1930	100	0.3 ± 0.3
Bleuler, 1941	100	1.1 ± 0.6
Grandchildren		
Juda, 1928	42	6.5 ± 3.1
Juda, 1928	30	1.8 ± 1.3
Oppler, 1932	95	2.5 ± 1.0
Kallmann, 1938		2.7 ± 0.5
Uncles and Aunts		
Bleuler, 1930	100	0.9 ± 0.4
Smith, 1936	200	1.3 ± 0.3
Galatschjan, 1937	214	3.6 ± 0.6
Bleuler, 1941	100	2.1 ± 0.6
Nephews and Nieces		
Schulz, 1926	76	1.4 ± 0.7
Brugger, 1928	85	3.6 ± 1.8
Walker, 1929	47	2.3 ± 0.9
Konstantinu, 1930	63	1.6 ± 0.6
Kallmann, 1938	328	2.6 ± 0.5

Table 6-11

Psychopathology in Offspring of Schizophrenic Couples

Study	Schizophrenia	Questionable Schizophrenia	Other Psycho- pathology	Normal	Total
Kahn, 1923	7	2	5	3	17
Kallmann, 1938	13	3	16	3	35
Schulz, 1940b	13	5	22	20	60
Elsässer, 1952	12	3	12	32	59
Lewis, 1957	4	0	3	20	27
Total	49	13	58	78	198

of recessiveness or dominance predicts an incidence of 100 or 75 percent, respectively, the risk figure obtained, like all others in this section, falls below expectancy for either theory. In Table 6-9, we had noted that the morbidity-risk estimate for the children of one schizophrenic parent was 9.7 percent. Thus, the risk when both parents are schizophrenic increases about fourfold. An increase is predicted by genetic theory, but not one of this particular magnitude. An increase would also be predicted by environmentalist theories that stress the contribution to schizophrenia made by rearing in a psychosis-ridden or turbulent home.

To summarize briefly the section on familial morbidity risk, we may make the following points:

1 We concerned ourselves only with diagnoses of certain schizophrenia in relatives so that we could make the most reliable comparisons regarding different degrees of blood relationship to schizophrenic index cases and the population at large.

2 There is a clear correlation between the degree of blood relationship and the incidence of schizophrenia in relatives, but the ratios do not correspond to any simple Mendelian pattern.

3 One finds a considerable amount of variation in the morbidity-risk estimates found in different studies of the same class of relatives. It is difficult to say whether this variation reflects random sampling error, systematic errors introduced by differences in case finding, diagnosis, or other factors, or whether real differences exist.

4 There appears to be a correlation between the reported incidence of schizophrenia in a general population and the incidence found among schizophrenics' relatives.

5 We cannot decide on the basis of the reported information whether a modified single-gene theory or a quantitative genetic theory is correct.

6 Since the rate of schizophrenia in relatives is always less than Mendelian expectancy, it may be that some cases called uncertain schizophrenia or other psychopathology represent gene carriers who should be included in the tallies of affected cases.

7 On the basis of the data summarized thus far, we cannot make any inferences regarding the role of environmental factors in producing schizophrenia, but the best estimate of its heritability, if the assumptions regarding its calculation by Falconer's method are met, is about 73 percent when environmental conditions are uncontrolled or unspecified.

TWIN STUDIES

The findings of the major twin studies of schizophrenia are summarized in Table 6-12. Three points are important in this table.

1 The concordance rate for MZ twins is always less than 100 percent, sometimes much less, which indicates that nongenetic factors are playing an important role with respect to who develops schizophrenia and who does not.

2 The concordance rate is always greater for MZ than for DZ pairs, with the possible exception of Tienari's study. The MZ-DZ concordance ratio is appreciable, mostly between 3:1 and 6:1. These findings afford strong but not conclusive evidence of a genetic contribution to schizophrenia. Since schizophrenia occurs about as frequently in twins as in singlets, a view which holds that being an identical twin may itself pose biological or psychological problems that foster schizophrenia will have to explain at the same time why these problems do not lead to an increased incidence of the illness among MZ twins.

3 There is a considerable range in the rates reported both for MZ and DZ pairs. Why should such differences occur and what do they imply?

Probably the main differences can be traced to factors like sampling procedure, diagnostic preferences, methods of zygosity determination, and possibly cultural-geographical differences. With respect to sampling, the three studies that sampled primarily from resident hospital

Table 6-12

Concordance Rates in the Major Twin Studies of Schizophrenia

Study	Sampling Method	Source	Zygosity Diagnosis	MZ Twins		DZ Twins	
				Number of Pairs	% Con-cordant	Number of Pairs	% Con-cordant
Luxenburger, 1928a, 1934	CA*, RHP	Germany	S	17–27	33–76.5	48	2.1
Rosanoff et al., 1934–35	RHP	United States and Canada	S	41	61.0	101	10.0
Essen-Möller, 1941	CA	Sweden	B, S	7–11	14–71	24	8.3–17
Kallmann, 1946	RHP*, CA	New York	S	174	69–86.2	517	10–14.5
Slater, 1953	RHP*, CA	England	F, S	37	65–74.7	115	11.3–14.4
Inouye, 1961	NSS	Japan	S	55	36–60	17	6–12
Tienari, 1963, 1968	TR	Finland	B, S	16	0–6	21	4.8
Gottesman and Shields, 1966	CA	England	F, B, S	24	41.7	33	9.1
Kringlen, 1967	TR	Norway	B, S	55	25–38	172	8–10
Fischer, 1968	TR	Denmark	S	16	19–56	34	6–15
Hoffer et al.	TR	United States veterans	B, S	80	15.5	145	4.4

CA = consecutive admissions   RHP = resident hospital population
TR = twins register   NSS = no systematic sampling
* = primary source   F = fingerprint analysis
S = similarity method   B = blood grouping

populations had the highest pairwise concordance rates: 61, 65, and 69 percent, respectively, for MZ twins. This finding could occur because: (1) a resident population is older, or more chronically and severely ill; (2) resident, concordant MZ pairs are more likely to be called to the investigator's attention; or (3) discordant pairs are missed. When one samples from consecutive admissions, cases are likely to be younger, and some pairs classified discordant could eventually become concordant. Also, problems of diagnosis may be more difficult with acute admissions. When Luxenburger first reported his concordance rate for MZ twins in 1928, he found it to be 76.5 percent. By 1934, he revised the rate to 33 percent, probably because he had changed his mind about some of the original diagnoses or zygosity determinations among his consecutively admitted twins. Essen-Möller had seven definitely schizophrenic MZ index twins, and four who had diagnoses that were "probably genetically related" to schizophrenia. Among the cotwins, none had been hospitalized for psychosis, but most had what Essen-Möller called a *characterological defect,* which he thought was the basically inherited factor that could be the antecedent of schizophrenia. Many years later, one or two of the cotwins did develop hospitalizable schizophrenic illness.

Investigators may employ "strict" criteria of schizophrenia, in which case they would lean toward a Kraepelinian view of the disorder, or a broader, more Bleulerian view. Fischer found the concordance rate in her sample to be 19 percent for strict schizophrenia but 56 percent if one counted disorders in the cotwin such as episodic schizophreniform, and paranoid or atypical psychosis. Gottesman and Shields analyzed their pairs in terms of different gradations of concordance, so that the concordance rate varied with the gradation used, ranging from 41.6 to 79.1 percent. Kallmann employed a very broad conception of schizophrenia which would be more in keeping with American than European tradition.

The striking difference between the United States rates of Kallmann and those of Hoffer are probably best explained in terms of sampling differences. Kallmann's rates are probably too high because he sampled primarily from resident hospital populations. Hoffer, in contrast, obtained his cases from a National Research Council twins register of males actively in military service or those who were veterans. This method ensures against possible selection bias or loss of registered cases, but qualification for military service already provides a screen which could have kept out a number of potentially concordant pairs who would never have been registered. Thus Hoffer's rates are probably too low, and a more representative figure probably lies somewhere between these extremes.

Zygosity determination could account for a smaller part of the variation in Table 6-12. Studies that relied only on the similarity method (which takes into account how much the cotwins look alike, and whether they are concordant for known genetic traits, such as eye color, type of earlobe, complexion, and the like) were more subject to error. Other studies have shown that when errors are made with this method, they tend not to be large, and errors that do occur are in the direction of classifying MZ pairs as DZ.

It has been suggested that there may be true differences in concordance rates for schizophrenia between Scandinavia and Britain and the United States. How could such differences be explained? On environmentalist grounds, one might consider the possibility that sociocultural pressures toward uniformity, sameness, and intense mutual identification of MZ twins are less in Scandinavia. On genetic grounds, Shields has proposed the following explanation. It is possible that the genes that lead to schizophrenia once had survival advantages in the Scandinavian climate. Through natural selection, the population developed other genes that prevented the undesirable manifestations of the schizophrenic genes so that the latter would not be eliminated on that account. Eventually, the population became more uniform with respect to these countergenes, and because of this genetic uniformity, environmental factors contribute relatively more to the observed variance regarding schizophrenia in twins and relatives. The population has also become more uniform regarding the pathological genes, so that one finds in it less of an association between severity of schizophrenic disorder and concordance rates.

We are not able to say which of the two explanations has merit, if either, but they represent very well the imaginative and provocative theorizing generated by the kinds of data with which we are concerned in this chapter.

Concordance and severity of the illness

Evidence exists to indicate an association between the severity of the illness in the index twin and the rate of concordance. That is, the more severely ill the index case, the higher the concordance rate. Rosenthal (1961) organized Kallmann's twin data as shown in Table 6-13 to demonstrate this point.

Kallmann had grouped his schizophrenic MZ twins according to three degrees of severity, based primarily on the degree of deterioration. When the index twin's illness was described as extreme or medium, the concordance rate was 100 percent. When the index twin's illness was mild, the concordance rate fell to 26 percent.

Table 6-13

Severity of Illness in Monozygotic Cotwin in Relation to Severity of Illness in Originally Ascertained Twin*

Severity of First Twin's Illness	Severity of Cotwin's Illness				
	Extreme	Medium	Little or No Deterioration	No Schizo- phrenia	Total
Extreme	29	10	9	0	48
Medium	0	33	20	0	53
Little or no deterioration	0	0	19	54	73
Total	29	43	48	54	174

* Data from Kallmann, 1946.

Similarly, Gottesman and Shields divided their index MZ twins into two classes of severity: those who had been hospitalized more or less than 52 weeks. For those hospitalized more than 52 weeks, the concordance rate was 67 percent, but for those hospitalized less than 52 weeks, it was only 20 percent. Rosenthal also pointed out that in Slater's series, the illness tended to be more severe among the concordant than among the discordant schizophrenic twins. Kringlen found that concordance for the cotwins of less severely ill index cases occurred about half as often as for cotwins of cases with more severe deterioration. It should be clear then, that if one obtains one's sample of twins from a more severely ill population—such as chronic hospital residents—the concordance rates found will be selectively high.

Relatively few cotwins of index cases with typical schizophrenia are found to be "normal." Kringlen finds such normality in 31 percent of his cotwins, with another 31 percent showing typical schizophrenia. Of the cotwins, 9 percent were said to have reactive psychosis or borderline states, while 29 percent carried a diagnosis of neurosis, including character disorders, anxiety states, depressive or somatic neuroses, and alcoholism. Tienari stressed introverted neurotic and borderline features among his cotwins, but found four of them to be "healthy."

Why does one MZ twin become overtly schizophrenic, whereas the other one does not? Usually, the investigator tries to answer this question by interviewing the twins and their relatives to learn about differences between the twins during their developmental years. Most often, the sick twin is the one who was described as neurotic in childhood and who never married. He has been described as more often submissive to his cotwin, sensitive, serious, worried, obedient, gentle, dependent, well-behaved, quiet, shy, and stubborn. More often, too, he was lighter in weight at birth, shorter, weaker, and slower in development, and less intelligent. For an intensive study of how such factors may be implicated in the eventual development of clinical schizophrenia, one can read the case history of the Genain quadruplets (Rosenthal, 1963), who were MZ girls concordant for schizophrenia, but discordant with regard to severity and outcome. Kringlen believes that the sick twin was more likely to have difficulties in relation to his father and to be closer to and overprotected by his mother. Pollin and Stabenau (1968) emphasize the fact that the twins are constantly compared with one another, that the less-favored twin's relatively greater weakness and vulnerability generalizes to become an essential component of his self-image and identity in relation to the entire world, and that these feelings about himself are incompatible with the family's expectations regarding his independence and achievement. The initial CNS (central nervous system) deficiency results in ego weakness and inability to cope with stresses, at which point the genetic factor, in the form of some endocrine or enzyme system abnormality, might play its role. Kringlen reports that his concordant pairs usually experienced a more stressful or pathogenic childhood, in that they came from a lower social class and were subjected to more frequent isolation, and that they tended to be closer to each other and to be less influenced by extrafamilial social contacts.

Sex and concordance

In the systematically sampled twin studies we find a small but consistent difference in the concordance rates for male and female twins, as shown in Table 6-14. In all studies, the number of pairs is rather small. Kallmann did not report concordance rates by sex, but did make it clear that the rates were very similar for both sexes, although just a trifle higher for the female twins. If we consider each sample of MZ or DZ twins as an independent test of the null hypothesis that there is no difference in concordance rates between male and female twins, we should expect that, by chance alone, the rate for males will be higher about half the time. We find instead that the female rate is higher in 12 out of 12 samplings.

It is difficult to say whether this finding is meaningful. By and large, the differences are small and would hardly reach statistical significance for any single study. In studies that sampled from resident hospital populations, there was an excess of female as compared with male index twins, and the higher concordance rates for females might be secondary to this fact. Also, Kringlen's rates are for hospital diagnoses. When he examined the twins personally, he revised the rates

Table 6-14

Twin Concordance Rates for Schizophrenia, According to Sex

	MZ Rates, %		DZ Rates, %	
Study	Female	Male	Female	Male
Luxenburger, 1928b	88	67		
Rosanoff et al., 1934–35	78	42	14	9
Essen-Möller, 1941	75	67	18	9
Slater, 1953	73	45	16	10
Gottesman and Shields, 1966	45	38	12	6
Kringlen, 1967	29	23	9	6
Fischer, 1968	71	44		

to 33 percent for females as compared with 42 percent for males.   This is the only instance of a trend reversal.   The rates in the Fischer study are based on a broad definition of schizophrenia.   Still, the figures may represent a slightly greater tendency for female twins to be (or to have been) drawn into psychosis together, possibly on psychological grounds. Other studies of personality traits and mental illness have pointed fairly consistently to higher concordance rates for females than males in first-degree family relationships.   This finding is most striking in *folie à deux,* a psychotic illness based on long isolated association of two people who eventually come to share the same delusions and other symptoms. Perhaps longer, closer, and more isolated associations between female as compared with male twins could have contributed to some of the differences in the rates found in Table 6-14.   In the past, at least two distinguished investigators considered the possibility that such differences might reflect some kind of sex linkage, but both ruled against it.

Concordance in twins reared apart

Many people have thought that twins reared apart could cast some light on the relative contributions of heredity and environment to schizophrenia.   Unfortunately, the number of such twin pairs is small and knowledge about the rearing circumstances is limited.   Still, the cases are informative.   They have been summarized by Slater, and are shown here as Table 6-15.

Of the 16 twin pairs in Table 6-15, 10 were concordant, 6 discordant.   The concordance rate of 62.5 percent is actually *higher* than the median rate for twins reared together, as summarized in Table 6-12. Why should this be so? It may be simply that whether MZ twins are reared together or apart makes no difference with respect to the eventual development of schizophrenia in one or both twins, and that the environmental factors that make for discordance have nothing to do with a common rearing.

Another possible explanation of the finding might have to do with sampling. For example, among the 5 earlier pairs reported, all were concordant. Among the 11 pairs reported later, 5 were concordant and 6 discordant. The Craike and Slater case was not obtained as part of a systematically selected sample. Neither were the 8 cases reported by Mitsuda. Such sampling tends to favor concordant pairs. The 3 pairs obtained from twin registers were all discordant, and of the 2 concordant pairs obtained through consecutive admissions, the twins' clinical pictures in Essen-Möller's pairs were markedly different. For such reasons, the data in Table 6-15 cannot be regarded as conclusive, but they do suggest again that genetic factors in the etiology of schizophrenia must be taken seriously.

That a common rearing cannot be dismissed entirely by these cases of MZ twins reared apart is supported by a comparison of concordance rates in DZ twins and siblings. Genetically, the DZ twins and sibs are similar in that they share about half their genes in common. Among three studies that provided concordance rates for these two types of relationship, all found a higher rate for DZ twins as compared with sibs in the same families. In Kallmann's study, the difference was negligible:

Table 6-15

Schizophrenia in Monozygotic Twins Reared Apart*

Study	Age at Separation	Concordant Pairs	Discordant Pairs	Source
Kallmann, 1938	Soon after birth	1		Daughters of a schizophrenic proband
Essen-Möller, 1941	7 years	1		Consecutive series of twins
Craike and Slater, 1945	9 months	1		Single case report
Kallmann and Roth, 1956	Not stated	1		An index pair in a series of twins with childhood schizophrenia
Shields, 1962	Birth	1		Consecutive series of twins
Tienari, 1963	3 years; 8 years		2	Register of twin births
Kringlen, 1964	22 months		1	Register of twin births
Mitsuda, 1965	Infancy	5	3	All investigated twins with psychiatric illness

* Data based on Slater, 1968.

15 percent for the DZ twins and 14 percent for sibs. Slater, however, found concordance rates of 14 and 5.4 percent for the DZ pairs and sibling pairs, respectively. This difference is very large. Similarly, Kringlen's rates for the two groups were 8.1 percent as contrasted with 5.2 percent, an increase for DZ twins over sibs of almost 60 percent, which is appreciable. Again, these data are not conclusive, but merely indicate that common rearing in a special relationship may also have etiological significance for schizophrenia.

ADOPTION STUDIES

Five studies have now been reported in which parents and children were separated early in the child's life and the incidence of schizophrenic disorder in the children or their families examined. In this way possible etiological factors related to a common association between parent and child were separated from genetic factors.

The adoptees' families method

One such study was carried out by Kety et al. (1968) in Denmark. Their starting cases included all children (about 5,500) given up for nonfamilial adoption at an early age between 1924 and 1947. All had reached the age of risk at the start of the study. Through a national Psychiatric Register, all adoptees who had been admitted to a psychiatric facility and diagnosed schizophrenic were selected as index cases. From among the remaining adoptees, the investigators selected a control group who had no psychiatric history and who were matched case by case to the index group for sex, age, age at transfer to the adoptive parents, pretransfer history, and socioeconomic status of the adopting family. All adoptive and biological parents, sibs, and half-sibs of both groups were identified through a nationwide People's Register. A search of the Psychiatric Register revealed who among these relatives had a psychiatric history. Their hospital records were examined and diagnoses made without the investigators knowing whether the case diagnosed was a relative of an index or a control case. The major findings of the study are shown in Table 6-16.

In evaluating relatives, the investigators subsumed a broad grouping of cases under what they called *schizophrenic-spectrum disorders*. In this way, no possibly schizophrenic cases were lost. The spectrum included chronic, certain schizophrenia, acute schizophrenia, borderline schizophrenia, and severely schizoid or inadequate personality. As

Table 6-16

Distribution of Schizophrenic-spectrum Disorders among the Biological and Adoptive Relatives of Schizophrenic Index Cases and Control Ss*

	Biological Relatives		Adoptive Relatives	
	Total	Schizophrenic Spectrum	Total	Schizophrenic Spectrum
All probands:				
Index cases (n = 33)	150	13	74	2
Controls (n = 33)	156	3	83	3
p (one-tailed)		0.0072		NS
Probands separated from biological family within one month of birth:				
Index cases (n = 19)	93	9	45	2
Controls (n = 20)	92	0	51	1
p (one-tailed)		0.0018		NS

* Data from Kety et al., 1968.

Table 6-16 indicates, there was a significantly greater number of schizophrenic-spectrum disorders among the biological relatives of schizophrenic index cases than among controls' relatives. Among adoptive relatives, there was no appreciable difference between the two groups. This was true whether the adoptees included only those who had been separated from their biological relatives in the first month of life, or all index adoptees, most of whom had been separated in the first year of life (two Ss had been separated in their second year, and two after age two). Genetic theory would predict such a finding. Most environmentalist theories would predict a higher incidence of such disorders among the adoptive parents of the index cases as compared with the controls, but the findings do not support this prediction.

A corroborative finding in a study carried out in Iceland was reported by Karlsson (1966). He compared the biologic and foster sibs of schizophrenics who had been adopted before age one. Among the biologic sibs, 6 of 29 were schizophrenic. Among the foster sibs, none of the 28 was schizophrenic.

The adoptees study method

Two studies have used this method. One was carried out in Denmark by Rosenthal et al. (1968) and complements the adoptees' families study by Kety et al. The investigators began this study with the approximately 11,000 biological parents who had given up their children for nonfamilial adoption. About 1,000 of the fathers could not be identified with reasonable certainty. Among the remaining 10,000, the files of the Psychiatric Register were searched to find out who among them had a psychiatric history. The hospital records of the latter group were reviewed, and the children of those diagnosed schizophrenic or manic-depressive constituted the index group. From among the remaining pool of approximately 5,500 adoptees, a group of controls was selected, matched on a case-by-case basis to the index Ss. The matching variables were sex, age, age at transfer to the adopting family, and socioeconomic status of the adoptive parents. The controls differed only in that neither of their biological parents was known to have any psychiatric history.

The two groups of subjects were given an intensive personal examination that lasted two days. One-half day was devoted to a psychiatric interview and assessment and one and one-half days to psychological evaluation by means of a variety of tests. The examiners did not know if the subject before them was an index case or a control. Since the adoptee seldom knew about the mental illness in his biological father or mother, he himself could not provide the information that might reveal his index or control status. This study is still in progress at this writing, but Table 6-17 shows some of the main findings that had been accumulated by 1967 regarding the diagnosis of schizophrenic-spectrum disorders in the index and control groups.

Table 6-17

Schizophrenic-spectrum Disorders in Adoptees Who Had a Biological Schizophrenic or Manic-depressive Parent, or Both Biological Parents without Psychiatric History*

Diagnosis of Adoptee	One Parent Schizophrenic or Manic-depressive (n = 39)	Parents without Psychiatric History (n = 47)
Schizophrenia:		
Hospitalized	1	0
Never hospitalized	2	0
Borderline schizophrenia	7	1
Near or probable borderline	0	2
Schizoid or paranoid	3	4
Not in schizophrenic spectrum	26	40

* Data from Rosenthal et al., 1968.

Among the 39 index adoptees examined, 3 were diagnosed schizophrenic, but only 1 of these had been hospitalized; 7 were diagnosed as borderline schizophrenic. Among the 47 control adoptees examined, none was schizophrenic, 1 was a clear borderline, and 2 were near or probable borderline cases. Among the index adoptees, 13 of 39, or one-third, were in the schizophrenic spectrum, as compared with 7 of 47 controls, or about 1 in 7. Moreover, the more severe cases cluster clearly among the index cases, with a ratio of 10:1. There could not have been any biasing tendency based on knowledge of which subject was an index case or a control, since the diagnostician did not have this information. Therefore, the data provide strong evidence indeed that heredity is a salient factor in the etiology of schizophrenic disorders.

The adoptees study method was also used in modified form by Heston (1966). Indeed, his was the first such study of schizophrenia to be reported. He began with actively schizophrenic women who had babies while hospitalized. The babies were separated from their mothers at birth and either placed in foundling homes or in the care of members of the father's family. A control group was selected from records of the foundling homes. The matching variables—on a case-by-case basis—included sex, age, type of eventual placement, and length of time in child care institutions. At the time of study, the age of the Ss averaged thirty-six years. Heston tracked down and personally interviewed most of them—both index cases and controls. He also obtained information about them from other sources, such as private physicians, psychiatric facilities, schools, courts, social agencies, friends, relatives, and employers. He also obtained their IQs and had them complete the Minnesota Multiphasic Personality Inventory (MMPI). Based on all this information, Heston and two other psychiatrists made diagnoses of the Ss and rated them on the Menninger Mental Health-Sickness Rating Scale (MHSRS). The major findings of the study are summarized in Table 6-18.

Most important in Table 6-18 is the fact that five index cases were diagnosed schizophrenic but no controls were. The difference is statistically significant. All five had been hospitalized; three were diagnosed as *chronic deteriorated*. The age-corrected risk for schizophrenia in the index group was 16.6 percent, a rate that falls in the upper reaches of rates reported for offspring who were *not* separated at birth from their schizophrenic parents (see Table 6-9). This finding again provides strong support for the genetic hypothesis. It is worth noting, too, that the index cases also had more mental deficiency, neurotic personality disorder, and sociopathic personality with long incarceration for major crimes. Why should such a finding occur at all? Later we will deal with this question in more detail.

Table 6-18

Characteristics of Adult Offspring Separated at Birth from Their Schizophrenic or Normal Mothers*

Characteristic	Normal Mother	Schizophrenic Mother	p
Number of offspring	50	47	
Males	33	30	
Mean age	36.3	35.8	
MHSRS: mean ratings	80.1	65.2	0.0006
Schizophrenia	0	5	0.024
Mental deficiency (IQ < 70)	0	4	0.052
Sociopathic personality	2	9	0.017
Neurotic personality disorder	7	13	0.052
1+ years in penal or psychiatric institution	2	11	0.006
Felons	2	7	0.054
Psychiatric or behavioral military discharge	1	8	0.021

* Data from Heston, 1966.

The adoptive parents method

A study using this method was carried out by Wender et al. (1968). It directed itself to issues raised by earlier studies, for example, that of Alanen et al. (1966), who had found that the parents of schizophrenics had more severe psychopathology than the parents of neurotics. What role does the degree of parental psychopathology play in the genesis of schizophrenia in the child? The parental psychopathology could reflect the possibility that the parents were carriers of the schizophrenic gene(s), or such psychopathology could have been instrumentally responsible for the development of the child's schizophrenia.

To place these two alternatives in their proper perspective, the investigators asked: What degree of psychopathology might we find in the adoptive parents of schizophrenics? If the genetic explanation is correct, adoptive parents should have less psychopathology than natural parents. If the instrumental explanation is correct, adoptive parents should manifest as much psychopathology as biological parents.

The study began with a search for schizophrenics who had been adopted by nonrelatives in the child's first year of life. Both adoptive parents had to be alive and available for examination. A control group consisted of schizophrenics matched with the index group for sex, age, and severity of illness, but who had been reared by their biological parents. The latter in turn were matched to the adoptive parents of the index group with regard to age, religion, education, and socioeconomic status.   The focus of study is the comparison of psychopathology in the adoptive versus the biological parents.   To control for the possibility that simply being an adoptive parent might be associated with degree of psychopathology, an additional group of adoptive parents was obtained, but their adopted children did not have any severe mental illness.   The three groups of parents were examined psychiatrically and by tests.   Psychopathology was rated on a seven-point scale of severity: the larger the number, the more severe the illness.   The major findings are shown in Table 6-19.

It can be seen from the table that the biological parents of schizophrenics have more severe psychopathology than the adoptive parents of schizophrenics ($p < 0.005$, all tests one-tailed).   This is true for both mothers ($p < 0.05$) and fathers ($p < 0.05$).   However, the adoptive parents of schizophrenics also had a higher degree of psychopathology than the adoptive parents of normals ($p < 0.05$).   Thus, these findings again provide strong evidence for the genetic hypothesis, but they also leave open the possibility that parental psychopathology could also have played some instrumental role in the induction of the child's schizophrenia.

From the traditional consanguinity and twin studies, much evidence had been accumulated that was consistent with a genetic etiology of schizophrenia.   However, such evidence was also consistent with environmentalist interpretations.   The main virtue of the adoption studies is that it enables us to separate the genetic and familial environmental variables.   In all the studies done so far that have used this research strategy, the evidence has turned up so consistently and so strongly in favor of the genetic hypothesis that this issue must now be considered

Table 6-19

Severity of Psychopathology in Adoptive and Biological Parents of Schizophrenics and in Adoptive Parents of Controls*

Parental Relationship	Child Status	Number	Severity of Parental Psychopathology						Mean
			1–2	2.5–3	3.5–4	4.5–5	5.5–6	6.5–7	
Adoptive	Schizophrenic	10 fathers	1	4	3	2	0	0	3.3
		10 mothers	1	3	4	1	1	0	3.5
Biological	Schizophrenic	10 fathers	1	1	1	6	1	0	4.2
		10 mothers	0	0	4	3	1	2	4.9
Adoptive	Normal	10 fathers	2	6	2	0	0	0	2.6
		10 mothers	2	4	4	0	0	0	3.0

* Data from Wender et al., 1968.

closed. Genetic factors do contribute appreciably and beyond any reasonable doubt to the development of schizophrenic illness. Any theory of schizophrenia must take this fact into account. We need to concern ourselves with the mode of genetic transmission and the biological-psychological mechanisms involved. We know too from the twin studies that nongenetic factors play an important role, and we must identify these and determine how they relate to expression of the genetic factors.

PREDICTION STUDIES

Prediction studies examine the proposition that people who eventually become schizophrenic show personality characteristics or behavioral patterns in early life that distinguish them from nonschizophrenics. If such distinguishing traits can be found, they may represent hereditary factors related to the subsequent illness. They may in fact reflect (1) early signs of schizophrenia or (2) personality or behavioral traits that make such individuals more vulnerable to the development of schizophrenia. Theoretically, it is important that the investigator try to decide which of the two possibilities is correct. If the second is correct, knowledge about such factors may eventually enable us to influence the vulnerable person's development in ways that might prevent the predicted clinical schizophrenia from occurring at all.

Retrospective postdictive studies

Beginning in the 1940s, a number of studies compared child guidance clinic records of index children who later became schizophrenic with control children who eventually developed some other disorder or none at all. Generally, the records indicated that the index children had been more often described as apathetic, dreamy, listless, uninterested, withdrawn, shy, seclusive, few or no friends, maladjusted in groups, and poor in social behavior. They had more "shut-in" personalities and fewer interests. In high school, index children showed less leadership, lower interest in the opposite sex and in their environment generally, poorer mental health, and poorer overall adjustment to school.

Many of these traits are representative of a characteristic social introversion, the latter having been reported to have a heritability as high as 0.69 in one study (Gottesman, 1963). However, among all children described as introverted, only a tiny fraction become schizophrenic. In at least one study, the morbidity risk among introverted children was consistent with rates usually reported for the general population. Moreover, we know that some people who become schizophrenic have been described as extroverted. Thus, it may be that the signs indicating social introversion in the index children who became schizophrenic were really early manifestations of the illness, and that these signs could not be distinguished retrospectively from traits descriptive of introversion generally. In support of this view, we may note the finding at one excellent children's clinic that almost 15 percent of future schizophrenics had been described as psychotic or schizophrenic, although the clinic opposed the recording of diagnoses.

Some studies also reported excessive eating and sleep disturbances and speech anomalies in their index cases' childhood. Some reported "acting-out" behavior, such as stealing, running away, truanting, and promiscuity.

Prospective, longitudinal studies

The longest continuing investigations of this type have been conducted by Dr. Barbara Fish. She began in 1952 to examine infants who were "genetically loaded for schizophrenia," that is, those born to schizophrenic mothers who were hospital patients. She also studied other infants picked at random at a well-baby clinic. Among the latter, some were thought to have signs indicative of schizophrenia. The signs were suggested by Bender, who in turn thought of them as characteristics paralleling those in the fetal infant as described by Gesell. Bender believed that "the pattern of growth is characterized by retardation and precocity, alternately and simultaneously . . . that childhood schizophrenia represents a lag in maturation within the embryological level of development in all the areas that are prerequisite of future behaviors in all fields—motor, adaptive, language, and personal-social."

The following are some characteristics exhibited by Peter, son of a schizophrenic mother, at various stages in his development, as described by Fish (1957):

$5\frac{1}{2}$ *weeks.* Cyanosis of the hands and circumoral zone after crying. Doughy muscle tone. Much less active than normal. Did not show usual brisk movements, but slow, writhing, fishlike motion of trunk and extremities. Development abnormally uneven, head control advanced, vasomotor control and muscle tone markedly immature. Diminished exteroceptive responsiveness.

$3\frac{1}{2}$ *months.* Sleeps all day and cries all night. Soft muscle tone. Postural tone regressed. Expression impassive. Vocal-social response diminished.

6 *months*. Disturbed sleep. Cranky. Constipated. Lagging body growth. Pale, waxy-looking. Flaccid trunk and legs. Tonic neck reflex persisting.

7 *months*. Expression serious, nonresponsive. Increased irritability, gastrointestinal symptoms, and lag in body growth.

9½ *months*. Wants to be held all the time. Unable to suck milk from a bottle. Body and cranial growth at lowest ebb. Inactive, apathetic. Reaching and manipulation slow, without vigor or enthusiasm.

10½ *months* (following return of mother from hospital). She is affectionate and responsive to his needs. He develops at a rapid rate. Holds own bottle. Body growth accelerated. Sleep difficulty only occasional. Now able to sit straight. This general acceleration continues at 11½ and 13½ months.

18 *months*. Locomotion and body growth now at normal levels. Spontaneous behavior, active, happy. Language and manipulative behavior advanced minimally. Shy. Turns away from strangers. Cries if he can't get something.

31 *months*. Speech level several months retarded. Talks only to mother, not strangers. Constantly sad, anxious expression. Clings to mother. Development still uneven. Now lagging in language and social adjustment more than manipulation and locomotion.

37 *months*. Mother back in state hospital four months. He is now even more anxious and withdrawn. Runs around aimlessly, plays poorly, throws and breaks toys. Very scared, shy. Bad temper tantrums, kicks and screams.

At this time, Fish considered Peter to be a schizophrenic child. In a later report, she stated that at age 5½, Peter was "clinically schizophrenic." The account of his development suggests that the symptoms and behavior he shows are influenced by the presence or absence of his mother. Some of the behaviors are common to children who are obviously not schizophrenic, and many investigators would be critical of applying the diagnosis of schizophrenia to Peter at these tender ages for these symptoms. Fish continues to report periodically on the children in her series, and we may some day learn whether Peter has been hospitalized with that diagnosis. Even if he does, we still will not know how much environmental factors—such as the repeated absences of his mother, or perhaps her intermittently psychotic behavior—may have contributed to his psychopathology. But the descriptions provided by Fish nevertheless afford us some valuable cues about what kinds of behavioral pathology may reflect the schizophrenic genotype, even in early childhood.

Sobel (1961) studied 8 infants whose *both* parents were schizophrenic. In 4 cases, the mother was hospitalized and the infants were placed in foster homes. The other 4 were reared at home by their schizophrenic parents. Of the 8 infants, 3 showed clear-cut signs of emotional disturbance in infancy. All 3 were home-reared. None of the 4 fostered children showed such disturbances. Such findings again emphasize the need to pay close attention to environmental factors. Unfortunately, Sobel was unable to continue the study of this unusual sample of children, but hopefully another investigator may be able to follow and report on their subsequent development.

Methodologically, the most sophisticated study of this type is the one carried out by Mednick and Schulsinger (1968) in Denmark. It successfully integrates theory and research design, and pays careful attention to the selection of index cases and controls, to the selection of examination procedures that are aimed at tests of the theory, and to the follow-up studies and diagnostic assessments of the subjects. Mednick's anxiety-generalization theory states that schizophrenia begins with high anxiety that habituates (extinguishes) slowly, a trait that could be hereditary or have an environmentally induced basis. When anxiety is high, stimulus generalization occurs so that more stimuli are able to potentiate the slowly habituating anxiety. The increased potentiation in turn leads to increasingly higher anxiety levels which lead in turn to increased stimulus generalization. This anxiety-generalization spiral culminates eventually in a schizophrenic break, which involves an attempt to find remote cognitive associations that serve to avoid or reduce the anxiety, but at the cost of the cognitive and affective dissociation seen in chronic schizophrenia.

Mednick and Schulsinger call their index cases *high-risk Ss* because they all have schizophrenic mothers. Control Ss with normal parents were matched to the index Ss for sex, age, social class, education level, years in children's homes, and rural residence. There were 207 index and 104 control Ss. Index Ss were also paired as controls for one another. The investigators chose not to focus on early infancy or childhood but on ages more proximal to those in which schizophrenia is usually thought to have its clinical onset, namely, the pubertal and post-pubertal periods. Therefore, the mean age of their Ss was 15.1 years. At that time, no S was thought to be psychotic. Table 6-20 shows some of the major variables that significantly discriminated the two groups.

It is not yet possible to say whether the birth and placental aberrations might contribute to personality deviations in the children. The

Table 6-20

Characteristics Differentiating High- and Low-risk Subjects*

Trait or Measure	High-risk Subjects	Low-risk Subjects
Mothers unwed	More	Less
Birth difficulties	More	Less
Longer birth process	More	Less
Abnormal placenta	11.3%	1.2%
GSR to stress stimulus	Shorter latency	Longer latency
GSR overgeneralized	More	Less
GSR amplitude response	Greater	Lower
GSR recovery from stress	Faster	Slower
Idiosyncratic, fragmented word associations	More	Less
Poor level of adjustment	24%	1%
Sees mother as scolding, unreliable, and not worthy of confidences	More	Less
In school:		
Gets upset easily	More	Less
Reacts to excitement by withdrawing	More	Less
Passivity in peer relations and challenges	More	Less
Rejected by peers	More	Less
A loner	More	Less

* Data from Mednick and Schulsinger, 1968.

test findings are consistent with a modified version of Mednick's original anxiety-generalization theory. Some of the behavioral characteristics noted primarily in the index Ss are in agreement with those reported in previous studies, namely, poor adjustment, easily upset, withdrawal, passivity, and social isolation.

By the fifth year of the project, 20 Ss manifested "severely abnormal behavior." All were index cases. Of these, 12 had been admitted to a psychiatric facility or placed under psychiatric care. The other 8 were severe schizoids, delinquents, or alcoholics, or manifested bizarre symptomatic behavior. The investigators compared these 20 Ss with matched high-risk Ss who had had the same level-of-adjustment rating at the original examination, but whose adjustment rating had not declined. The two groups were called *sick* and *well*, respectively.

Interestingly, mothers were more often absent from the home earlier and permanently in the case of the sick group. The absence was always the result of the mother's psychiatric illness. When the illness of all schizophrenic mothers was rated with regard to two degrees of severity (very severe versus moderately severe) 3 of 4 mothers were rated "very" severely ill in the sick group, as compared with 1 of 3 mothers in the well group.   Thus, absence of the mother from the home was correlated with her severity of illness, and it cannot be said whether the environmental factor of absence or the possible genetic factor of illness severity in the mother was associated with the psychiatric disorders in the sick group.   On tests and in school behavior, the well group had frequently appeared to be similar to the control Ss, whereas the sick group had contributed largely to the group differences shown in Table 6-20.

Anthony (1968) has organized a study that combines some of the features in the Fish and Mednick-Schulsinger studies, and has added some features of his own.   His index groups span three ages: (1) preschool up to five years, (2) elementary school to eleven years, (3) high school to seventeen years.   Each index child has a schizophrenic parent, but both parents must be alive and living together—except for interruptions by hospitalization.   Half the schizophrenic parents are mothers, half are fathers.   One control group had parents with no history of serious mental or physical illness, but the major comparison group has one parent undergoing hospitalization for a subacute or chronic physical illness.   The study is not yet very far along and few data are available.

One unusual feature in Anthony's study is the enduring and relatively close association between the index child, his family, and the research staff.   This closeness has enabled the staff to observe *micro-paranoidal episodes* in some index children, as in the following account by Anthony.

> The precursive, micro-paranoidal episode may last anything from 3 days to 3 months and then seems to disappear almost completely with the child resuming normal reality testing and ego functioning.   Peggy, aged 8, is an example of one of these "little madnesses."   She is a girl of superior intelligence who is doing extremely well at school.   She was always regarded as sensitive, given to taking life over seriously, but at the same time remaining fairly popular with her classmates.   She was always extremely well behaved, and her teacher referred to her as "trustworthy."   (One would place her in group 4 of the Kasanin groupings of the prepsychotic state.)   One day, on the playground at school, she was asked by a boy to throw him a rock so that he could bat it with a stick.   Before she could bring herself to realize that this was against the rules, she had done so, and immediately she was overcome with guilt and remorse.   When they went into the classroom again, she felt as if everybody was staring at her and that the teacher was paying special attention to her.   All of a sudden, the boy involved in the situation went

up to the teacher's desk, whispered to her and went out.   (He had asked
to go to the bathroom.)   She immediately felt that he had taken it upon
himself to report her and had been told to go to the headmistress and
give a full account of the incident.   She became more and more terror
stricken until eventually she could bear it no longer and broke into loud
wailing.   Nothing the teacher could do was able to reassure her.   She
felt that she was trapped and that they were going to do something
terrible to her.   She was no better at home, and since she could not be
induced to return to school again, I admitted her to hospital.   When
first seen, she was intensely suspicious and felt that I had been in touch
with school and was simply trying to get her to confess.   As a result,
she was uncommunicative and wary.   Naturally, of its own accord, the
intensity of the reaction subsided, and within a period of 3 months she
resumed her normal, pleasantly cooperative behavior and was even able
to laugh at the silly ideas, she had once had.   She returned to school and
continued to do very well.   A year and a half later, I saw her for a minor
episode involving some pimples on her skin; she felt that some of the
children might have been making offensive additions to her diet when
she was not looking.   This little episode subsided without admission.
The relevant information in her case is that her mother had been hospitalized on two occasions with a diagnosis of paranoid schizophrenia.

It is clear that the prediction studies can be designed in many
ways and that they can do much to elucidate the personality and behavioral precursors of hospitalizable schizophrenia.   Although they have
not as yet been designed to differentiate the etiological contributions
made by heredity and by environment, it is likely that in the future
they will throw light on this issue as well.

THE BIOLOGICAL UNITY
OF SCHIZOPHRENIA

For many years, genetically minded psychiatrists have wondered
whether all schizophrenic disorders have the same genetic origins and
whether other psychiatric disorders are genetically related to schizophrenia.   They have referred to this issue as one involving the *biological
unity* of schizophrenia.   For several decades, many psychiatrists and
psychologists did not believe that schizophrenia had any genetic basis
at all, and were inclined to ignore the issue.   Now that it has been
demonstrated beyond any reasonable doubt that heredity plays an important role indeed in the etiology of schizophrenia, the issue of biological
unity must be taken seriously, and we will do so here.   However, for
the sake of clarity it is best to divide the problem into two separate

parts. In the first, which we shall continue to call the biological-unity problem, we shall concern ourselves with whether those disorders commonly subsumed under, or clinically related to, schizophrenia share a common genetic identity. These disorders include the various subtypes, borderline cases, schizoid or paranoid personalities, reactive or other benign forms of schizophrenia or schizophrenia-like disorders, and pre-adolescent schizophrenias.

The second part of the issue we shall call the *specificity of the schizophrenic genotype*. Here we shall ask whether other psychiatric disorders are genetically associated with or distinct from schizophrenia. This matter could be of fundamental importance to the larger problem of nosology in the functional-behavioral disorders. If they are all genetically related, this fact could provide support for the popular claim that nosology is useless and that there is only mental illness of more or less degree. If they are genetically distinct, then we have a firm case for proclaiming the validity of nosological distinctions.

Subtypes

Kallmann (1938) found a rate of schizophrenia among the children of hebephrenic and catatonic patients that was twice as high as the rate among the children of patients with simple or paranoid schizophrenia. Such a finding might suggest that the subtypes were genetically related, but that genetic factors were stronger in the case of hebephrenia and catatonia. However, Kallmann also found a positive association between subtype diagnoses in index patients and in their relatives, and the results of his findings are shown in Table 6-21.

If we simply count the number of instances in which relatives were

Table 6-21

Subtype Associations in Index Cases and Their Relatives

Index Cases	*Hebephrenic*	*Catatonic*	*Paranoid*	*Total*
	Relatives			
Hebephrenic	49	10	21	80
Catatonic	6	31	15	52
Paranoid	5	10	13	28
Total	60	51	49	160

concordant with index cases as to subtype, the figures in Table 6-21 may be rearranged as follows:

Index-case Subtype	Concordant	Discordant	Percent Concordant
Hebephrenic	49	31	61
Catatonic	31	21	60
Paranoid	13	15	46

Thus the association is appreciable, and tends to be somewhat stronger in the hebephrenic and catatonic than in the paranoid subtype. Actually, the first investigator to find subtype associations in family members was Schulz (1932), who had divided his cases into hebephrenic, catatonic, and paranoid groups, much as Kallmann did later, but Schulz's *n*'s were considerably smaller. Garrone, dividing his S*s* into a paranoid and a hebephrenic-catatonic group, found 60 percent subtype concordance and 40 percent discordance among pairs of relatives of both first and second degree. M. Bleuler (1941) also found a strong correlation among relatives with respect to clinical course. Ödegaard (1963) found subtype associations between first-degree family members as follows:

Probands	Relatives		
	Paranoid	Hebephrenic	Catatonic
Paranoid	19	8	8
Hebephrenic	6	7	4
Catatonic	5	1	6

In contradiction with Kallmann's findings, the subtype association appears in Ödegaard's first-degree relatives to be strongest for the paranoid form and weakest for the hebephrenic subtype. However, the overall concordance as to subtype is statistically significant.

If the association with respect to subtype is genetically based, it should be revealed even more strikingly in MZ twins. In Table 6-22, we see that this is probably so. In fact, the association in Kringlen's table is almost perfect. Gottesman (1968) reports similar findings in his study with Shields. In their MZ twin series, 7 pairs were concordant for hebephrenia, and 2 for paranoid subtype; 2 pairs were discordant as to subtype. Different heritability for subtypes is indicated by the fact that 7 of 8 MZ twins were concordant for hebephrenia, but only 2 of 6 MZ twins were concordant for the paranoid subtype. We must be cautious in evaluating such figures, however, because the reliability of subtype diagnosis, when tested carefully, has not been notoriously high. Investigators making the diagnosis in the cotwin should not know the subtype diagnosis of the index twin so that they may not be unduly influenced by that knowledge. Kringlen could not keep himself blind in this respect, but Gottesman and Shields could.

Further evidence of a genetic determination of subtype was found in the case of the Genain quadruplets. The fact is that schizophrenics usually have several hospital admissions, and their subtype diagnosis may differ with each admission or may change with time. This was the case with the Genain girls, whose history of subtype diagnosis is shown in Table 6-23. Diagnoses of Myra were made at one hospital, of Hester at two hospitals, and of Nora and Iris at three hospitals. By and large, their illness begins as a catatonic syndrome, goes through periods where it is called *undifferentiated*, and progresses toward a hebephrenic outcome in those girls who become more severely and chronically ill. Myra, who was hospitalized primarily for research purposes, though she was clearly ill, never developed hebephrenic features. Nora, with the second best premorbid history, did develop some hebephrenic features. Iris was called hebephrenic twice, and Hester, who had the poorest premorbid history, was called hebephrenic four times.

Subtypes are based on specific behaviors, some of which are more

Table 6-22
Subtype Association in MZ Twins Concordant for Schizophrenia*

Index Case	Cotwin					
	Hebephrenic	Catatonic	Paranoid	Catatonic-Paranoid	Others	Total
Hebephrenic	2					2
Catatonic		1			1	2
Paranoid			2			2
Catatonic-paranoid				7		7
Others, mixed syndrome					1	1
Total						14

* Data from Kringlen, 1967.

Table 6-23

Subtype Diagnoses of the Genain Quaduplets (Arranged Chronologically)

Nora	*Iris*	*Myra*	*Hester*
Acute	Catatonic	Catatonic	Catatonic
Acute	Undifferentiated	Undifferentiated	Catatonic
Undifferentiated	Catatonic	Catatonic	Hebephrenic
Catatonic	Undifferentiated		Undifferentiated
Catatonic	Undifferentiated		Undifferentiated
Catatonic	Catatonic		Undifferentiated
Hebephrenic features	Catatonic		Paranoid features
Hebephrenic features	Catatonic		Hebephrenic
Hebephrenic features	Hebephrenic		Undifferentiated
Undifferentiated	Catatonic and hebephrenic features		Hebephrenic
Undifferentiated	Catatonic and paranoid features		Hebephrenic
Undifferentiated	Hebephrenic		Hebephrenic
	Hebephrenic or undifferentiated		Hebephrenic features
	Hebephrenic or undifferentiated		Hebephrenic features

prominent in some subtypes but less so in others. If genes influence subtypes, they should influence the degree of pathology in some behaviors relative to others. In a study of the Genain quadruplets at the National Institute of Mental Health, the girls were rated daily for two months by many different trained observers with respect to a variety of behaviors. A summary of the findings is shown in Table 6-24. In this table, a rank of 1 indicates the greatest degree of pathology. In section (1) of the table, the *girls* are ranked with respect to pathology in each behavior. It is clear that Hester is consistently ranked most pathological, regardless of the behavior rated, while Myra shows least pathology with equal consistency. Section (2) is of more immediate interest because here the *behaviors* are ranked according to degree of pathology. All four girls are described as most pathological with respect to activity; that is, they tend to be very underactive. The second area of greatest pathology involves speech, the girls tending to talk too little and too softly. And so on down the list. Kendall's coefficient of concordance w equals .91, indicating almost perfect homogeneity of behavioral ranks despite the clear and significant difference among the girls with respect to overall degree of pathology.   If underactivity is the most pathological characteristic for Hester, it tends to be so for Myra as well.   These findings suggest strongly that such patterning of behavioral pathology is influenced by heredity, and affords further support for a genetic basis with respect to subtype patterning.

In the case of the quadruplets, their father had paranoid traits (but was not overtly schizophrenic), and their paternal grandmother had once been hospitalized for what was probably paranoid schizophrenia.   However, the girls had a catatonic-hebephrenic form of the illness.   Elsässer (1952) describes a case where two parents with paranoid subtypes had two children who were hebephrenic.   In Table 6-21, we saw that different subtypes commonly occur in the same family.   If subtype patterning is inherited, how can we explain such phenomena?

The most parsimonious explanation implicates a polygenic mode of inheritance.   The fact that the subtypes distribute themselves in the same family provides testimony for the biological unity of schizophrenia.

Table 6-24

Rank Orders of the Genain Quadruplets with Respect to Pathology of Day-to-day Behaviors

Categories	(1) Rank of the Girls				(2) Rank of the Categories				Total
	N	I	M	H	N	I	M	H	
Activity	3	2	4	1	1	1	1	1	4
Loudness of speech	3	2	4	1	3	3	3	2	11
Amount of speech	3	1	4	2	2	2	2	3	9
Cooperation	4	2	3	1	6	4	7	4	21
Sociability	2	3	4	1	5	6	5	5	21
Speech integration	3	2	4	1	8	7	9.5	6	30.5
Mood content	1	3	4	2	4	5	4	7	20
Mood changes	4	2	3	1	10	9	6	9	34
Eating desire	2	3	4	1	7	8	8	10	33
Temper control	2	3	4	1	11.5	12	9.5	8	41
Tidiness (clothes)	2	3	4	1	9	11	11	11	42
Eating habits	2	1	4	3	11.5	10	12	12	45.5
Total	31	27	46	16					
	$n = 4, m = 12,$				$n = 12, m = 4, w = 0.91,$				
	$w = 0.64, p < 0.01$				$p < 0.01$				

The fact that MZ twins almost never have different subtypes, as far as we now can tell, suggests, however, that the subtypes are genetically different. We may therefore assume that the pathological genes tend to cluster more in some families and that those who have most of these genes will show hebephrenia and/or catatonia; whereas those who have fewer of these genes will show paranoid, simple, atypical, or possibly borderline forms of the disorder. Since MZ twins will have exactly the same number of pathological genes, they are much more likely to show the same subtypes. Of course, nongenetic factors, both biological and psychological, could help to blur the overall picture.

Preadolescent schizophrenia and early infantile autism

Since dementia praecox was originally thought to be associated with the onset of puberty and the biological changes that occur in the transition from childhood to maturity, it seemed neither convenient nor appropriate to consider severe mental illnesses of the prepubertal ages in the same diagnostic category as illnesses with later onset. Nevertheless, that such disorders existed had long been recognized, as well as the fact that there were many similarities between the prepubertal and postpubertal psychoses. Kraepelin himself called the prepubertal disorders *dementia praecocissima.* The very name indicated his own recognition of a basic association between the two diagnostic groups, at least on phenomenological grounds. To determine whether this association reflects the biological unity of both disorders we must be able to show that: (1) preadolescent schizophrenia is attributable in good part to genetic factors, and (2) preadolescent and postadolescent schizophrenias cluster together in the same families.

Between 1948 and 1952, known hospital admissions for schizophrenia in children below age fifteen comprised 1.9 percent of all admitted schizophrenics and 0.6 percent of all first admissions in New York State. In the single major twin study of preadolescent schizophrenia, Kallmann and Roth (1956) reported "difficulties in obtaining a statistically representative and diagnostically uniform sample of early schizophrenia cases." They nevertheless were able to find in New York 52 twins and 50 singletons below age fifteen who were diagnosed schizophrenic by one of the investigators who had no knowledge of family background. Diagnostic criteria and major symptoms included early apparently normal development followed by a distinct behavioral change, diminished interest in the environment, peculiar conduct, especially in motor activity, diffuse anxiety with phobias and vague somatic complaints, bizarre thinking with a tendency toward exaggerated fantasies, and hallucinations. The observed parental consanguinity rate was 3.0 percent for the entire sample and 5.8 percent for the twins. Zygosity determination was based on the usual similarity method, and by blood group and dermatoglyphic analyses. The twins were observed for an average of 10 years from the time of onset. The salient twin data are shown in Table 6-25.

The expected predominance of male cases occurred both in twins and singletons. The male-female ratio was 12:5, 15:10, and 37:13 for MZ, DZ, and single-born index cases, respectively. Of the 17 MZ pairs, 12 cotwins also had preadolescent schizophrenia, but 3 cotwins developed schizophrenia *after* age fifteen. The remaining two cotwins had a *schizoid personality*. The uncorrected concordance rates were 70.6 percent for preadolescent schizophrenia and 88.2 percent for *total schizophrenia*. It is difficult to know what age correction to use with respect to preadolescent schizophrenia, but clearly any plausible correction would bring the concordance rate to 100 percent.

Among the 35 DZ pairs, 6 cotwins had preadolescent schizophrenia and 2 developed schizophrenia *after* age fifteen. The uncorrected concordance rates were 17.1 and 22.9 percent for preadolescent and total schizophrenia, respectively. An additional 25.7 percent of the cotwins had a schizoid personality.

The very high concordance rates suggest strongly that genetic factors underlie the disorder. The virtually 100 percent MZ rate and almost 25 percent DZ rate are figures that one would expect for a recessive trait if one used the proband method to calculate concordance. Indeed it was a recessiveness theory to which Kallmann held. However, he employed the pairwise method to calculate concordance, and with this method one expects a DZ concordance rate of 14 percent for a simple

Table 6-25
Distribution of Schizophrenia by Sex, and Concordance Rates in Preadolescent Twins*

	MZ Twins			*DZ Twins*		
Age	*Male*	*Female*	*Concordance Rate*	*Same Sex*	*Opposite Sex*	*Concordance Rate*
5–9	2	0	?	0	0	
10–14	7	0	?	8	4	?
15+	3	5	?	16	7	?
Total	12	5	88.2	24	11	22.9

* Data from Kallmann and Roth, 1956.

recessive trait with complete penetrance, and a DZ rate of 33 percent for a simple dominant. Thus Kallmann's rate falls between these values.

The fact that the MZ rate is so high suggests that if preadolescent schizophrenia has the same genetic basis as adult schizophrenia, it is a more virulent form which has virtually complete penetrance. Since Kallmann's postulated recessive gene would be the same in both the preadolescent and postadolescent disorders, the factors making for the almost complete penetrance in preadolescents would most likely be attributed to other modifying genes. A straightforward polygenic theory would simply postulate that individuals with preadolescent schizophrenia had more of the pathological genes than did individuals with the adult forms of the illness. The increased number of pathological genes would not only explain the earlier onset, but the increased concordance rates as well.

However, we must consider the alternative possibility that, since the investigators did not have strict control over sampling, extraneous factors could have led to a disproportionate number of concordant pairs coming into the sample and discordant pairs being overlooked or missed. If true, this would reduce the actual concordance rates to levels more like those in adult schizophrenia, but even so, the reduction would in all likelihood not be sufficient to alter the inference of a genetic basis for preadolescent schizophrenia.

Does adult schizophrenia cluster in the families of these child schizophrenics? We have already seen that five of the cotwins developed schizophrenic illness postpubertally. Among the 204 parents of the twin- and single-born index cases combined, 18 (9 mothers and 9 fathers), or 8.82 percent, were schizophrenic. This rate of parental illness is consistent with the rates we noted earlier regarding schizophrenia in the parents of postadolescent index cases. Among the sibs of the combined index cases, 102 were aged five to fourteen, and 97 were over fourteen. Of these 199 sibs, 16 had childhood schizophrenia and 2 developed schizophrenia after age fifteen. Thus, although the heaviest concentration of cases takes on preadolescent forms of the illnesses, adult forms occur in MZ and DZ cotwins, sibs, and parents as well. The findings considered collectively make a strong case for the biological unity of these age-based diagnostic groupings.

Other studies provide additional support for this view, most notably those of Bender (1953, 1955). In a study of 143 schizophrenic children, 57 (40 percent) had one schizophrenic parent and 15 (11 percent) had *both* parents schizophrenic. The overall rate was 30.4 percent of all 286 parents, a figure that is extraordinarily high. Yet, in a second study of 30 schizophrenic children less than seven years old (Bender and Grugett, 1956), the investigators found 14 mothers and 12 fathers to be schizophrenic, that is, 26 of 60 parents, or 43.3 percent. The authors included cases classified "ambulatory schizophrenia," based on social maladjustment, and this may account for some of the difference between these rates and the rates usually reported for parents of adult schizophrenics. However, these findings may also indicate additional support for a polygenic theory in that the high genetic loading in the parents could contribute to the probability of higher than usual concentrations of pathological genes in the children, who in turn suffer more serious forms of the illness with earlier onset.

The issue with respect to early infantile autism is less clear. Unlike childhood schizophrenia, as described above by Kallmann and by others, in which a period of apparent normality exists before the illness has its onset, the autistic child as described by Kanner manifests withdrawal virtually from the beginning of life. Kanner thinks the trait may be thought of as *aloneness* rather than withdrawal. Other distinctive features of the illness as the child develops include muteness or failure to use language for communication, an obsessive insistence on the maintenance of sameness, with paniclike reactions when environmental changes do occur, an inability to relate to people, and rather good intellectual potential, including skill in manipulating objects, and often a phenomenal memory. In a follow-up study made nine years (on the average) after initial evaluation, among 63 children who had been autistic in their adolescence, 3, 14, and 46 later achieved a good, fair, and poor adjustment, respectively. The best prognostic sign was useful speech by age five (Eisenberg, 1956).

Among 973 parents, grandparents, uncles, and aunts of the autistic children in his original series, Kanner (1954) found only 1.3 percent who were psychotic. This is only slightly higher than the rate for the general population. Of 131 sibs, 3 were also autistic. However, Kanner found an extremely high proportion of the parents who were cold, obsessive, and very intelligent. Later Eisenberg (1957) reported that 85 of the fathers had a totally mechanical attitude toward child rearing and a formalistic approach to marriage. The other 15 were warm, giving, and devoted. If early infantile autism is biologically homogeneous with adult schizophrenia, we should have found an elevated incidence of schizophrenia among the probands' parents, and, in line with the polygenic theory proposed above, an incidence at least as great as that found among the parents of preadolescent schizophrenics.

As a matter of fact, the characterizations of the autistic children's parents suggest that the parental attitudes and behaviors to the child might have actually caused the disorder. Twin studies could provide some indication of whether the disorder is inherited or not, but its incidence is low and only a scattered sprinkling of twin cases has been reported. Of these, 8 are MZ, 1 is questionable MZ, and 2 are DZ. Not only are the numbers small, but they also reflect the usual bias in favor of reporting MZ pairs when sampling is not systematically controlled. Among the 8 MZ pairs, 7 were concordant, and 1 discordant. The questionable MZ pair was discordant. Of the 2 DZ pairs, 1 was discordant and 1 concordant. The figures suggest a genetic factor in the disorder, but there may well have been a bias in favor of reporting instances of concordance in MZ pairs. Thus, we can have little confidence in any inferences based on the sparse twin data.

The problem is complicated further by the fact that some children diagnosed "autistic" have signs of neurological damage that may be congenital but not genetic. Goldfarb (1968) has devoted considerable attention to this problem. His subjects seem to resemble rather closely those described by Kanner and Eisenberg, but Goldfarb prefers the term *early-childhood psychosis*. Among the parents of 58 psychotic children in his series, in only two families did he find the kinds of parents described by Kanner. He attributed these differences to sampling artifacts. Among 45 mothers and 39 fathers, only 1 mother and 1 father had been hospitalized for psychiatric reasons. But on the basis of a psychiatric examination including history and mental status, 29 percent of the mothers and 13 percent of the fathers were classified as schizophrenic. The latter finding suggests again the difficulty for genetic purposes of using only hospitalized cases in studies of schizophrenia. The finding is also in line with what a theory of biological unity predicts, except that we would expect the rates of schizophrenia to be higher if we accept Bender's findings in families of preadolescent schizophrenics and if we pursue the argument for a polygenic mode of transmission.

The rates do become somewhat higher if the children are divided into groups classified *organic* and *nonorganic*. Children diagnosed organic manifest any of a number of neurological abnormalities indicating central nervous system impairment. These include the generally accepted ones, such as reflex changes, abnormal reflexes, and sensory or motor dysfunctions; "soft" signs, such as nonlocalizing disturbances of gait, posture, balance, coordination, muscle tone, perception, and speech; EEG deviations; congenital stigmata; and aberrations in head size. Among the parents of the psychotic children diagnosed nonorganic, 44 percent of the mothers were classified as schizophrenic, and 8 percent of the fathers. Thus the rate of schizophrenia is somewhat higher for the parents of a relatively "purer" group of psychotic children than for the parents of all organic and nonorganic children combined.

However, the figures are still puzzling. From a genetic point of view, why should there be $5\frac{1}{2}$ times more schizophrenic mothers than fathers?   Perhaps there are some sampling or diagnostic factors that are contributing to this biased ratio.   An environmentalist could argue that the predominance of psychosis in the mothers indicates that it is parental—especially maternal—rearing that is responsible for the psychotic behavior in the children.   Moreover, if we assume that the psychosis in the organic children is a phenocopy caused by other congenital disturbances of central nervous system functioning, we should not expect to find an elevated incidence of schizophrenia among their parents.   Yet Goldfarb reports that 21 percent of the mothers and 15 percent of the fathers of the organic children were schizophrenic.

Thus, although some of the evidence indicates support for considering early infantile autism to be genetically related to schizophrenia, the overall picture is hardly clear.

The more benign schizophrenic-like conditions

Since Kraepelin's diagnosis of dementia praecox was based on prognostic indications of a deteriorative end state, problems arose immediately when many cases so diagnosed remitted or recovered.   The assumption was often made therefore that these cases had been misdiagnosed.   If so, what should be done nosologically with these more benign psychoses that had so closely resembled dementia praecox as to be mistaken for it?   Many investigators began to pay special attention to these psychoses, and later assigned different names to them.   These names included schizophreniform psychosis; symptomatic schizophrenia; psychogenic psychosis; atypical, peripheral, or reactive schizophrenia; and schizo-affective psychosis.   The first three names suggest that these psychoses are in an entirely different category from schizophrenia; the latter four suggest that they are variants of schizophrenia.   From a genetic standpoint, which view is correct?

Moreover, what should be done with the many cases that were not clearly schizophrenic, but which could conceivably be less severe forms of the illness?   Some were called borderline schizophrenia, and others schizoid or paranoid states.   Pseudoneurotic and pseudopsychopathic schizophrenia were terms applied to other conditions that seemed to defy the earlier accepted classifications.   Are all these part of one genetic family?

First, let us address ourselves to the benign schizophrenic-like psychoses.   Because most studies are in German and because American psychologists have paid much attention to these disorders, we will review a number of the relevant studies in some detail.   By now these psychoses are almost always classified as *reactive schizophrenia* in the United States, whereas the more traditionally accepted Kraepelinian forms of the illness are classified as *process schizophrenia*. An excellent, probing review of this process-reactive distinction has been provided by Garmezy (1965).

In the first studies designed to test whether the more benign psychoses are genetically different from true, typical, nuclear, endogenous, or process schizophrenia, the investigators employed the following research strategy:

1 They collected a series of patients diagnosed schizophrenic.

2 They examined the family histories of these patients, and on this basis divided the proband sample into *tainted* and *untainted* groups.

3 They then compared the tainted and untainted probands to see if the latter contained the more benign forms of schizophrenic illness.

The first study was that of M. Bleuler (1930). He collected 100 cases of schizophrenia admitted to New York's Bloomingdale Hospital for the first time. He had known each case personally for at least four months, and accepted only those whose case histories had sufficient information to help classify the patient diagnostically and the family history according to taint. He also questioned patients' relatives. There were 69 male and 31 female probands, divided into three groups:

1 Tainted family histories loaded with schizophrenia, other psychoses, and psychiatric illnesses of significant degree ($n = 76$)

2 Questionably tainted families with suspected schizophrenic loading, or loaded with other disorders pertaining to mental health ($n = 16$)

3 Untainted families without taint or suspected taint ($n = 8$)

He then rated the probands on a continuum of severity, from *recovered* to *severe defect*. The severe-defect group included 30 probands. The main findings are given in Table 6-26.

If we combine all the tainted groups, we see that there are *fewer* cases observed (17) than expected (23.1). If we collapse the remaining two groups, we find that there are *more* cases observed (13) than expected (7.2). Chi-square equals 5.13, which is significant at the 0.05 level. Thus the findings are actually opposite from the expected direction.

Schulz (1932) began his study with 660 cases that had been diagnosed dementia praecox 20 years earlier by Kraepelin and Rüdin, elimi-

Table 6-26

Cases of Severe Defect in Schizophrenics with Tainted and Untainted Family Histories*

Family History	Expected Cases	Observed Cases
Tainted:		
With schizophrenia	9.9	7
With noteworthy psychiatric illnesses	9.9	7
With other psychoses	3.3	3
Questionably tainted	4.8	6
Untainted	2.4	7

* Data from M. Bleuler, 1930.

nating 42 cases as "uncertain." He followed each proband by searching all available records and sources for at least 10 years after the first admission, seeing many probands and relatives personally. As a measure of taint, he employed the morbidity-risk estimate for schizophrenia in the sibs and parents of probands. All probands in turn were divided into a group of cured cases, which concerns us most here, and eight other groups, as shown in Table 6-27.

Table 6-27

Morbidity Risk for Schizophrenia in Sibs of Cured and Not-cured Schizophrenics*

Proband Group Defined	n	Sibs' Morbidity Risk, %	
		Certain Schizo- phrenia	Certain and Probable Schizo- phrenia
Fully cured: outside institution 10+ years	67	4.2	5.4
Slight defect: outside institution 10+ years	32	9.9	10.8
Clearly ill: outside institution 10+ years	83	4.1	7.7
Repeated remissions for 10+ years	55	6.0	7.8
Defect: in institution	123	5.2	7.1
Severe defect more than 10 years	141	7.6	7.6
Died before 10 years, in institution	137	8.0	9.6
Died before 10 years, outside institution	10	9.1	12.1
Suicide before 10 years, outside institution	12		

* Data from Schulz, 1932.

As can be seen from the table, the sibs of the fully cured cases do indeed have the lowest morbidity risk, with the exception of *certain schizophrenia* among the sibs of the clearly ill group that stayed out of the hospital for over 10 years. Thus, here the trend is in the predicted direction. However, the cured cases, which are the ones most clearly representative of the reactive type, also have more schizophrenic sibs than would be expected in a normative sample. Both the Schulz and the Bleuler studies support the hypothesis of biological unity, since schizophrenia occurs at a higher-than-general-population rate in the families of the reactive or benign cases as well as in the process group. However, Bleuler's study suggests that hereditary factors are more salient in the more benign forms of the disorder, whereas Schulz's study suggests the opposite. In a later study using much the same type of strategy and index group, Wittermans and Schulz (1950) reported findings and conclusions similar to those of Schulz.

In a study by Leonhard (1936), the author began with a sample of 530 schizophrenics. Of these, 440 were classified as "typical," and 90 "atypical." The atypical cases showed a defect state (which was deemed necessary by the author for the diagnosis of schizophrenia) but manifested a periodic course and an apparently enduring remission of at least 10 years, and often the defect was mild. Unfortunately for our purposes, he excluded cases classified as "degeneration psychosis," which are schizophrenic-like but without deterioration. Such a group may have included exactly the kinds of cases that many investigators today think of as reactive schizophrenia.

From among his starting cases Leonhard isolated a group of 55 probands who had at least one institutionalized case of endogenous nonorganic psychosis in the family. These probands were considered tainted. Among the 55 cases, 22 were typical and 33 atypical. Thus a much larger proportion of the probands came from the atypical group. Moreover, most of them had cases of atypical rather than typical schizophrenia in their families.

On the basis of these findings, Leonhard concluded that he had isolated two schizophrenic groups: (1) typical, which is recessive and has low penetrance, and (2) atypical, which is dominant and has high penetrance, although it requires environmental factors to achieve expression. Thus, with respect to the more benign forms of schizophrenia, Leonhard's conclusions are more like M. Bleuler's in that he ascribes greater heritability to them than to clear process schizophrenia.

Langfeldt (1939) began his study with cases of doubtful rather than clear-cut schizophrenia. These consisted of 100 consecutive admissions (53 male, 47 female) so diagnosed at the clinic, and confirmed by the author who reviewed the records. In the diagnosis "doubtful schizophrenia," unmistakable schizophrenic signs occurred, but these did not dominate the clinical picture and various alternative diagnoses had been offered as well. The families of the probands were divided into those indicating taint or no taint, based on the indication of familial mental illness in the case histories. Langfeldt personally examined the probands several years after their hospital admission and divided them with respect to four types of outcome. The main findings are shown in Table 6-28.

As can be seen in Table 6-28, there were no significant differences between the two groups with respect to outcome. In retrospect, Langfeldt divided his patients into two groups. The first he classified as typical, and of the 45 so labeled, 36 were "uncured." The second he classified as atypical, or *schizophreniform*. These he described as preponderantly endogenously conditioned reaction forms, including the neurosislike, more psychogenically precipitated disorders, symptomatic psychoses, manic-depressive type of psychoses, and cases diagnosed real atypical schizophrenia. Of the 55 cases so labeled, 7 were uncured and 32 were cured.

Unfortunately, this study throws little light on the genetics issue in these disorders, although the selection of doubtful or borderline cases for study may be one worth repeating with different research methods. It is noteworthy in any event that about one-third of these "doubtful" cases were thought to be cured and another one-fourth improved, whereas slightly less than one-half eventually became clear-cut schizophrenics. Such data as that in Table 6-28 point to a continuum of outcome severity, which, at least by Langfeldt's research methods, appears to be independent of the hereditary factors he used to define taint.

In a very well-designed and well-executed study, Welner and Ström-

---

Table 6-28

Types of Outcome in Doubtful Schizophrenics with or without Hereditary Taint*

Hereditary Taint	Type of Outcome				
	Cured	Improved	Defect	Uncured	Total
Present	16	9	14	8	47
Absent	16	16	12	9	53
Total	32	25	26	17	100

* Data from Langfeldt, 1939.

gren (1958) followed 72 patients (32 male, 40 female) who had had a benign schizophreniform psychosis with a good prognosis at the initial examination. The main clinical criteria included the absence of autism, the presence of features called katathymic (in which an unconscious complex has sufficient affective charge to produce effects in consciousness) and the presence of cure (allowing for nonschizophrenic abnormalities) at the follow-up examination. The examinations occurred 1.5 to 20 years after onset, the average being 8.8 years. Detailed reports were obtained from hospitals, physicians, and relatives for those cases that could not personally be examined. The examinations revealed that 16 were apparently normal; for 8 cases information was insufficient to classify them as normal; 41 were classified as severely neurotic or character deviant, including 5 diagnosed schizoid; and 6 were diagnosed psychotic but not schizophrenic.

The probands had 315 sibs. Morbidity expectancy rates among them included 1.3 percent for schizophrenia, 1.7 percent for schizophreniform psychosis, 1.6 to 2.5 percent for manic-depressive psychosis, or 4.9 percent for all psychoses. The authors compared their findings with Strömgren's 1938 material regarding the sibs of "certain" schizophrenics. The expectancy of psychoses, especially schizophrenia, was significantly lower among the benignly ill probands' sibs, but expectancy was significantly higher for nonpsychotic abnormalities such as neuroses and character deviations. Based on their findings, the authors concluded that the benign psychoses were not manifestations of a specific, distinctive genetic factor, but that cases so affected suffered from a relatively unspecific mental vulnerability, which under certain conditions could lead to a schizophrenic-like psychosis.

In additional studies, Rohr (1961) reported a lowered expectancy of schizophrenia in the parents and sibs of 44 probands (23 male, 21 female) diagnosed as "schizophrenic reaction" by the author. As a control for the reactive group, he compared the rates with "accepted" incidences in families of schizophrenics. Nevertheless, among 86 parents, the expectancy was 4 to 6 percent; and among 136 sibs, 6 percent. Thus, the rates fall in the range of expectancies for schizophrenia generally. Zolan and Bigelow (1950) had 21 male and 29 female probands diagnosed functionally psychotic (43 schizophrenia and 7 manic-depressive psychosis), who had evidence of hospitalized mental illness in their families. For control, they had an "untainted" group of 50 unselected functional psychotics from the same hospital. Among the schizophrenic probands, those who made a subsequent adjustment called satisfactory or better numbered 22 tainted and 19 untainted of the 43 cases in the respective groups. The difference was not significant. Vaillant (1962) studied 30 recovered schizophrenics. A comparison group had remained schizophrenic for at least two years. He found schizophrenia in 26 percent of the index group's families as compared with 33 percent of the controls'. The difference was not significant. However, he also found depressive psychosis in 67 and 11 percent of the index and control groups' families, respectively. This difference was significant at the 0.001 level.

What conclusions can we draw from these studies? First, it seems clear that most of the more benign forms of schizophrenic-like illnesses belong in the same genetic spectrum as the more malignant forms, since the occurrence of schizophrenia often occurs in relatives at rates that are comparable for both groups, and is always more frequent in the families of the benign cases than in the population at large.

If there is a difference with respect to the heritability of the more benign or malignant disorders, the trend of the findings in the Schulz, Wittermans and Schulz, Welner and Strömgren, and Rohr studies suggests a slightly higher heritability for the more typical forms of schizophrenia. However, the Bleuler and Leonhard findings seem to point in the opposite direction. A methodological factor might account for the difference. In the two latter studies, "taint" was defined not in terms of schizophrenia alone, but included other psychoses and disorders as well. Welner and Strömgren's and Vaillant's study suggest that reactive schizophrenia may indeed have a higher heritability for psychiatric disorders other than schizophrenia, and the Bleuler and Leonhard studies might have reflected this fact.

If the inference of biological unity with respect to the more benign psychoses is correct, we might expect to find both process and reactive schizophrenia occurring with the same genotype. This is the case. Fischer found in her series of 16 MZ pairs that 3 cotwins had typical schizophrenia, whereas 9 cotwins had psychoses diagnosed as episodic, schizophrenic, paranoid, or atypical. Gottesman and Shields had one MZ twin pair with one twin atypical, and the other paranoid-schizophrenic. Kringlen found one MZ pair in which the index case had typical schizophrenia and the cotwin had a reactive psychosis. However, among 10 index cases diagnosed as schizophreniform psychosis, no cotwin had typical schizophrenia but 3 also had schizophreniform psychosis. Among the MZ Genain quadruplets, Myra is reactive, Nora is questionable, and Iris and Hester are clearly process schizophrenics.

If the inference of a higher heritability for process than reactive schizophrenia is correct, the genetic picture here may be similar to the picture regarding subtypes. There we found a higher heritability for catatonia and hebephrenia than for the paranoid and simple forms of schizophrenia. The parallel may be more than accidental. Langfeldt's process cases were described as serious catatonic, paranoid-catatonic, and pure hebephrenic. On the other hand, he stated that the paranoid psychoses especially are often merely schizophreniform psychoses. Held and Cromwell (1968) found that reactive cases (defined by premorbid social history, which predicts outcome quite well) tend to be either paranoids or nonparanoids, but process cases tend to be nonparanoids. They cite another study in which 44 percent of the reactive cases (as defined by premorbid social history) were paranoids but only 8 percent of the process cases were paranoids. Thus, there may be some overlap between the paranoid versus catatonic-hebephrenic distinction and the reactive versus process distinction. E. Bleuler had already noted in his classic monograph that paranoid cases had the best prognosis. The higher heritabilities for the process and the catatonic and hebephrenic disorders suggests that they may have a greater number of pathological genes if a polygenic explanation of these differences is correct.

Unfortunately, one major difficulty in comparing the genetic studies regarding process versus reactive schizophrenia arises from the different definitions of the index cases used by the various authors. These differences prevent one from drawing anything more than loose generalizations based on the collective findings. Psychologists often hypothesize that process schizophrenia is caused by genetic-organic factors and reactive schizophrenia by psychogenic factors. The inferences we have drawn suggest that it is better to think of both as extremes along a continuum; that is, they are genetically related, but the role of genetic factors is stronger in the process group. From the polygenic point of view, the process cases would be thought to have more of the genes or the more pathological genes.

Further support for this inference may be obtained from an examination of the offspring of dual matings in which both parents have atypical schizophrenia. Lewis (1957) carried out a study that bears on this point. He had 4 couples with typical schizophrenia and 3 couples with atypical schizophrenia. Among 12 children of the "typical" couples (age-corrected $n = 8.5$), 3 were schizophrenic. Among 15 children of the atypical couples (age-corrected $n = 9$), 1 was schizophrenic. Thus, the only type of psychosis to occur among all offspring was schizophrenia, but the rate was approximately three times higher for the offspring of the typical than of the atypical schizophrenic couples. Of course, the numbers are small, and it is possible that environmental factors were worse in the families where the parents had typical schizophrenia.

Additional relevant data come from studies by Schulz (1940b) and Elsässer (1952). They found that among the offspring of 11 marriages in which one parent was a typical schizophrenic and the other had an atypical psychosis, 4 children were schizophrenic, 3 had an atypical endogenous psychosis, and 1 had a questionable psychosis. These findings could be interpreted either in favor of or against homogeneity theory.

At the very extreme of the reactive end of the continuum, it is possible that cases exist in which no specific genetic factors are involved at all. How could one demonstrate convincingly instances of schizophrenic illness that have no genetic basis? Such cases might most likely occur in a schizophrenic twin who had a nonschizophrenic MZ cotwin and who had no history of schizophrenia among his relatives. In fact, Rosenthal (1959) identified a group of such cases in Slater's twin series. Interestingly, the schizophrenic twin was most often diagnosed paranoid.

It is difficult to say what role different environmental factors may play with respect to the etiology of process or reactive schizophrenia. Alanen (1958) divided his series of 100 schizophrenics into process and reactive types, with 6 cases excluded because of organic complications. He found that the mothers of the process cases more frequently held "firmly and aggressively dominating attitudes toward the child," whereas the mothers of reactive cases were "warmer" and "more softly overprotective." A number of psychological studies have found differences regarding the behavior of parents of process (poor premorbid) and of reactive (good premorbid) schizophrenics, and differences between the two groups of patients in regard to their perceptions of and responses to parents or parent figures (Garmezy, 1965). These findings in toto indicate that parents' behavior may influence to a considerable extent the psychological history and clinical outcome of gene carriers. The detailed case history of the Genain quadruplets lends further support to this view.

Before leaving this subject of the relation between genetic etiology and type of outcome in the schizophrenic disorders, it is worth presenting a unique and imaginative approach to the problem. Mitsuda (1967) carried out pedigree surveys on a large series of hospital admissions, both for inpatients and outpatients. Based on the survey, families were grouped according to the mode of inheritance suggested by the pedigree: dominant, recessive, or intermediate. Among 88 of the families so classified, the author evaluated the probands' course and outcome, and then related these clinical factors to the three suggested transmission patterns, as shown in Table 6-29.

Mitsuda divided clinical course into two major categories: *recovered,* including "social remissions," and *chronic.* Among the dominant cases, more than half recovered. Among the recessive cases, about one-fourth recovered. Mitsuda also classified outcome with respect to four degrees of defect. Not a single case of the dominant group had the most severe form of defect, as compared with about half of the intermediate cases and slightly less than one-fourth of the recessive cases.

Table 6-29

Relationship between the Suggested Mode of Genetic Transmission and the Course and Outcome of Illness*

	Dominant	*Intermediate*	*Recessive*	*Total*
Course:				
Recovered	12(8)	4(2)	12(6)	28(16)
Chronic	10(6)	9(8)	41(27)	60(41)
Total	22(14)	13(10)	53(33)	88(57)
Extent of defect:				
No defect	7(5)	3(1)	8(4)	18(10)
Psychic rapport well preserved	10(6)	1(1)	14(6)	25(13)
Psychic rapport almost completely absent	5(3)	3(3)	19(11)	27(17)
Severe defect ("vegetation")	0(0)	6(5)	12(12)	18(17)

* Data from Mitsuda, 1967.
Note: Figures in parentheses denote cases with more than five years since the onset of illness.

The differences are clearly significant.   They suggest that the possibility of biological heterogeneity in the schizophrenic disorders cannot be completely discounted.   Mitsuda also found that among the psychoses in families of 182 typical schizophrenics, 39.6 and 7.1 percent were chronic and recovered schizophrenics, respectively, whereas among families of 102 atypical schizophrenics, he found 13.7 percent chronic and 49.0 percent recovered schizophrenics.   Such findings could support heterogeneity theory, but they are also consistent with a unitary polygenic theory.   However, since all the other analyses that we have presented support a theory of genetic unity, there may be some way to integrate all of Mitsuda's findings within a unity model.

Schizoid or paranoid personality and borderline states

In almost all genetic studies of schizophrenia, the investigators based their evaluations of the mode of inheritance on cases diagnosed as clear-cut schizophrenics.   With respect to the selection of probands, this was easily done and highly desirable.   With respect to the evaluation of secondary cases, problems appeared.   For example, many family members were not overtly schizophrenic according to accepted diagnostic standards, but neither were they normal.   Should they be counted or ignored?

Many such individuals show symptoms or behaviors that may be regarded as signs of schizophrenia, but in mild degree.   Eugen Bleuler referred to milder schizophrenic cases with manifestations that, although not healthy, would not be regarded as mentally ill.   They included character anomalies, indifference, lack of energy, unsociability, stubbornness, moodiness (whimsicality), and hypochondriacal complaints. Bleuler pointed out that to be considered schizophrenic, such signs had to be evaluated in terms of their intensity, expressiveness, and especially their relation to the psychological setting.   For example, drawing doodles during a boring lecture is common, but including them as part of a serious written communication would be pathognomonic of schizophrenia.   Bleuler classified cases with the above signs as *latent* schizophrenics.   Their symptoms existed in varying degrees and shadings from pathological to normal and fluctuated over time.   But most important for our purposes here, Bleuler maintained that these milder latent schizophrenics with far less manifest symptoms were "many times more common than the overt, manifest cases."

Clearly, Bleuler regarded latent schizophrenia as the same basic illness as clear-cut schizophrenia, but one that is "less advanced."   However, to *demonstrate* that the two disorders are biologically homogeneous is no easy matter, primarily because the diagnosis is so difficult to make with good reliability in many cases.

By and large, the term *latent schizophrenia* never gained wide acceptance, but the concept has always remained very much alive.   Most of the cases that fit Bleuler's description of the disorder are now called borderline or doubtful schizophrenics or schizoid personalities.   Some investigators have used the term *schizoidia* as a separate diagnostic category.

As an illustration of the likelihood of obtaining diagnostic inconsistency among investigators with respect to schizoidia, we may refer back to Table 6-11 in which we examined the rate of schizophrenia among the offspring of schizophrenic couples.   The percentage of all offspring diagnosed schizophrenic was 41, 22, 20, 15, and 37 percent, respectively, for the five studies.   However, the percentages for the diagnosis of schizoid personality (excluding cases called questionable schizophrenia) were 24, 8, 0, 4, and 46, respectively.   Thus, the variation increases considerably for the latter diagnosis, probably, in good part at least, because of the relatively vaguer and more varied criteria used by the different investigators in making the diagnosis.

With this reservation in mind, let us see if there is sufficient evidence to decide on whether these schizoform abnormalities, as they have been called, are genetically related to schizophrenia.   Table 6-11 suggests that cases called *questionable* schizophrenia do belong in the schizophrenia family, since they occur with fair frequency among the children of schizophrenic couples. However, we do not have any good information about the incidence of similar cases in the general population. Similarly, we have no reliable information for cases classified *schizoid* either. Kallmann's (1938) category of schizoidia included two groups:

1 *Eccentric personalities.* These were "borderline cases" who were "abnormal types . . . with schizophrenic defects following unusually mild or hidden psychotic episodes."

2 *Schizoid psychopaths.* These cases showed "autistic introversion, emotional inadequacy, sudden surges of temperament and inappropriate motor responses to emotional stimuli, and in whom such symptoms . . . as bigotry, pietism, avarice, superstition, suspicion, obstinacy, or crankiness" occurred in "disproportionate degree, dominating the personality."

This definition of schizoidia transcends Bleuler's already broad concept of latent schizophrenia to a considerable extent and gives pause to the cautious investigator. Yet Kallmann felt that his concept of schizoidia was not only practical and useful for diagnostic purposes, but, in fact, "almost indispensable."

Among the offspring of schizophrenics, Kallmann found schizoidia in about one-third. Interestingly, whereas schizophrenia occurred twice as often in the children of hebephrenics and catatonics as in the children of patients with the simple or paranoid subtype, schizoidia occurred with approximately the same frequency among the children with respect to the four parental subtypes. The reported figures are shown in Table 6-30.

Kallmann also estimated the morbidity risk for schizoidia to be

Table 6-30

Expectancy of Schizophrenia and Schizoidia in Children of Schizophrenics, According to Parental Subtype*

Parental Subtype	Expectancies, %		
	Schizophrenia	Schizoidia	Total
Hebephrenic	20.7	31.9	52.6
Catatonic	21.6	30.2	51.8
Paranoid	10.4	35.6	46.0
Simple	11.6	31.7	43.3

*Data from Kallman, 1938.

22.8 percent for grandchildren, 10.5 percent for sibs, and 7.9 percent for half-sibs of schizophrenics. Based on all his findings, he concluded that schizoid individuals were heterozygous carriers of a recessive pathological gene, whereas schizophrenics were homozygous. His attempts to fit such findings and others into a theory of recessiveness often lead him to strained explanations which do not hang together well. But his findings suggest that at least some schizoid types of personality are genetically related to schizophrenia.

Of course, it is possible that the family members with schizoid personalities developed their behavioral disturbances as a consequence of rearing in a family with a schizophrenic member. However, in the adoption studies, biological relatives separated from schizophrenic family members also developed borderline schizophrenia or schizoid personality (see Tables 6-16 and 6-17). Additional evidence to suggest that some such personality disturbances are on a graded continuum with schizophrenia can be gleaned from the prediction studies. There we learned that children who later became schizophrenic had traits that are currently accepted as prototypical of the schizoid personality: apathetic, dreamy, listless, shy, seclusive, friendless, socially maladjusted, shut-in, and uninterested. Thus, the early schizoid personality and the later schizophrenia can actually occur in the same person.

In the Kallmann-Roth study of preadolescent twins, 25.7 percent of the discordant MZ cotwins of the schizophrenic index cases were diagnosed as having schizoid personality. Tienari described 6 of his discordant MZ cotwins as introverted, 1 as "primitive," and 4 were thought to have borderline features. Kringlen found that 3 discordant MZ cotwins of typical schizophrenics had "borderline states." Essen-Möller described all his discordant MZ cotwins as having a "characterological defect." Gottesman and Shields (1966) found a considerable proportion of their discordant MZ twins to have a gradation of traits that could be called schizoid or subschizophrenic. As a matter of fact, all investigators found only a small percentage of cotwins of MZ schizophrenic probands that could be called normal. Thus, individuals with the same genotype as schizophrenics usually show personality aberrations that can be classified as schizoid, indicating again that such disorders are probably biologically homogeneous with schizophrenia. The research task of the future will require that we distinguish among all schizoid characters those that reflect the genotype in good part and those that arise from other causes.

What implications do the borderline and schizoid cases have for theories regarding the mode of inheritance? Kallmann, in attempting to justify his theory of a single recessive gene, maintained "that the constant occurrence of schizoidia in the descendants of schizophrenics gives only an illusion of a dominant hereditary pattern." He tried to explain away the "illusion" by asserting that the schizoid personalities were heterozygous carriers of the pathological gene. However, the figures in Table 6-30 indicate that the difference between the hebephrenic-catatonic and paranoid-simple subtypes regarding the incidence of schizophrenia in children does not occur with respect to schizoidia. Kallmann postulated "constitutional" factors to account for the different expectancies regarding schizophrenia but held that these did not apply to schizoidia. One might question why these constitutional factors might protect individuals who are homozygous for the pathological gene but fail to protect the heterozygous carriers. In point of fact, the gradation of schizoidia, and borderline, moderate, and severe schizophrenia, strongly suggest a continuum of degree which is most simply accounted for by a polygenic theory, probably in conjunction with environmental factors of various kinds.

THE SPECIFICITY OF THE SCHIZOPHRENIC GENOTYPE

In this section, we will review the possibility of a genetic association between schizophrenia and some of the other common behavioral disorders. We will examine the genetic studies of these disorders themselves in the next chapters. Here we will be concerned primarily with concurrent elevated frequencies for familial schizophrenia and each of the other disorders, and we will propose possible explanations of such concurrences where indicated.

Manic-depressive psychosis and schizophrenia

The great appeal of Kraepelin's nosology stemmed from his reducing a plethora of diagnostic categories to two major ones. Since then, most clinicians and investigators around the world have accepted these as two distinct entities, that is, two different diseases, in the etiological as well as the clinical sense. Table 6-31 presents data bearing on a possible association between the two diagnoses—schizophrenia and manic-depressive psychoses.

Our present concern with Table 6-31 involves the number of children found to be schizophrenic. In one study, the rate for schizophrenia was about the median rate found in the general population, but in the other four studies the rate was appreciably higher than the population incidence—more than two to three times higher. The ratio of manic-depressive to schizophrenic children among the five studies combined

Table 6-31
Morbidity Expectancies among Children of a Manic-depressive Parent

Study	Total Number of Children	Age-corrected Number	Manic-depressive n	Manic-depressive %	Schizophrenic n	Schizophrenic %	Ratio Manic-depressive– Schizophrenic
Hoffmann, 1921	139	94.5	13	13.8	3	2.5	4.3:1
Weinberg and Lobstein, 1936	158	94.5	6	6.3	1	0.8	6:1
Röll and Entres, 1936	132	82.5	8	9.7	2	2.0	4:1
Slater, 1938	491	204	26	12.8	8	3.1	3.3:1
Stenstedt, 1952		149	9	6.0	5	3.1	2:1

is 3.26:1. From the genetic point of view, why should schizophrenia have occurred at all in these families? Three possible explanations come readily to mind:

1 Schizophrenia and manic-depressive psychosis are genetically related.

2 Rearing by a manic-depressive parent can produce either schizophrenia or manic-depressive psychosis in children.

3 The marital partners of the manic-depressive parents may have been carriers of schizophrenic genes, even if they were not overtly schizophrenic.

From such data, we cannot evaluate the rearing hypothesis. However, it is possible to get some leverage on the genetic hypotheses by finding couples where both parents are manic-depressive. If schizophrenia is genetically related to manic-depressive psychosis, the offspring of such couples should show a proportionate increase in both disorders. If a decrease in the rate of schizophrenia occurs in the children, or if the illness does not occur at all, this finding would provide support for the hypothesis that the spouses of the manic-depressives in Table 6-31 were carriers of schizophrenic genes.

Schulz (1940) and Elsässer (1952) examined the offspring of manic-depressive couples. Elsässer combined all couples in both studies, excluding those in whom he thought the illness was atypical. Among his own cases, the age-corrected number of offspring was 13.63, but he found no schizophrenia among them (one case was classified atypical endogenous psychosis; the other psychoses were manic-depressive). In Schulz's series of nine couples acceptable to Elsässer, one child was schizophrenic. The morbidity risk for schizophrenia was 2.7 percent. Elsässer believed that this one case afforded no compelling reason to postulate a genetic association between the two disorders, especially since the incidence of manic-depressive psychosis in the children was very high. The crude manic-depressive–schizophrenic ratio in both studies combined was 20:1, which is six times higher than the ratio based on Table 6-31, thus affording support for the hypothesis that a number of spouses of the manic-depressive parents had been carriers of schizophrenia-causing genes. The possible contribution of environmental factors, such as behavioral identification with the parental forms of illness, cannot be entirely excluded, based on these findings alone. However, in the adoption studies of schizophrenia, where the child never had a parental model of psychosis with which to identify, no case of a child with manic-depressive psychosis has as yet been reported.

What happens when a schizophrenic marries a manic-depressive? Will the illnesses segregate equally in their children, will one predominate, or will clinically mixed psychoses occur? Elsässer again compared his own cases and those of Schulz (1940*c*) in which such matings occurred. In his own series of four such couples, no child had manic-depressive psychosis, but three were definitely schizophrenic, one was probably schizophrenic, and a fifth had an undetermined endogenous psychosis. However, the picture differs in Schulz's series of 15 such matings. There the morbidity expectancy was about equal for the two disorders. Combining all 19 matings, Elsässer calculated the rates to be 16.5 percent for manic-depressive psychosis, 11.4 percent for schizophrenia, and 3.3 percent for atypical or undetermined endogenous psychosis.

How can we explain such findings? We should expect to find a number of cases among the offspring in which there occurred various admixtures of schizophrenic and manic-depressive symptoms. This expectation would obtain whether each disorder was a single-gene dominant or recessive, or was polygenic. However, at least in these two studies, this hardly appears to be the case. One might wonder whether the investigators simply favored one diagnosis over another in any particular patient, while deemphasizing the concurrence of both types of symptoms in at least some cases. The authors publish the clinical pictures and case histories, however, and it does appear from a reading of the cases as presented by the authors that the diagnoses are ones in which most clinicians would concur.

To illustrate the point at issue, let us assume that both disorders involve dominant single genes. An individual who has the genotypes *Mm* and *Ss* might be expected to manifest both manic-depressive and schizophrenic symptoms, yet he might show only one of the disorders. This could occur if, for example, *Ss* suppressed manifestation of *Mm*, or vice versa.   In the combined Schulz and Elsässer series there occurred a slightly higher rate of manic-depressive than of schizophrenic offspring, and the difference might reflect some suppressed manifestation of Ss by Mm.

However, many cases occur in the general population in which individuals do have both manic-depressive and schizophrenic symptoms, and these cases are properly diagnosed as schizo-affective psychosis. One might well expect such clinical pictures to occur commonly in offspring of matings between a manic-depressive and a schizophrenic. Why they do not occur in the combined Schulz and Elsässer series is hard to explain on simple genetic grounds.   The same reasoning applies if we assume that both disorders are recessive.

If both disorders are polygenic, it may be that where the number of genes for one disorder predominates over the other, the predominant ones will achieve manifestation in most cases.   One could assume that different sets of polygenes cause each of the disorders, and that if the relative number of genes in each set determines the type of clinical manifestation, then, based on the Schulz-Elsässer combined findings, the numbers of genes in each are approximately equal to one another.

Another possibility exists, namely, that essentially the same genes are causing both disorders.   Such a view would hold that some of the genes have a qualitatively different effect than others and that the type of clinical manifestation that occurs depends on the particular number and combination of genes present.   In a modification of this view, we assume again that the same set of genes leads to the clinical pathological condition, but that their manifestation as schizophrenia or manic-depressive psychosis depends mostly on other genes.   For example, the genes that cause one body type, for example, pyknic, could modify the expression of the pathological genes in the direction of manic-depressive psychosis, whereas genes causing a leptosomic body type might foster a schizophrenic type of manifestation.   However, these polygenic models still do not explain why, by and large, the two disorders tend to run true in families, why the offspring in the Schulz-Elsässer series do not develop schizo-affective psychoses, and why the offspring of manic-depressive parents sometimes develop schizophrenia whereas the offspring of schizophrenics seldom develop manic-depressive psychosis.   In any event, the above studies provide no clear evidence of a genetic association between schizophrenia and manic-depressive psychosis.

Among the offspring of 11 marriages between a manic-depressive and a spouse with an atypical endogenous psychosis, the Schulz and Elsässer studies yielded a morbidity expectancy rate of 14.9 percent for manic-depressive illness and 10.7 percent for "other endogenous psychoses."   No case of "pure" schizophrenia was found, although one daughter was called atypical schizophrenic. These findings, although relevant to the problem under discussion, do not help us to decide for or against a theory of genetic relatedness between the two disorders.

As stated above, however, schizophrenic and manic-depressive symptoms can and do occur in the same patient, and such cases are diagnosed schizo-affective or "mixed" psychosis. Since they tend to have a good prognosis and recovery rate, such cases are often included as reactive or atypical schizophrenics. Vaillant (1962) compared the families of 30 recovered and 30 chronic schizophrenics. Among the recovered cases he found depressive psychosis in the families of 67 percent of his recovered probands, as compared with 11 percent in the families of his chronic cases. The very high incidence of depressive psychoses among the families of recovered cases suggests that a considerable number of these probands may have had schizo-affective or mixed psychosis. Such a high rate was not reported in other studies of the families of atypical or reactive schizophrenics.

Moreover, Welner and Strömgren reported a morbidity expectancy of 1.6 to 2.5 percent for manic-depressive psychosis in the siblings of their probands with schizophreniform psychosis. This rate is similar to the expectancies in sibs of 1.3 and 1.7 percent for schizophrenia and schizophreniform psychosis, respectively. Other studies report modest admixtures of schizophrenia and manic-depressive psychosis in the same families. An illustration is shown in Table 6-32.

Unfortunately, Ödegaard does not say how many relatives he had in his total sample, and so we do not know the morbidity expectancies for the diagnostic groups shown. But among the relatives of schizophrenics there was one case of manic-depressive psychosis for every five cases of schizophrenia, and among the relatives of manic-depressives,

---

Table 6-32

Psychoses in First-degree Relatives of Schizophrenic and Manic-depressive Probands*

Diagnosis of Proband	*Diagnosis of Relatives*		
	Schizophrenia	*Manic-depres-sive Psychosis*	*Other Functional Psychoses*
Schizophrenia	55	11	19
Manic-depressive psychosis	5	26	4

* Data from Ödegaard, 1963.

there was one case of schizophrenia for every five cases of manic-depressive psychosis. Thus, although there is a clear concentration of the same disorder in families, the other disorder may occur to an appreciable extent as well.

Let us review again some findings of theoretical interest:

1 Among children who had two schizophrenic parents, Schulz found two who had manic-depressive psychosis.

2 Manic-depressive parents sometimes have schizophrenic children, but schizophrenic parents rarely have manic-depressive children.

3 No instance has ever been reported of clear-cut schizophrenia in one twin and clear-cut manic-depressive psychosis in his MZ cotwin.

How is it possible to reconcile all these findings theoretically? The first point that we can make with fair confidence is that there is a pronounced familial separation of the two disorders. This suggests that they represent two different genetic entities. How then can we account for the findings that suggest genetic overlap? Several explanations are possible.

One possibility is that some cases are misdiagnosed. It is well known that differential diagnosis between the two disorders is sometimes difficult and that diagnostic differences between investigators occur. A second possible explanation is that in the cases where genes for both schizophrenia and manic-depressive psychosis occur in the same individual, one or the other may be sufficiently predominant with respect to manifestation that the investigator will diagnose the predominant symptoms and minimize the others. Third, it may be that constitutional or other genetic factors modify clinical expression sufficiently to mask the usual genetic manifestation and permit alternative clinical diagnoses. And, fourth, environmental influences might also affect symptom formation sufficiently to modify or alter the clinical picture. This last point might explain why schizophrenia sometimes occurs in the children of manic-depressives, but why the reverse almost never happens.

From a methodological standpoint, any future investigations of this issue (and in fact all genetic issues in this field) ought to institute four standard procedures:

1 The authors should specify clearly the criteria they employ with respect to the diagnoses made.

2 The individual making the diagnosis of relatives should not know whether they are related to probands with one particular diagnosis

or with another. Ideally, he should not know the disorders under study at all.

3 All diagnoses should be based on personal examination.

4 There should always be a control or comparison group.

Whether studies that meet all four criteria will clarify the specificity issue or not, we cannot say. But we could at least be assured that the probability of error would be reduced.

Psychopathy (sociopathy) and schizophrenia

If schizophrenia is defined as a disorder characterized by social withdrawal, psychopathy may be defined as a disorder characterized by antisocial behavior. Since schizophrenia was first recognized as a disease entity, both clinicians and psychiatric geneticists have noted the common occurrence of psychopaths among the families of schizophrenics. Kallmann (1938), for example, reported that in the families of his schizophrenic probands, he found that psychopathy occurred in 12.8 percent of their parents, 17.0 percent of their children, and 10.7 percent of their sibs, as compared with a rate of 3.5 to 10 percent for the general population. The figures for family members are as high or higher than the expectancy rates for schizophrenia. The rate for the general population, however, is extraordinarily high. By contrast, Hallgren and Sjögren (1959) reported a rate of 1.1 to 1.3 percent among sibs of schizophrenics and 1.7 to 2.5 percent among parents. Part of the difference may be that these authors used age twenty as the *upper* limit of the risk period. The general population incidence was 0.20 to 0.35 percent for psychopathy. Thus, national differences between Germany and Sweden with respect to psychopathy may also contribute to the markedly different rates in the two investigations. But in both instances, the rate of psychopathy was appreciably higher for the first-degree relatives of schizophrenics than for the population at large. Do such findings imply a genetic association between the two disorders?

Both Kraepelin and E. Bleuler recognized that at least a symptomatic overlap of both disorders could occur in the same individual. As a matter of fact, it was well known that schizophrenia occurred commonly among incarcerated criminals. Kraepelin noted the contribution of the prison environment to the disorder, but believed that those who developed this "prison psychosis" were markedly schizoid or latent schizophrenic individuals. Bleuler pointed out that "the intense hatred of society and the utter failure of any means of escape . . . leads to outbursts of destructive fury" in these cases "as in other psychopaths."

The attack may be brief, but the prison environment may also lead to delusions of being tortured, of enemies holding the victim prisoner and poisoning him, of his being a second Savior, and so on. He may then be transferred to a psychiatric hospital where the episode subsides in a few weeks, but he harbors some residuals of chronic schizophrenia thereafter. Bleuler felt, like Kraepelin, that "the thrust of schizophrenia . . . in most cases was present already before imprisonment" and "was the very cause of the antisocial behavior." He added that "many disorders regarded as 'moral insanity' must be included" in the group of schizophrenias.

Such phenomena continue to occur. Hamburger (1967) reported that among the 2,200 prisoners at the Leavenworth Penitentiary, whose average sentence was 10.8 years, a high incidence of paranoia occurred. He found that of 132 consecutive admissions to the psychiatric inpatient hospital unit, 82 percent had significant paranoid features. Almost 60 percent suffered from paranoid schizophrenia or paranoid reaction. Of the inmates who had had MMPI examinations and were subsequently hospitalized, 80 percent had elevated paranoia scale scores. Of *all* penitentiary admissions, 18 percent had elevated scores on this scale, but on subsequent testing, abnormally high paranoia scores had spread to 32 percent of the retest group. The author concluded that many inmates had a premorbid paranoid personality that decompensated in the prison milieu, but that the milieu also increased the paranoid feelings of individuals who had had little of these tendencies before. Thus it seems as if at least some antisocial, presumably psychopathic, offenders are also schizophrenic, and, at least in the view of Bleuler, the antisocial behavior may actually be an expression of the schizophrenic illness.

Among the family members of schizophrenics, some have been described as eccentric, repressed, markedly reserved and cool, sometimes cold and inconsiderate, sometimes hypersensitive, aesthetic people. They have been called *schizothymic*. According to Zerbin-Rüdin, if these traits intensified toward overtly expressed abnormality, they would be diagnosed schizoid psychopaths. Presumably, it would be such schizothymic individuals who would develop the paranoid reactions and the prison psychoses described above. It is likely, too, that many, if not most, of Kallmann's cases of schizoidia in Table 6-30 were schizoid psychopaths. We can see in that table that, among the four subtypes, the one somewhat elevated rate for schizoidia occurred among the offspring of paranoid schizophrenics. This is what we might expect if we assumed a more direct genetic association between the paranoid schizophrenic subtype and schizoid psychopathy. We must have reservations about this hypothetical association, however, especially since Kallmann's definition of schizoid psychopathy is so sweeping, and is

far broader than that of Europeans generally as, for example, the one
given by Zerbin-Rüdin.

Further evidence of the symptomatic overlap between the psychopathic and schizophrenic disorders is provided by Bender (1959). She
describes a syndrome that she calls *pseudopsychopathic schizophrenia*.
This disorder is most characteristic of late childhood, puberty, and early
adolescence. Of 10 cases presented, she traces the onset from infancy
in 8, whereas the other 2 had severely disturbed early environments,
having been abandoned as infants and deprived. The latter two had
low IQ and showed negativism, anxiety, social conflict, vagrancy, stealing, sex offenses, and general maladjustment. Half had been considered
retarded in their early school years, but later their IQs ranged from
91 to 126. Bender describes them as regressed, dependent, and unable
to get along with other children. They had motility disturbances, were
anxious, preoccupied with their body and identity, felt disliked, and
developed paranoid attitudes.

Their maximal schizophrenic symptomatology developed between
age eight and ten; they had auditory hallucinations, showed impulsive
negativistic behavior and acute panic states, and often could not attend
school. All 10 were diagnosed as schizophrenic. Their psychopathic
behavior included delinquency, homosexuality, attacking women with
knives, murder, pyromania, impulsivity, hostility and negativism, and
other acts of violence. According to Bender, their behavior is classified
as psychopathic until it reaches explosive degrees or chronic psychotic
states during which there occurs schizophrenic disorganization with
withdrawal, autistic, or catatonic behavior, or neurotic symptoms that
mask the basic paranoid attitudes.

Further evidence of a genetic association between psychopathy and
schizophrenia can be found in the adoption studies. Heston, as shown
in Table 6-18, found nine cases of sociopathic personality among the
children of schizophrenic mothers, as compared with only five cases
of schizophrenia. There were only two cases of sociopathic personality
among the controls, the difference between groups with respect to this
disorder reaching a high level of statistical significance. Seven of the
index cases had committed felonies or major crimes for which they were
imprisoned with long sentences. In the study by Kety et al., the investigators found a significantly higher prevalence of cases diagnosed psychopathy or character disorder among the biological relatives of schizophrenic adoptees than among control adoptees. However, such findings
do not occur in the study by Rosenthal et al., where the only subject
diagnosed as a psychopath was a control case. Kaufman et al. (1963)
distinguished two separate diagnostic groups among juvenile delin-

quents.   One they classify as schizophrenic delinquents, and the other, impulse-ridden, character-disordered delinquents.

The findings of an elevated frequency of psychopathy and schizoid psychopathy among families of schizophrenics, of elevated rates of paranoid schizophrenia among psychopaths, and high frequencies of sociopathy or character disorder among individuals who have had no personal contact with their index schizophrenic relatives, taken together, suggest that a genetic association between psychopathy and schizophrenia does exist.

However, such findings could be explained on other bases as well. The psychopathic behavior in the family members of schizophrenics could represent the behavior of despair and frustration that could occur as a reaction to living with a psychotic relative.   Both the schizophrenia and psychopathy could be induced by living conditions commensurate with a low social class.   The criminals who develop prison psychoses with paranoid-schizophrenic reactions may be genetically conditioned schizophrenics, who, out of environmental and perhaps constitutional considerations, behave antisocially as well as asocially until the relevant environmental stresses elicit more clearly the basically schizophrenic personality.   The pseudopsychopathic schizophrenic children described by Bender provide parallels to those cases with prison psychosis: their disorganized, twisted psyches impel them to gross, often peculiar antisocial acts which color them psychopaths at first blush, but whose schizophrenia eventually reveals itself as the underlying, unleashing force behind the antisocial behavior.

The findings by Heston might reflect the fact that his index children were conceived and carried during pregnancy by mothers who were actively schizophrenic, who were perhaps catatonically immobile with no exercise or physical activity, poor diet, intense prolonged anxiety with concomitant circulatory effects, various medications or shock treatments, and who otherwise subjected the fetus to conditions that result later in disorganized, uncontrolled, acting-out kinds of behavior.   Perhaps, too, some adoptive parents knew of the biological mother's schizophrenic illness and this knowledge may have influenced their own behavior to the child, and the child's consequent response to his environment.   In the study by Kety et al., some of those diagnosed as psychopathy or character disorder may have had association with the index case's biological parents who carried diagnoses in the schizophrenic spectrum.   If there really is a genetic association between the two disorders, findings of such an association should have occurred in the studies by Rosenthal et al., and by Karlsson, but did not.

That the disorders are separate and independent, from the genetic standpoint, is also suggested by the study of Kaufman et al. They found that the families of their schizophrenic delinquents tended to reveal similar underlying pathology in at least one family member. There is less antisocial acting out in these families than in the families of the delinquents with impulse-ridden character disorder. The parents of the latter group, moreover, tend to be impulse-ridden character-disordered personalities themselves. In addition, there is no clear case in MZ twins where one is typically schizophrenic and the other typically psychopathic. Slater reports two MZ pairs where one was schizophrenic and the other diagnosed as a psychopath, but in one pair the schizophrenic twin had similar psychopathic features, and in the other pair, both twins had congenital syphilis. Finally, it is possible that psychopathy is not genetically determined at all. Later we will examine the evidence regarding this point. But with respect to the question of a possible genetic unity between schizophrenia and psychopathy, we are not able to draw any firm conclusions without further studies of this issue.

We may mention one further point. Among both psychopaths and schizophrenics, we usually find a higher incidence of electroencephalographic abnormalities than that in the general population. If such abnormalities tend to occur in families, this factor may serve as a common link between the two disorders and could account for some of the familial association between them. Some of these abnormalities are heritable.

Neurosis and schizophrenia

Although Freud and many of his followers often referred to schizophrenia as a neurosis, many psychiatrists and psychologists have accepted the idea that neurosis and psychosis are distinct and separate forms of mental illness. Others have held that neuroses are merely milder forms of mental disturbance that could exacerbate to become the more serious psychoses. Support for the latter view can be found in studies of the premorbid personality of individuals who later became schizophrenic. Many report various neurotic symptoms in the childhood of such patients. The findings of one such study are shown in Table 6-33.

The subjects in Table 6-33 had been referred to the Judge Baker Guidance Center by schools, courts, and social agencies. The subjects in the table were 60 boys and 48 girls who subsequently were hospitalized for schizophrenia, and 28 boys and 29 girls who subsequently made a socially adequate adjustment. The author reviewed the records, including a checklist of presenting symptoms, without knowing the subject's subsequent fate. With respect to the males, the preschizophrenic group was significantly higher than the controls with respect to three

Table 6-33
Neurotic Symptoms in Children Who Became Schizophrenic and
Controls Who Did Not*

Symptom	Male Schizophrenics		Male Controls		Female Schizophrenics		Female Controls	
	n	%	n	%	n	%	n	%
General anxiety	35	58	9	32	31	65	15	52
Phobias	11	18	0	0	8	17	6	21
Obsessive-compulsive traits	18	30	1	4	13	27	4	14
Hysterical traits	2	3	1	4	6	12	5	17

* Data from Gardner, 1967.

of the four symptoms. The groups did not differ with regard to hysterical traits. The highest level of statistical significance occurred for the obsessive-compulsive traits. However, the female groups did not differ significantly in regard to any neurotic category. The author points out that neurotic symptoms occur more commonly in girls than boys and are less in conflict with their cultural sex role. For such reasons, it is important to control for sex in studies of the possible etiological relationship between neurosis and schizophrenia.

In any case, Table 6-33 does indicate that neurotic symptoms do occur more often at least among male preschizophrenics then among controls. These symptoms could indicate (1) early *signs* of the developing schizophrenic illness, (2) indications of the subject's attempts to deal with a vaguely sensed intrapsychic disorganizing process, (3) neurotic behaviors—induced by life stresses—that could, if exacerbated, culminate in schizophrenic reactions. It is well known that high anxiety levels and fears of various kinds precede or are concomitant with an acute schizophrenic onset. Moreover, many clinicians have known for decades that there is an elevated incidence of obsessive-compulsive symptoms in schizophrenics. Sometimes these symptoms are prominent in the total clinical picture and are long-standing as well, so that these patients may be diagnosed obsessive-compulsive neurotics for years before they are diagnosed schizophrenic. As we saw earlier, such symptoms are prominent among autistic and schizophrenic children as well.

If these symptoms have a common genetic basis with schizophrenia, we should find an elevated incidence of schizophrenia among relatives of patients with obsessive-compulsive neurosis. As a matter of fact, Luxenburger (1930) reports just this finding. E. Bleuler (1930) expressed his clinical conviction that obsessive-compulsive neurosis belonged with the schizophrenias. However, Lange (1935) and Rüdin (1953) both found an elevated incidence of manic-depressive psychosis as well as schizophrenia among relatives of obsessive-compulsive neurotics. If we accept the hypothesis that schizophrenia and manic-depressive psychosis are genetically distinct, the finding that obsessive-compulsive neurosis is related to both makes no sense genetically, except in the most strained sense. Perhaps some cases diagnosed as manic-depressive psychosis should really be called schizophrenia.

It is possible too that the neurotic symptoms seen in the preschizophrenic and acute schizophrenic are only superficially the same as the symptoms found in the neuroses themselves. That is, from the genetic standpoint, they may be phenocopies. Would we find these neurotic syndromes in the relatives of psychotics? A study to answer this question was carried out by Cowie (1961). Though she carried out the research with great care, it is perhaps unfortunate that the author was unable to observe and examine the relatives personally. The relatives are the offspring of psychotics. She obtained information about their neurotic traits from a parent, sometimes both parents. Psychotic parents and their spouses may not be the best observers or informants with respect to such matters. However, supplemental information was also obtained from psychiatric social workers, children's officers, hospitals, clinics, and general practitioners. Where possible, a teacher filled out a rating form, and offspring who had reached school-leaving age completed the Maudsley Personality Inventory (MPI).

The psychotic parents were of three main types: obsessional, affective, and schizophrenic. A control group of parents was obtained from nonpsychiatric hospitalized patients, some of whom were clearly neurotic. The author found no differences among the offspring of the four groups of patients with respect to the distribution or degree of neurotic symptomatology. Among the 96 offspring of 39 schizophrenic parents, 26 showed signs of neurosis. The author states that these signs were exaggerations of personality qualities rather than specific behavioral disturbances. Among these neurotic offspring, she also found traits such as undue sensitivity, irritability, overexcitability, solitariness, timidity, excessive daydreaming, and a tendency to retreat into a fantasy world. Thus, the findings here tend to support the view that the neurotic signs in these subjects were secondary to the primary schizoid disorder, but several explanations of their origin are possible. The mean neuroticism score for 17 offspring of schizophrenics was 19.65. This was actually *lower* than the mean neuroticism score for 122 offspring of controls, which was 24.76.

The overlap of neurotic and schizophrenic symptoms in the same subject may be found in cases diagnosed as *pseudoneurotic* schizophrenia (Hoch and Polatin, 1949). It would be highly advantageous for our purposes if we could study the psychiatric disorders of relatives of such cases in a systematic, well-controlled study, but no such studies are as yet available.

Additional information that might help to unravel our problem comes from twin studies. Slater (1953) had four diagnostic groups of index twins: (1) schizophrenia, (2) affective illness, (3) organic states, and (4) psychopathy/neurosis. The incidence of psychopathy/neurosis among sibs was the same for the first three groups, but twice as high for the fourth. There was no such elevation among sibs of the schizophrenic probands. Moreover, according to the author, there was a marked tendency in all diagnostic groups for the more severely affected DZ twin to have been the more neurotic child. But MZ twins differed very little in the degree of neuroticism in childhood, and this trait was not related to the subsequent severity of illness in these twin pairs. The author inferred that the neuroticism was associated with constitutional features resulting from genetic differences.

However, the twin studies differ greatly with respect to whether neurosis is found in the discordant partner of an MZ schizophrenic twin. For example, Kringlen (1967) reports that among *all* cotwins of index cases with typical schizophrenia, 13 of 45, or 29 percent, had a diagnosis of neurosis; when the index twin had atypical schizophrenia, 4 of 10 cotwins, or 40 percent, had neurosis. In fact, neurosis was the most common diagnosis among all his cotwins. Similarly, in Tienari's study, among the 16 cotwins of his schizophrenic index cases, 6 carried a primary diagnosis of neurosis, mainly character neurosis. In contrast, Slater reported only 2 MZ pairs in which the cotwins of the schizophrenic index case were diagnosed reactive depression and chronic anxiety state respectively. Fischer did not report any neurosis at all in the MZ cotwins of her 17 schizophrenic index cases.

The differences between studies arise from differences with respect to the number of discordant pairs found and probably the diagnostic predilections of the investigators as well. With regard to the problem under discussion, however, the finding of a substantial number of MZ twins in which one is schizophrenic and the other neurotic is consistent with the findings in Table 6-33. Both indicate that in the same genotype, neurosis and schizophrenia may occur. They also suggest that the neurosis is an earlier manifestation which may or may not progress toward eventual schizophrenia. Clearly, environmental factors must be implicated with respect to whether such a progression does or does not occur. Whether the kinds of neurosis that occur with this genotype differ both clinically and genetically from other neuroses remains an open question. Among Tienari's cotwins, most had character neuroses, with features he called *borderline*.

The entire problem, however, is clouded further by the extraordinarily high prevalence of neurosis in the general population. For example, Shields (1954) obtained a series of twin pairs from a normal school population. Of the 124 individuals, 42 showed moderately severe psychiatric abnormalities, 25 showed mild abnormalities, 35 showed some neurotic traits, and only 22 were well adjusted in every way. Shields examined the possibility that such findings might be peculiar to twins, but concluded that his twin sample was representative of all the school population. The neurotic symptoms were of a kind to which most children are subject, and some investigators believe that these symptoms must be regarded as part of the normal experience of childhood.

Because of the high prevalence of neurotic traits in the general population, it is not surprising to find a high prevalence of neurotic disturbances in the families of schizophrenics. Alanen (1958), for example, reports that among the 100 mothers of schizophrenics, 16 had slight neurotic disturbances or were normal, 21 were psychoneurotically disturbed, and 40 had disturbances "more serious than psychoneurotic," but not bordering on the psychotic. Mitsuda et al. (1967) believe that there is a genetic association between some forms of neurosis and schizophrenia. Their relevant findings are shown in Table 6-34.

The degree of association between schizophrenia and all neuroses combined is not large. Among 672.0 age-corrected sibs, only 9 developed schizophrenia. The morbidity risk is not much different from that of the population at large. However, if we excluded some forms of neurosis which seem clearly to have no association with schizophrenia at all (for example, hysteria and depressive reaction), the morbidity risk for schizophrenia would be somewhat higher. Moreover, if we included only certain types of neurosis, such as the anxiety reactions and oversensitivity neurosis, the morbidity risk for schizophrenia becomes appreciable indeed. Thus, the findings of Table 6-34 lend considerable support to the hypothesis that some forms of neurotic disturbance are genetically linked to schizophrenia, whereas others are not, and that these forms should not be called neuroses but should carry another nosological classification. However, further confirmatory studies of such issues should be conducted before we generate new diagnostic categories to add to an already overpopulated nosology.

Other disorders and schizophrenia

MENTAL DEFICIENCY. Some investigators have purported to find an elevated prevalence of mental deficiency among families of schizophre-

Table 6-34
Familial Association between Types of Neurosis and Schizophrenia*

Proband Diagnosis	Number of Probands	Families with One or More Schizophrenics		Schizophrenia Morbidity Risk for Sibs
		n	%	
Hysteria	36	0	0	0
Depressive reaction	20	0	0	0
Neurasthenia	40	3	7.5	0
Hypochondriasis	59	8	1.63	1.38
Anxiety reaction	23	5	21.7	4.08
Obsessional states	65	14	21.5	1.03
Depersonalization	23	3	13.0	4.88
Oversensitivity	12	4	33.3	5.71
Total	278	37	13.3	1.34

* Data from Mitsuda et al., 1967.

nics and among schizophrenics themselves. The clinical observation that both mental deficiency and schizophrenia commonly occurred in the same individual led diagnosticians to give special names to these cases. In Germany, they are classified as *Pfropfschizophrenia*. In the United States, they have sometimes been classified *psychosis with mental deficiency,* or the two diagnoses of mental deficiency and schizophrenia have been made separately. Psychologists have a long history of trying to establish whether the intelligence levels of schizophrenics are different from those in the population at large. Although the literature is uneven, there is no certain evidence to indicate that mental deficiency is more common among schizophrenics than among well-matched controls. When differences in IQ levels between the index and control groups have been found, it has often been difficult to state whether the apparent deficit in the schizophrenic group may not have been due to the effects of the illness itself, including reduced interest or motivation in the task, heightened distractibility, or related factors.

In studies that reported an elevated prevalence of mental deficiency among family members of schizophrenics, two methodological factors could have led to the authors' conclusions:

1 The investigator may not have had a well-matched control group. Since schizophrenics tend most often to come from families of lower socioeconomic status, and since such status is correlated

with educational level and cultural deprivation or enrichment, finding low IQs among many schizophrenics should occasion no surprise.

2 The investigator's diagnosis of mental deficiency was often based on his clinical judgment rather than on standardized tests of intellectual functioning. Thus it is not surprising that in some investigations, no association between schizophrenia and mental deficiency has been found.

However, psychologists have established clearly that schizophrenics have a definite tendency to perform better on verbal than on nonverbal or performance tests. It is quite possible that this difference may be related to the schizophrenic genotype itself. Evidence to this effect was presented by Rosenthal and Van Dyke (1968).

Whatever the cause, lower levels of intellectual functioning may play some role in the symptomatic expression of schizophrenia, and perhaps even determine whether clinical schizophrenia does or does not occur. For example, among MZ twins concordant for schizophrenia, the one who becomes more severely ill is likely to have had lower IQs during his formative years. Among the Genain quadruplets, premorbid IQ levels were correlated with eventual outcomes and severity of the clinical disturbance. Also in cases of MZ twins discordant as to schizophrenia, the sick twin is likely to be the one who had a lower level of intellectual functioning during his earlier years. Since IQ differences among MZ pairs are usually associated with differences in birth weight which are in turn associated with prenatal factors, the latter may play some etiological role with respect to schizophrenia. This role may primarily be one in which resistance to clinical manifestation is reduced, or where the ability to cope with stresses, interpersonal problems, or psychological conflicts is impaired.

SEXUAL DISTURBANCE. Sexual problems are prominent in all the functional psychiatric disorders, but perhaps especially so in schizophrenia. E. Bleuler had noted a strong homosexual component in schizophrenics, and Freud proposed a specific psychological mechanism underlying paranoia, in which latent homosexual desires were projected onto others. Lang (1941) examined 92 adult sibs of 33 male homosexuals and estimated their morbidity risk for schizophrenia to be 7.1 to 10.0 percent. Kallmann (1952*a,b*) found a series of 40 male homosexual MZ twins. In 6 pairs, the twins were concordant for schizophrenia as well as homosexuality. Of the remaining twin probands, he found at least 22 others to be schizoid, labile personalities.

Several investigators have questioned the importance of the relationship between homosexuality and schizophrenia, especially paranoid schizophrenia. The best-known study of this issue was for a long time that of Kolle (1931). He reported a thorough study of 127 typical paranoid cases and found only 2 or 3 men with definite homosexual problems. This is the lowest rate reported. One study reports homosexual content in the delusions of 5 of 24 paranoid schizophrenics. Another study finds homosexual conflict pertinent in a number of paranoids, but concludes that the paranoid mechanism cannot be explained solely by homosexual conflict. Another study reports more actual homosexual experiences among paranoid schizophrenics than nonpsychotic controls.

An exceptionally careful and well-done study was carried out by Planansky and Johnston (1962). By various means they determined the incidence of sexual problems in a sample of 150 hospitalized, schizophrenic male veterans. They also divided their sample into four degrees of paranoidness, based on the number of paranoid symptoms observed. The authors found that 72 percent of all subjects had heterosexual problems, 51 percent manifested overt homosexual concerns while they were actively psychotic, 24 percent had had recorded homosexual experiences, 44 percent revealed sexual problems on psychological tests, and 15 percent directly expressed their confusion of sexual identity. The figures do not add up to 100 percent, since each patient could be included in more than one category, but they suggest that virtually every case had some manifest sexual difficulties.

The authors concluded, however, that paranoid development and homosexuality as found in schizophrenia are not specifically related to each other. The conclusion was based primarily on finding no significant relationship between degree of paranoidness and heterosexual problems or homosexual concerns in psychosis. However, the rejection of an association between paranoia and homosexuality ought to be held in reservation. The concept of *degree* of paranoia, as determined by the *number* of paranoid symptoms, may not be entirely relevant to the basic hypothesis. Moreover, the authors do find an association between clearly recorded homosexual experiences and degree of paranoia that is significant beyond the 0.10 level, using a two-tailed test, whereas a one-tailed test could have been justified.

There is no question about the prominence of sexual problems in schizophrenia, or the fact that homosexual concerns predominate among such problems. If homosexuality has a genetic basis, the genetic relation between it and schizophrenia is hardly clear. Perhaps the same genotype that leads to schizophrenia also provokes sexual or psychosexual disturbances of one kind or another, and the latter, depending on the individual's ability to cope with and master them, may exert psychological pressures that are instrumental in the progression toward clinical schizophrenia.

EPILEPSY. A group of patients with temporal-lobe epilepsy has been shown to have symptoms very much like those of schizophrenia. In fact, many authors have long discussed whether some schizophrenia-like conditions and epilepsy, especially the epileptic twilight states, have a common bond. However, in major studies by Kallmann (1938) and Hallgren and Sjögren (1959), the estimated morbidity risk for epilepsy among the first-degree relatives of schizophrenics was about the same as the risk for the general population. Nevertheless, some investigators still believe that there is some connection between these two disorders. The most prominent among them is Mitsuda, who has evolved an interesting theory that we shall present in more detail later. Mitsuda (1967*b*) studies families in which he finds both schizophrenia and genuine epilepsy in the same pedigree (first-degree relatives, grandparents, aunts, uncles and cousins). Thus far he has accumulated 612 such pedigrees, among which 408 probands are schizophrenic and 204 epileptic. In his report, he has selected 25 pedigrees, not to determine how often schizophrenia and genuine epilepsy occur together, but to consider the symptoms of both sorts of patients in detail.

After examining the clinical features of the schizophrenics and the epileptics, Mitsuda, who believes that schizophrenia is genetically heterogeneous with respect to nuclear and peripheral schizophrenia, comes to this conclusion:

> Nearly all cases of schizophrenia and epilepsy that occur in the same pedigree have characteristics of the peripheral group of each psychosis as distinct clinically and genetically from the nuclear group. In other words, if there is a genetic relationship between schizophrenia and epilepsy in terms of a common criterion, such a relationship must be found exclusively between the peripheral groups of both psychoses, while between schizophrenia and genuine epilepsy in the narrow sense (i.e., between their nuclear groups) there is probably no close relationship, either genetic or clinical.

On the other hand, Meduna (1937) proposed that schizophrenia and epilepsy were "biologically antagonistic" diseases. This hypothesis provided the rationale for the introduction of the convulsive therapies in schizophrenia (initially insulin and metrazol, later electroconvulsive shock). Hoch (1943), in a careful review of the relevant literature, concluded that the two diseases were neither pathogenically related nor antagonistic. He thought that most cases could be considered symptomatic epilepsy in schizophrenia, or symptomatic schizophrenia in epilepsy. This conclusion is similar to Mitsuda's.

Bender (1961) reported on 51 cases who were considered schizophrenic in childhood but who also had some form of convulsive disorder. She divided the sample into five groups:

1 Ten autistic, nonverbal children, treated unsuccessfully, developed severe *grand mal* convulsions. She thought this group was basically organic.

2 Eight children, initially normal, later showed motoric, impulsive, and behavioral disorders, and then, in puberty, deteriorating intelligence and temporal-lobe disorders.

3 Thirteen disturbed children with dramatic psychotic features developed *grand mal* convulsions but responded to anticonvulsant drugs and some could return to normal life.

4 Nine children showed both typical epilepsy and schizophrenia.

5 Thirteen children were typically schizophrenic with isolated atypical convulsive behavior. They did not respond to anticonvulsant drugs but responded very well to treatment programs for schizophrenic children.

Thus, Bender's groupings reveal the complexities involved in theorizing about possible genetic associations between the two disorders, but she also indicates how, with careful clinical analysis, it is possible to sort out the relevant variables and make both clinical, therapeutic, and genetic sense of heterogeneous material. Bender thought the first three groups were basically organic, and she could find no family history clearly schizophrenic among them. In group 4, there were strong schizophrenic family histories, but also known brain damage. In group 5, eight children had close relatives with known schizophrenia.

In all probability, the lessons to be learned from Hoch, Bender, and Mitsuda are that one must define one's phenotype as carefully and thoroughly as possible, from several vantage points when feasible, before one can hope to make sound genetic inferences regarding human clinical material.

FERTILITY, MUTATION, AND SELECTIVE ADVANTAGE

From an evolutionary standpoint, since schizophrenia and other behavioral disorders are clearly maladaptive, why should they persist at all if they are genetically conditioned? In Chapter 1 we noted that maladaptation in the cultural sense may not be the same as maladaptation in the evolutionary sense. The latter involves a diminution in the ability to survive and reproduce. There is little question that schizophrenia impairs the affected individual's ability to survive without help and protection in Western society, and in times past the mortality of hospitalized schizophrenics, who often died in periods of heightened excitement, committed suicide, or contracted fatal diseases of various kinds, especially tuberculosis, was considerably higher than the mortality of the population at large. Schulz (1949/50) estimated that their mortality was elevated threefold. With respect to reproduction, all well-done studies indicate that schizophrenics generally are inferior in this respect as compared with the general population.

An exemplary study was carried out by MacSorley (1964). Her probands were 187 male and 203 female psychotic patients. The psychoses were diagnosed as schizophrenic, affective, organic, and atypical. The celibacy rates of all patients were more than 50 percent higher than that of the general population and that of an independent control population taken from the medical and surgical wards of a general hospital and from local industrial firms. The number of children produced by the patients who did marry was considerably less than that of the control group, and the percentage of childless marriages among patients was considerably higher. The atypical patients resembled the schizophrenic groups very closely with respect to the low marriage and reproductive rates. Sibs of the psychotic patients fell between the patient and control groups with respect to not marrying, number of children per marriage, and percentage of childless marriages. Such findings turn up consistently in the various studies done.

Since all knowledge indicates incontrovertibly that schizophrenics fail to survive and reproduce at the same rate as the general population, we have reason to expect that the proportion of schizophrenics in the population should be constantly decreasing. However, there is no evidence to indicate that such a decrease has occurred. Most investigators believe that the rate of schizophrenia in the population remains constant and some have suggested that an actual increase seems to be occurring. If other family members, who might be gene-carriers, even if not psychotic, were *more* fertile than the average population, they could be putting enough of the pathological genes back into the common gene pool to counterbalance those lost through the relative infertility of the schizophrenics themselves. However, MacSorley and others find that schizophrenics' sibs also have a somewhat decreased fertility rate and if anything, should contribute further to the gene loss. No increased fertility has been found among other relatives of schizophrenics.

To accentuate the problem further, it is likely that matings are not random with respect to schizophrenia. If we estimate the frequency of schizophrenia in the general population to be about 1 percent, we would expect by chance alone that the frequency of two schizophrenics marrying would be $0.01 \times 0.01 = 0.0001$, or once in every 10,000 marriages. However, Erlenmeyer-Kimling and Paradowski (1966) found that 2 percent of all marriages among 2,706 index cases were assortative matings. Such matings do not by themselves produce any changes in the gene frequency except insofar as they produce fewer children and a proportionately greater number of affected individuals who, in turn, are selected against because of reduced fertility.

Some investigators have tried to solve this dilemma by postulating a mutation rate for the pathological gene that is sufficiently high to maintain a constant rate of schizophrenia in the population by compensating for the genes lost through diminished fertility. The indirect methods used to calculate the mutation rate required to maintain a constant incidence of the trait are based on the Hardy-Weinberg law. For exposition purposes, let us assume that the trait is a partial dominant. For such traits, an appreciable number of heterozygotes will show the trait, whereas virtually all homozygotes will show it. The fraction of all heterozygotes who show the trait is called penetrance. Let us make the following designations with respect to alleles at a given locus.

p = frequency of the dominant gene
q = frequency of the recessive gene
m = penetrance
w = fitness, or reproductive capacity as compared with a control
  population, expressed in percent
n = number of individuals in the population

In each generation, $p^2 + 2pqm$ individuals will get the disease, and $2pq(1 - m) + q^2$ individuals will escape it. The number of eliminated genes is

$$\frac{2p^2n(1 - w) + 2pqmn(1 - w)}{2n}$$

This value represents the mutation rate if equilibrium, or the relative frequencies of the p and q alleles, is to be maintained. By simplifying the value above, the mutation rate becomes

$$mu = (1 - w)(p^2 + pqm)$$

Böök (1953b), using his study of a north Swedish isolate population which included about 9,000 individuals over a 48-year period and using the partial dominant model, estimated m to be 20 percent, $p = 7$ percent, $q = 93$ percent, and $w = 70$ percent. He calculated the mutation rate to be 5×10^3. This means that 1 of every 5,000 of the normal alleles in the population mutates to the allelic pathological gene in each generation. Such a rate is very high. Previous estimates of the mutability of other human genes have mostly resulted in rates of about 10^{-5}, or 1 in 100,000.

Penrose (1956), assuming recessivity, a 1 percent incidence of schizophrenia, and a reproductive fitness of 95 percent, estimated the mutation rate to be 5×10^{-4}, which is still quite high. Kishimoto (1957), using four different estimation formulas for three different Japanese isolates, obtained mutation estimates that were mostly in the order of 3 to 5×10^{-3}. Böök is not discouraged by the high mutation estimate he finds, but defends the view that we should not be surprised to find some instances in man of high mutation rates. Others believe that such high estimates are unrealistic.

Erlenmeyer-Kimling and Paradowski (1966) have provided the most thoughtful consideration of an alternative explanation for the seemingly constant rate of schizophrenia in the face of reduced fertility. They explore the possibility that schizophrenia may have a compensating adaptive value, and examine three kinds of adaptational hypotheses that have been proposed.

1 *Social-advantage hypothesis.* Schizophrenic behavior may have achieved high social status for affected individuals in past times. They may have been revered as visionaries, mystics, shamans, or saints. However, the authors point out that saints and prophets are not renowned for their high fecundity, and that their social benefits were hardly accompanied by reproductive advantages of the required magnitude.

2 *Sibling-advantage hypothesis.* Heterozygosity (or heterosis) may confer superiority and selective advantage. Heterozygotes or unaffected gene carriers may have favorable psychological attributes which lead to higher reproductivity. Heston found that unaffected children of schizophrenic mothers were more artistic, spontaneous, and interesting than a control group. Karlsson believed that he found a higher than expected number of creative individuals in the pedigrees of schizophrenics. For generations it has often been maintained that there was some association between creativity or genius and schizophrenia. Some have conjectured that relatives may have higher flexibility or sex drive, or lower thresholds of sexual arousal. However, it has never been demonstrated that such individuals have an elevated reproductivity, irrespective of whether they really possess such traits or not. We have observed, in fact, that neither sibs nor other relatives of schizophrenics reveal such an elevation.

3 *Physiological-advantage hypothesis.* The implicated genetic factors may confer increased viability on gene carriers (Huxley et al., 1964). They may be more resistant to diseases, wounds, and infections. No such relative immunity has been found, but proponents of this view stress that the possible selective advantage on this basis would have been conspicuous only during eras antedating modern medicine, in which the advantage dwindles. However, mortality data regarding infants born to schizophrenic parents lend no support to this view. Some data (Rosenthal, 1966) actually suggest increased mortality and congenital malformations.

Erlenmeyer-Kimling and Paradowski propose a fourth hypothesis. They raise the possibility that schizophrenia is not a single genetic entity, but a heterogeneous collection of genotypes that produce similar phenotypes. If so, the estimations of mutation rates would have to be based not on a single locus, but on several. Therefore, the mutation rate for any particular locus would be more in keeping with rates usually found, and the summed mutation rates could replenish the gene loss through reduced fertility. The hypothesis must be taken seriously, but our own examination of the genetic unity or heterogeneity of schizophrenia provides strong support for homogeneity theory. The burden of proof must rest with those who would demonstrate heterogeneity in the sense of several pathological major genes.

However, if the authors use the word *heterogeneity* to refer not to clinical syndromes but to different gene loci in a polygenic system, their hypothesis is compatible with the findings reviewed here that suggested a quantitative view of schizophrenia. According to such polygenic theory, a number of genes at different loci produce effects that are both similar to one another and cumulative. If the normal allele at each of these loci mutated to one of the schizophrenic-spectrum pathological genes, the mutation rate at each locus could be consistent with usual human mutation rates and consistent as well with most of the findings reported in this chapter.

Let us raise a fifth hypothesis. It may be that the environmental factors that interact with hereditary ones to produce clinical schizophrenia are increasing in number and intensity at a rate that approximately counterbalances the reduced fertility. For example, it could well have been true that schizophrenia occurred less often in simpler, more pristine societies. However, as cultures, or some particular aspects of them, became more complex, specialized, industrialized, or whatever it is that the relevant environmental variable involves, more psychonoxious forces evoked more schizophrenic reactions, which led to more gene loss, which was temporally accompanied by further increase in the environmental stresses, and so on. Of course, one would not have to exclude the probability of some gene replenishment through mutation, in this view, but one would still have to explain how the pathological-gene frequency became so high in the first place.

A sixth hypothesis is that the rates for schizophrenia are not constant, and in fact, that the rate may be increasing in some areas and decreasing in others. We saw earlier that there was considerable variation in the frequency of schizophrenia in different populations. These differences could reflect variations in gene frequencies, environmental factors, or both; they might be the result of differential migration, or they might be statistical artifacts. They could also be influenced by varying fertility rates in the different populations studied.

A seventh hypothesis is that genetic factors are not important in schizophrenia at all, and that the entire problem arises only because a false assumption has been made. However, the evidence presented in this chapter so strongly reinforces the probability of a genetic contribution to schizophrenia that such a view no longer appears tenable.

One additional point bears making before closing this section. Erlenmeyer-Kimling and her associates have compared the fertility of schizophrenics in 1934–1936 and in 1954–1956. They find that, probably because of modern therapeutic efficacy, the reproductive rate of schizophrenics is increasing and approaching that of the general population. Moreover, the reproductivity of the unaffected siblings is also increasing and even surpassing that of the general population. These findings suggest that we will have increased incidences of schizophrenia in the future, whether the transmission occurs primarily through genetic or environmental mechanisms. Many individuals have expressed consternation at the prospect. Some states have passed laws permitting the "eugenic" sterilization of schizophrenics and other psychotics. The wisdom or ethics of such actions deserves widespread thought and discussion.

THEORIES OF THE ETIOLOGY
OF SCHIZOPHRENIA

It is not possible to summarize all the theories that men have proposed with regard to what causes schizophrenia. So many environmental, biochemical, or physiological "causes" have been postulated over the years that it is almost easier to list factors that have not been proposed than those that have. All metabolites that have been suspected and tested failed the tests. Physiological, psychophysiological, psychological, sociological, and ecological hypotheses are difficult to rule out or confirm. If, however, the theories are classified into broad groups, without specifying particular hypothesized etiological agents, it is possible to form a conceptual framework. When this is done, the myriad theories can be reduced to three main types: *monogenic-biochemical, diathesis-stress,* and *life-experience theories.*

According to monogenic-biochemical theory, a single gene leads to a specific metabolic error which causes the disease. In fact, a two-gene theory that proposes a specific genotype involving four alleles on two loci also belongs here if the theory assumes that this particular genotype produces a specific metabolic error that alone causes the illness. The multitude of studies that have searched for the twisted molecule that produces a twisted mind are all based on this theory. Diathesis-stress theory is more loosely formulated and more difficult to test, but its looseness gives it a broad cover that enables it to blanket most research findings regarding the causes of schizophrenia. In the main, it holds that it is not a particular biochemical abnormality that is inherited, but rather a *predisposition* to develop the illness. Environmental stresses of certain kinds may potentiate processes involving the predisposition, culminating in clinical schizophrenia. With a benign environment no overt psychopathology need become manifest, and, indeed, the carrier may have traits that are unusual, desirable, and adaptive. Although single-gene theories could fit here, this theory best accommodates a polygenic mode of inheritance. Life-experience theory denies any important role to specific genes. Although we believe that the mass of genetic studies presented here invalidates this type of theory, the many investigations by its proponents who attempt to elucidate environmental causes of schizophrenia could point up the kinds of stresses that may be implicated in diathesis-stress theory. Interested readers will find a more detailed discussion of the three classes of theory in *The Genain Quadruplets* (Rosenthal, 1963, section on theoretical overview). A comparative summary of the three theories' views of some different aspects of schizophrenia is presented in Table 6-35.

Models of monogenic-biochemical theory

Is it possible to fit the data on schizophrenia into a theoretical model of single-gene dominance? Of course it cannot be complete dominance, since we do not find the Mendelian ratios and pedigrees that such a model implies. However, we can assume partial dominance and proceed from there. Slater (1965) has done just that. First, he makes the assumption that all individuals homozygous for the pathological gene manifest the illness, whereas only some of the heterozygotes do. He then assumes the best estimate of the population incidence of schizophrenia to be 0.8 percent. With this assumption, it is now possible to calculate

Table 6-35

Comparison of Three Major Classes of Theory Regarding the Etiology of Schizophrenia

Aspects of the Illness	Monogenic-Biochemical Theory	Diathesis-Stress Theory	Life-experience Theory
Biological unity	Homogeneity: one gene, dominant, recessive, or intermediate. Trait is qualitative, discontinuous.	Homogeneity or heterogeneity. Trait may be qualitative or quantitative.	Neither homogeneity nor heterogeneity. Some question whether it should be considered a disease at all. Trait is quantitative.
"What" is inherited?	A specific but as yet unknown error of metabolism due to a mutant gene.	(1) A single gene. (2) Several major genes. (3) Polygenes. In either case, a "constitutional predisposition."	No special genotype necessary. Anyone could be a potential victim if subjected to certain experiences.
Manifestation	Very high: almost everyone (67 to 86 percent) with the genotype, but some have constitutional resistance to expression.	Considerably lower than monogenic-biochemical. Depends on whether predisposed schizophrenic encounters sufficient stress and how predisposed he is.	Depends on whether an individual is overexposed to certain noxious experiences or deprived of some benign "necessary" ones.
Role of environment	No special environments needed to precipitate illness. Incidental or minimal. Proponents like to cite a constant rate of schizophrenia in all cultures.	Necessary to precipitate the illness. The stressors are seldom defined: head trauma, disease, alcohol, parturition, exhaustion, etc., but usually psychological.	All-important: usually intrapersonal or interpersonal, but also sociological and even ecological.
Clinical subtypes	Of secondary interest, usually thought to reflect other inherited or constitutional factors which influence the form in which the illness is expressed.	Usually holds that they represent different predispositions interacting with different kinds of stressors.	Represent the consequences of different kinds of conflicts or conflict resolutions, or indicate modal types of attempted communication by the patient, or different patterns of learned disordered behavior.

Table 6-35

Comparison of Three Major Classes of Theory Regarding the Etiology of Schizophrenia (Continued)

Aspects of the Illness	Monogenic-Biochemical Theory	Diathesis-Stress Theory	Life-experience Theory
Severity of illness	Reflects the degree of metabolic disturbance.	Reflects the amount of inherited predisposition and the intensity of the stressor.	Reflects the intensity of the conflicts or of the configurational stimuli involved in the maladaptive learning, or of noxious response-reinforcement contingencies.
Remission	For some reason, the effects of biochemical disturbance clear, but personality defect remains.	Either the physiological aspects of the disease process are reduced or the stressors are reduced.	(1) Abatement of conflict intensity. (2) Modification of configuration of stimuli which maintain the illness, or of schedules of reinforcement.
Premorbid personality	Varies in usual ways. When aberrant, the deviations are thought to be early signs of the metabolic disturbance.	Can provide clues about the nature of the predisposition inherited, as introversive personality or high anxiety.	Reveals the kinds of early conflict or learning patterns which eventually culminate in psychosis.
Research strategy	(1) Search for the biochemical aberrancy and its corrective. (2) Estimate gene frequency in population, mutation rate, mode of inheritance, etc.	Learn about the nature of the predispositions, the stressors, and the nature of the interaction.	Elucidate the conflicts or learning patterns leading to schizophrenia and the kinds of interventions most effective in counteracting the morbid process.
Example of problems posed by previous findings	Why does the distribution of illness in kindreds vary so markedly, for example, showing dominant, recessive, or intermediate patterns?	Why does the illness continue when the ostensible stressor has been removed?	(1) Why do patients get better with drugs or physical therapies? (2) How explain the genetic findings?

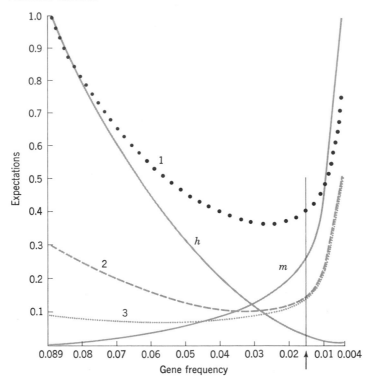

Figure 6-4. Theoretical expectations of incidence of schizo-phrenia in relatives of schizophrenics (*broken lines*), with vary-ing gene frequency and varying penetrance.   1 = children of two schizophrenics; 2 = sibs of schizophrenics; 3 = children of one schizophrenic; h = proportion of all schizophrenics who are homozygous; m = manifestation rate of gene in heterozygote. Reprinted with permission, from E. Slater, Clinical aspects of genetic mental disorders, in J. N. Cummings and M. Kremer (eds.), *Biochemical Aspects of Neurological Disorders*, 2d series, Blackwell Scientific Publications, Ltd., Oxford, 1965.

the proportion of heterozygotes who manifest the illness as a function of different possible gene frequencies in the population.   The results of Slater's calculations are shown in Figure 6-4.

Slater found that Kallmann's figures for sibs and for the parents of one schizophrenic, and Elsässer's figure for the children of two schizo-phrenic parents agree well with expectation for a gene frequency of 0.015 (shown by the arrow) and a corresponding manifestation rate of 26 percent in heterozygotes.   Homozygotes account for 3 percent, and heterozygotes 97 percent, of all schizophrenics.

The elegance of the model is apparent from Figure 6-4, but it pre-sents problems.   The population incidence of 0.8 may be too low, and the risk figure for Kallmann's sibs may be too high. The borderline cases and schizoid relatives are excluded in the calculations, and Slater found it difficult to fit the known twin data into the model.

A model for a single, recessive gene is provided by Kallmann (1953), and is shown in Figure 6-5. Kallmann's model is illustrative only, and makes no attempt to account for specific rates of schizophrenia in the population or among relatives of different degree. It involves, in addition to the assumption of a single recessive gene, only one other variable: constitutional resistance to manifestation. For illustrative purposes, he divides this continuous variable into four degrees of intensity. Kallmann's intent is to show how different combinations of genotype and constitutional resistance can account for different degrees of illness severity—from normal to deteriorative schizophrenia. It can thus account for all cases in the schizophrenic spectrum. However, since constitutional resistance is itself presumed to be a polygenically determined trait, Kallmann offers in effect a single-gene theory with modifying poly-

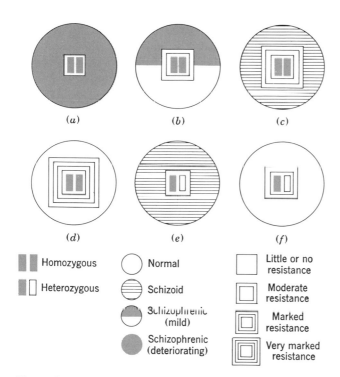

Figure 6-5. Possible variations in the expressivity of, or the resistance to, a recessive factor for schizophrenia. Reprinted, with permission, from F. J. Kallmann, *Heredity in Health and Mental Disorder*, W. W. Norton & Co., Inc., New York, 1953.

genes. Such a theory is difficult to distinguish by test from a straightforward polygenic theory, but it provides greater encouragement for those seeking the metabolic error in schizophrenia. A major difficulty confronting the theory comes from the twin studies that find relatively low concordance rates in MZ twins, both of whom share the same modifying genes that are presumed to influence manifestation. However, Kallmann points to other factors that could contribute to reduced constitutional resistance, such as lower birth weight or weight loss, both of which may be related to increased manifestation in the sicker twin.

Mitsuda (1967) proposes a model that is both unusual and imaginative. It is based on a different approach to psychiatric genetics, one that he calls the *clinico-genetic* approach. He states that "genetic studies in the field of psychiatry have tended to resort merely to assembling huge amounts of material and pursuing complicated mathematical treatments. From the viewpoint of clinical genetics, it seems more important to collect step by step individual cases which can be studied in detail clinically as well as genetically." Based on this orientation, he has examined the pedigrees of typical, atypical, and intermediate schizophrenics to determine the mode of inheritance among them. His findings are given in Table 6-36.

Mitsuda finds that the majority of cases of typical schizophrenia are recessive, while both the recessive and dominant modes of inheritance are about equally represented in atypical schizophrenia. Based on such data and on his finding epileptic and manic-depressive psychoses among the family members of schizophrenics, he has evolved the following model of the major psychoses, which subsume a monogenic-biochemical theory for both typical and atypical schizophrenia. The model is illustrated diagrammatically in Figure 6-6, and relies upon what Mitsuda calls the *three-entities principle*. The three entities are

---

Table 6-36

Mode of Inheritance in Typical, Atypical, and Intermediate Schizophrenia (by Percentage) *

Proband	*Mode of Inheritance*			
	Dominant	*Intermediate*	*Recessive*	*Combined*
Typical	8.2	17.6	72.5	1.6
Intermediate	37.5	15.6	34.4	12.5
Atypical	42.2	11.8	42.2	3.9

* Data from Mitsuda, 1967.

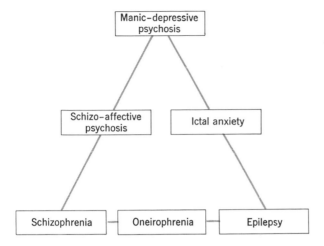

Figure 6-6. Schematic representation of relationship between various clinical types of atypical psychoses and the typical major psychoses. Reprinted, with permission from H. Mitsuda, *Clinical Genetics in Psychiatry*, Igaku Shoin, Tokyo, 1967.

schizophrenia, manic-depressive psychosis, and epilepsy. Each entity has both typical and atypical (nuclear or peripheral) forms. In the nuclear groups, there is hardly any overlap in the manifestational range, indicating complete genetic independence among them. But considerable overlap exists between the different peripheral groups, as shown schematically in Figure 6-6. The atypical psychosis takes a schizo-affective form in the overlap of typical schizophrenia and manic-depressive psychosis, a form classified as *ictal anxiety* or *ictal depression* when in the borderline area between epilepsy and manic-depressive psychosis. It is not clear how the genetics of the intermediate forms can be worked out with this model, but it does attempt to account for a wide variety of manifestations of psychosis, many of which are ignored, slighted, or simply included in one of the major diagnostic groupings, and it places a heavier emphasis on clinical analysis of cases than do most other genetic studies of the behavioral disorders. Such studies, however, demand strict methodological controls, especially with respect to the independence and reliability of the investigators' diagnoses.

Models of diathesis-stress theory

One of the models best known to psychologists was first publicly presented by Meehl in his presidential address to the American Psychological Association Convention in 1962. Meehl proposes that the old European notion of an inherited "integrated neural defect" may well be correct. The defect involves an aberration of some aspect of single-cell function which may or may not be manifested in the functioning of the more molar CNS systems. He calls this defect *schizotaxia*. Meehl, following Bleuler, also proposes that there are four core characteristics of schizophrenia, which he calls cognitive slippage, anhedonia, interpersonal aversiveness, and ambivalence. Though all schizophrenics have them, they are not innate. Rather, they are universally learned by schizotaxic individuals. The learning is *social* learning, and it will occur regardless of the social-reinforcement regime—whether very good or very poor. Consequent to social learning, the schizotaxic individual develops a form of personality organization that Meehl calls *schizotypy*. If the individual also inherits a "low anxiety readiness, physical vigor, general resistance to stress, and the like," and if the social-reinforcement regime is favorable, he will remain a well-compensated schizotype who shows no mental disease. This is what happens to most schizotypes. But a minority, who have other constitutional weaknesses that are mostly polygenically determined and who undergo a noxious social-reinforcement regime—by schizophrenogenic mothers, for example—develop clinical schizophrenia. Meehl speculates imaginatively about the nature of the inherited defect and outlines three possibilities, but they are not essential for demonstrating the model.

The model that has been most subjected to empirical test is the one proposed by Mednick (1958). We have mentioned it earlier and need not detail it here. It presupposes the possibility, but does not require, that the future schizophrenic inherits high-anxiety responsiveness which is slowly habituated. With respect to the question of what is inherited in schizophrenia, this is the most simplistic model of all. With respect to the environmental aspects in the theory, namely, the process of learning that culminates initially in acute schizophrenia and subsequently in chronic conditions, it is the most elegantly formulated diathesis-stress theory of all. Experimental findings have forced Mednick to modify the role of habituation in the theory, but it is otherwise still viable and promising (Mednick and Schulsinger, 1968).

Many other researchers have suggested alternatives with regard to the nature of the inherited diathesis: an introversive personality, a characterological defect, a constricted personality, a brittle ego, a conglomeration of traits, and the like. The point we want to make here is that Meehl's theory is one in which the diathesis involves a single gene, either dominant or recessive, that leads to a specific defect in CNS neural integration. However, it is essentially a diathesis-stress theory that requires environmental stresses to produce the clinical illness. Nor does the theory suggest that a particular biochemical abnormality, apart from the misguided genetic programming of the neural integrative defect, will be found in schizophrenics, any more than it will be found in the "normal" schizotypes. Mednick's theory also reveals the accommodative breadth of diathesis-stress theory in that, although the diathesis is specific with respect to anxiety and habituation, Mednick leaves open the possibility that it could result from one gene or many genes, or that it may be produced solely by environmental factors.

POLYGENIC THEORY. In the main, the diathesis is thought to be polygenically determined. Throughout this chapter we have discussed data where polygenic theory seemed to be most consistent with the findings. Now let us focus on polygenic theory itself and see what kinds of data are needed to fit it. We will review briefly how we can identify such multifactorial or quantitative inheritance and examine its implications for schizophrenia.

1 Traits that are determined by multiple factors, whether genetic, environmental, or both, tend to be continuously and normally distributed in the population. By definition, schizophrenia is itself not normally distributed, but schizophrenic-spectrum pathology of the types that we considered to be biologically homogeneous might be. We do not have reliable studies of this point, but they could be done. In such a model, schizophrenia and normality would comprise the opposite tails of the distribution. The continuously graded characteristics of "schizoidness" could be measured once they were defined, and we could see if they followed the normal curve.

However, we are equally concerned with whether the diathesis is itself polygenically determined. In Meehl's model, the diathesis was a single-gene effect, but he also postulated—like Kallmann and all other theorists—some polygenically determined traits that influence trait manifestation. Since there is no reliable information on what the nature of the schizophrenia diathesis might be, we cannot say anything about its distribution. But this, too, could be determined. For example, Mednick can easily determine whether the diathetic traits of anxiety responsiveness and habituation, as he measures them, are normally distributed in his index and control Ss or not, and they very probably are. The same could be done for other hypothesized diathetic traits as well.

2 In simple polygenic inheritance (where there is strict additivity of genes, that is, no dominance or recessiveness) the incidence in first-degree relatives of an index case should be approximately the square root of the trait's incidence in the general population (Edwards, 1960). We may use the data in Table 6-5 to compare the morbidity risk for

Table 6-37

Comparison of Morbidity Risk for Schizophrenics' Sibs and Risk Predicted by Polygenic Theory

Study	Observed Morbidity Risk for Sibs	Predicted Risk $(\sqrt{p})$	Morbidity Risk for the Population (p)
Brugger, 1928	10.3	12.4	1.53
Schulz, 1932	6.7	8.7	0.76
Luxenburger, 1936	7.6	9.2	0.85
Strömgren, 1938	6.7	6.9	0.48
Kallmann, 1938	7.5	5.9	0.35
Bleuler, 1941	10.4	12.4	1.53
Böök, 1953	9.7	16.9	2.85
Hallgren-Sjögren, 1959	5.7	9.1	0.83
Garrone, 1962	8.6	15.5	2.40

schizophrenics' sibs with that of the population at large. The figures are shown in Table 6-37. The study that comes closest to the expected approximation is that of Strömgren. The only study in which the rate for sibs is higher than expectation, based on population incidence, is Kallmann's. Three studies are far below expectation, but the remainder do not deviate seriously from what polygenic theory predicts. Thus, the data are not entirely consistent, but six of the nine studies suggest that a simple polygenic model may be appropriate.

3 The correlation between relatives should be approximately equal to the proportion of genes they share in common. The data presented earlier in this chapter rather consistently meet this criterion.

4 In twin studies, if MZ concordance is more than two times higher than that of DZ twins, the trait is not a simple dominant; if it is more than four times higher, it is not a simple recessive. We saw in Table 6-12 that the MZ-DZ ratios vary appreciably in the twin studies reported, with most occurring in the 3:1 to 6:1 range. The figures rule against simple—but not intermediate—dominance. If the differences between studies are not entirely the result of errors of various kinds, they could reflect differences in population incidences of the pathological genes, environmental differences, or both.

5 Parental consanguinity can signify that pathological genes with additive effects are involved if we can rule out recessive inheritance. The latter can be achieved by demonstrating that the parent-offspring correlation is similar to the sib-sib correlation.

6 The mean for the offspring is halfway between the mean for the parents and the mean for the general population.

Criteria 5 and 6 require that we have a suitable measure of the core traits—or diathesis—in schizophrenia. At this time, we are not in a position to test a polygenic theory of schizophrenia against these criteria.

MODELS OF THE DIATHESIS-STRESS INTERACTION. In a model such as Meehl's, the imposition of social learning—which must inevitably occur—upon the schizotaxia leads inexorably to the schizotype. Then the schizotype, if subjected to a noxious mother, develops into schizophrenia. Thus Meehl proposes a two-stage process. By and large, unless we are able to discover the biological nature of the defect that we call the diathesis, we are unable to come to grips with how it relates ultimately to the genesis of schizophrenia. Stating the point differently, we declare that we are not in a position at the present time to generate tests of first-stage hypotheses. However, prospects are brighter with respect to the second stage. If diathesis-stress theory is correct, it should be possible to identify, describe, and measure the schizotype in its various aspects and then to examine its further development under different environmental conditions. With respect to this second stage, it is possible to outline six general models of how the schizotype-stress interaction may be conceptualized. Since the term *schizotype* is now closely identified with Meehl's theory, and since for all practical purposes the schizotype may well be equated with the diathesis, we will speak here of the diathesis-stress interaction rather than the schizotype-stress interaction.

1 *Variance analysis.* This is the model that holds out the greatest promise for immediate research. It does not aim to say what the diathesis is, but only to indicate how much of the phenotype it accounts for in a direct sense, and as a consequence of its interaction with different environmental or stress factors. To illustrate the model, let us take the two variables that have been so often proposed as causal agents in schizophrenia: the schizophrenic genotype and the rearing by schizophrenic parents. Let us assume that it is possible, for example, through adoption, to design the following study:

	Type of Rearing Parent	
Biological Parent	Schizophrenic	Normal
Schizophrenic	25	25
Normal	25	25

According to the design, we have 50 children with a biological schizophrenic parent, half of whom are reared by a schizophrenic parent, half by normal parents. We also have a matched group of 50 children whose both biological parents are normal, half of whom are reared by a schizophrenic parent and half by normal parents. Let us assume that we are interested in the four core characteristics of schizophrenia described by Meehl: cognitive slippage, anhedonia, interpersonal aversiveness, and ambivalence. We measure these traits in each of the 100 Ss, and these measures are entered in the appropriate cells. We carry out the analysis of variance with respect to each trait separately and determine how much of the variance is attributed to the genotype, how much to type of rearing, and how much to the genotype-rearing interaction. The same model may be used repeatedly, with different environmental or stress variables being substituted for the one shown in the design here. From many such studies, we may be able to infer the nature of the diathesis.

2 *Activation.* In this model, the stress serves as a trigger that sets off or activates the diathesis so that a force or process is generated that impels the individual toward schizophrenia. Meehl's schizophrenogenic mother serves as the activator in his model.

3 *Augmentation.* The diathesis and the stress are somehow cast in the same mold or dimension. They compound the same phenotype. The imposed stress simply piles up on the diathesis, in a sense providing more of the same, the overload leading to schizophrenia. In the Genain quadruplets, it was thought that the girls inherited constricted personalities, on top of which was heaped a severely constricted upbringing. The combination culminated in different degrees of schizophrenia, depending on each girl's ability to circumvent the imposed constriction.

4 *Facilitation-resistance.* This is the model usually applied by theorists advocating monogenic-biochemical theory, but it could apply to diathesis-stress theory as well. For example, in Kallmann's model and in Meehl's, constitutional factors could facilitate or impede the development of a schizophrenic reaction. Kallmann and others have reported that an athletic or mesomorphic body build provides resistance to trait manifestation, whereas a leptosomic or ectomorphic body build makes the individual with the genotype especially vulnerable. How such factors influence the diathesis is not specified.

5 *Reciprocal escalation.* This model is best exemplified by Mednick's theory. Here the diathesis increases the stress, which increases the intrinsic diathetic reaction, which further increases the stress, and so on, the process intensifying until the schizophrenic break occurs. According to Mednick, the high anxiety leads to increased stimulus general-

ization, which increases the anxiety still further, the spiral continuing to the breaking point.

6 *Contradictory tendencies or opposed forces.* In this model, the diathesis predisposes toward one type of behavior, but the environment tries to impose a contradictory or opposed behavior. Depending on the nature of the diathesis and of the environmental pressure, the individual subjected to these opposing forces may develop various kinds of behavioral and psychological difficulties. A concrete illustration is provided by right- or left-handedness, which is clearly an inherited trait that does not conform to a strict Mendelian distribution. Falek (1967) believes that some behavioral deviation in left-handed children stems from parents' attitudes and behavior toward them. The children may provoke embarrassment, require special seating arrangements at the table, become the butt of unpleasant jokes, face problems in handwriting at school, be at a disadvantage regarding vocational opportunities, and so on. Some parents may resort to various degrees and types of coercion to induce a change of handedness in their children, and the consequences may involve various kinds of motoric and psychological difficulties. Presumably, an analogous confrontation of opposed pressures could be implicated in schizophrenia.

CLOSING COMMENTS

We will not discuss life-experience theories here, since they are so widely known and since they belong more appropriately in books dealing with such variables. There are many, and they are of great interest. Neither will we attempt to tie all the material we have covered in this chapter into a neat package with a cogent conclusion. The attempt would be forced at best. The reader can bring the bodies of data together in different ways to see what order he can bring to them, what research they suggest, or what new theories they generate. It should, however, be clear that the author leans toward a diathesis-stress theory of schizophrenia.

In the diathesis-stress theory, the mode of inheritance for most cases of schizophrenia is most likely to be either polygenic or a single dominant gene, with variable penetrance depending on multiple gene modifiers and environmental factors. As of now, the known data do not permit us to choose between these two competing hypotheses, but future research may help us to resolve the problem. We all have reason to desire a simpler solution to this disorder, but it is difficult to predict such a solution, given all the available data.

As a matter of fact, diathesis-stress theory may be even more complicated than implied here. The diathesis, for example, may have multiple genetic origins. This possibility is suggested by recent findings of an increased incidence of aneuploidy among schizophrenics. This finding in turn suggests that aneuploidy can either simulate the diathesis or lead directly to clinical schizophrenia without benefit of special stresses. It cannot by itself be a major factor in schizophrenia, however, because it accounts for only a tiny fraction of all cases, and because the same kinds of aneuploidy are more often found in nonschizophrenic subjects.

Diathesis-stress theory provides implications for research that may lead to important practical as well as theoretical results. Perhaps the first order of business is to determine the nature of the diathesis, both at the first-stage biological level and at the second-stage schizotypic level. Once we achieve the latter, which at the moment seems an easier task, we could conduct experiments to see what kinds of stresses interact in what ways with the diathesis to lead to pathological clinical manifestations. We could as well determine what kinds of environment lead not only to benign outcomes but to the realization of the artistic or creative potential that may be lying fallow in the diathesis. And once we know the nature of the diathesis-environmental stress interactions that lead to schizophrenia, we should be able to inaugurate rationally based therapeutic procedures in a preventive program of mental hygiene to assure that a large number of the predisposed individuals never develop schizophrenic illness at all.

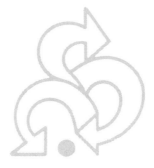

Chapter Seven

Genetic Studies of Manic-depressive Psychosis

Although in Chapter 6 I did not examine the data on the genetics of schizophrenia in an exhaustive way, I did present most of the studies that contributed prominently to an exposition and understanding of the major findings regarding the genetics of that disorder. At the same time, it was possible to examine the basic theoretical issues in the light of the findings. Virtually all the same issues apply to the other behavioral disorders that cause such great concern to mankind, but the amount and variety of research done with respect to them is much less. In this chapter, and Chapters 8 and 9, I will present some of the major findings regarding these disorders without delving as deeply into their explanations and implications as I did with regard to schizophrenia. Nevertheless, I hope to impart to the reader a proper understanding and appreciation of our current state of knowledge regarding the role of heredity in these disorders.

MANIC-DEPRESSIVE PSYCHOSIS

As noted earlier, the second major diagnostic category in Kraepelin's classification scheme was *manic-depressive psychosis*. Previously, although manic, excitatory conditions and depressive, melancholic states had sometimes been considered as manifestations of a single illness, it was not until Kraepelin described the conditions with great detail and clarity that they were lastingly combined into a single diagnostic category. From the prognostic point of view, which was so primary in Kraepelin's thinking, this disorder was especially contrapuntal to schizophrenia in that affected individuals did not suffer the deteriorative effects which were thought to characterize schizophrenia. The course of the illness is variable. An individual may have one attack or many, and the attacks may be of short or long duration, but they are always self-limiting; they may be primarily manic attacks in some cases, depressive in others, or cyclically alternating in still others.

In attacks of mania, the patient feels a sense of elation. If the attack is mild (hypomania), he manifests increased activity, cheerfulness, energy level, talkativeness, and liveliness, or he may be irritable and impatient, and unable to stick to a topic. Thoughts seem to flow randomly through his head and pour out into a stream of speech. When the attack is more severe, he may be entirely incoherent, the irritability, excitement, speech, and activity may be extreme, and the mood state may fluctuate markedly and precipitously.

Depressive states may range from listlessness, indifference, sluggishness, low energy level, poor appetite and concentration, and disturbed sleep pattern, to tearfulness, feelings of worthlessness or of being evil, agitation with constant pacing and hand-wringing, despair, and bitter self-abnegation.

Although these patients are fully oriented, they may manifest delusions in either the manic or depressive state. However, the delusions are compatible with the affect expressed, so that in a severe depression, the patient may feel that his internal organs are rotting, or that he has polluted the world, whereas in mania he may attribute many great deeds to himself. Eventually, the patient recovers, and between attacks he appears to be quite normal.

INCIDENCE AND DISTRIBUTION

Although we saw that the estimated morbidity risk varied considerably across populations with respect to schizophrenia, the variation is even greater with respect to manic-depressive psychosis. Some of the reported figures are shown in Table 7-1. The preparation of this chapter has been greatly facilitated by the literature review of Zerbin-Rüdin (1967), and we acknowledge our indebtedness to her.

Table 7-1

**Morbidity Risk for Manic-depressive Psychosis
in General Population**

Study	Location	Morbidity Risk, %
Early studies	Germany	<0.4
von Tomasson, 1938	Iceland	7.0
Sjögren, 1948	Sweden	0.6–0.8
Fremming, 1951	Denmark	1.2–1.6
A. Stenstedt, 1952	Sweden	About 1.0
Slater, 1953	England	0.5–0.8
Böök, 1953	Northern Sweden	0.07
Kallmann, 1959	New York	0.4
Helgason, 1964:	Iceland	
Males		1.8–2.18
Females		2.46–3.23

Böök (1953), who reports the lowest incidence, found only two clear cases of manic-depressive psychosis in a population of 9,000 inhabitants of a province in north Sweden. By contrast, von Tomasson (1938) reported an incidence of 7 percent in Iceland! The latter rate is 100 times as large as the former. In Table 6-3, the largest rate for schizophrenia was only 10 times larger than the smallest. Other studies range in between, the median value in Table 7-1 being about 0.7 percent (which is almost the same as the 0.8 percent in Table 6-3 for schizophrenia). What do these differences imply? Perhaps they represent national or climatic differences, isolate versus nonisolate breeding effects, sampling artifacts, hospitalization practices, environmental factors, and differences in diagnostic practices. One might assume that the clinical descriptions of manic-depressive psychosis and schizophrenia are sufficiently distinctive to make for highly reliable differential diagnoses between them. However, it has been reported that the ratio of schizophrenic to manic-depressive diagnoses varies considerably among psychiatrists in the same hospital or the same geographic region, and may well vary even more between individuals in different countries. Rosenthal (1963) pointed out that such ratios varied considerably in the major twin studies that collected systematic samples of hospitalized twins. The ratios are shown in Table 7–2.

Variations of such marked degree suggest that investigators do indeed employ different criteria in classifying a fairly good-sized number of psychotic cases. The variation cannot be attributed solely to national

Table 7-2

**Number of All Cases Diagnosed Schizophrenia and
Manic-depressive Psychosis in Twin Samples**

Investigator	*Schizophrenia*	*Manic-depressive*	*Ratio* *Schizophrenia–* *Manic-depressive*
Luxenburger	106	38	2.8:1
Essen-Möller	69	23	3.0:1
Rosanoff et al.	142	90	1.6:1
Slater	158	23	6.9:1
Kallmann	953	75	12.7:1
Chi square = 174.9, $p < 0.001$			

differences, since the highest and lowest ratios in Table 7-2 are both based on United States samples. Such findings serve to reinforce the conviction that investigators engaged in genetic studies of the behavioral disorders should not know the diagnosis of the index case when they are evaluating a relative, that they should specify their diagnostic criteria, and publish case histories, when possible, for subsequent comparisons between studies. Moreover, the findings in Table 7-1 suggest that the reliability of the diagnosis of manic-depressive psychosis may be less than that of schizophrenia.

The study by Helgason (1964) reports an appreciable difference between the sexes in the incidence of manic-depressive psychosis, with a higher rate occurring in females. Most investigators, beginning with Kraepelin himself, have noted a higher incidence among females than males in the samples of manic-depressive cases they collected, the modal ratio being about 1.5:1 to 2:1. For an illustration of sex-by-age first-admission rates, we may refer to Landis and Page (1938), as shown in Figure 7-1. The data in the figure are directly comparable with the sex-by-age first-admission curves for schizophrenia shown in Figure 6-2. The two sets of curves are almost complementary. In Figure 7-1, we see that the rate of manic-depressive psychosis is higher for females in the earlier ages, especially from their twenties through their forties. From their fifties on, the rate is somewhat higher for males, but the difference does not reach the magnitude of the earlier differences. For the entire group of first admissions, females outnumbered males 126.8 to 108.5 per 100,000. With respect to schizophrenia, males had the higher admission rates in the earlier ages, while females had higher rates after their middle thirties.

From an environmentalist point of view, one might consider that the incidence of psychotic reactions is similar in the two sexes, but that in the crises of earlier ages, males tend to react with schizophrenic patterns of behavior, whereas females react more affectively. In the later ages, the environmental situations and the corresponding reaction patterns are reversed in the two sexes. From a geneticist's point of view, the opposite directions in the sex-by-age admissions curves provide additional evidence that the two disorders are distinct, separate entities.

The finding by Landis and Page of a higher admission rate for women than men was confirmed and augmented by Merrell (1951). He examined United States Census reports and found a steady increase in the percentage of all manic-depressive cases in state mental hospitals who were women—from 54.2 percent in 1932 to 64.8 percent in 1946. Although this trend was statistically highly significant, Merrell doubted that it had any biological significance. He also pointed out that, during this same period, the proportion of persons with manic-depressive psychosis among all first admissions, and among readmissions as well, showed a steady decline. Thus, whereas the total number of first admissions for manic-depressive psychosis remained stable between 1922 and 1946, the total number of first admissions for schizophrenia doubled during the same period. Although one cannot rule out other possibilities on these grounds alone, there seems to be little doubt that the diagnostic

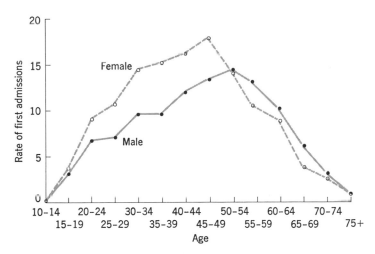

Figure 7-1. First admissions for manic-depressive psychosis to state mental hospitals in the United States during 1933, expressed as rates per 100,000 of the corresponding general population (Based on C. Landis and J. D. Page, *Modern Society and Mental Disease,* Ferrar & Rinehart, Inc., New York, 1938.)

habits of American psychiatrists were undergoing change during that quarter-century—schizophrenia had caught the psychiatric eye, whereas manic-depressive psychosis evoked no parallel excitement.

Interestingly, the number of first admissions for cases diagnosed *involutional psychosis,* a depressive type of disorder that occurs at about the time of life when menopause takes place, increased more than threefold during the same quarter-century. Later we shall discuss whether this disorder is genetically related to manic-depressive psychosis. It is also worth noting that from 1934 to 1946, the percentage of cases with manic-depressive psychosis who recovered *declined* from 56.3 to 45.0 percent. Since, by definition, the prognosis for this disorder is good, why should only half the cases recover, and why should the recovery rate decline at all? Again, the most likely explanation of such findings is probably best found in the difficulties surrounding the diagnostic process.

The distribution of manic-depressive psychosis also differs from schizophrenia in that one does not find an excess of such cases among the lower social and economic classes. As a matter of fact, some investigators have reported an excessive clustering among the higher classes, especially among people in positions of responsibility, but others have found the distribution to be evenly spread over the socioeconomic class range. Rin and Lin (1962) found no manic-depressive psychosis at all in three Formosan villages with a total population of more than 6,000 people. In a fourth village, they found 10 cases, 4 of which were in a single family that had assumed a leading role in the village for generations.

FAMILIAL
MORBIDITY RISK

Table 7-3 shows the morbidity risk for the illness in first-degree relatives of manic-depressive probands. Only cases in which the diagnosis was certain are included, except where the investigator has included "uncertain" cases in his calculations. Sometimes the number of uncertain cases is as large or larger than the number of certain cases, the rates varying considerably with respect to the less clear diagnostic group.

Again we see the considerable degree of variation across studies with respect to the risk rates reported. The ratio of the highest to the lowest rate is approximately 7:1, 9:1, and 4:1 for parents, siblings, and children, respectively. The median rates for the three groups in the same order are 7.6, 8.8 (which includes uncertain cases), and 11.2 percent. Such rates suggest that if the disorder is attributable to a single gene, its penetrance is quite low. Had we included doubtful

Table 7-3

Morbidity Risk for Manic-depressive Psychosis in First-degree Relatives of Manic-depressive Index Cases

	Parents		Siblings		Children	
Study	n	%	n	%	n	%
Hoffmann, 1921					139	13.8
Banse, 1929	160	3.4	292	9.0		
Röll and Entres, 1936	166	10.4			132	9.7
Weinberg and Lobstein, 1936	98	9.9	249	7.2	158	6.3
Slater, 1938	504	10.2			491	12.8
Strömgren, 1938:						
Longitudinal	154	4.1	335	10.7†		
Cross-sectional	110	4.5	216	8.0†		
Luxenburger, 1942			1,018	12.7	380	24.1
Sjögren, 1948	88	3.4	165	2.7		
Kallmann, 1952c	122*	23.4	184	22.7		
Stenstedt, 1952	381*	5.3	579*	6.0	149*	6.0
Slater, 1953	76	13.6†	136.5*	8.8†		

* Indicates the age-corrected n.
† Includes "uncertain" cases.

cases, the respective rates would have been 11.6, 11.7, and 12.5 percent.

With respect to relatives who share approximately one-fourth their genes with a manic-depressive proband, the following morbidity-risk estimates have been reported: half-sibs: 1.4 (Rudin, 1923) and 16.7 percent (Kallmann, 1950); aunts and uncles: 4.22 percent (Weinberg and Lobstein, 1936); nephews and nieces: 1.3 (Weinberg and Lobstein, 1936) and 2.3 percent (Röll and Entres, 1936); grandchildren: 1.9 (Schaedler, 1938) and 3.3 percent (Schmidt-Kehl, 1939). As in schizophrenia, there seems to be a correlation between the degree of consanguinity and the morbidity-expectancy rate. This finding is required by genetic theory, but does not account for the possible contribution to it by environmental factors.

Three investigators evaluated the morbidity-risk estimates for sibs of a manic-depressive proband when one parent also has manic-depressive psychosis. The relevant findings are shown in Table 7-4. In the first two studies shown in the table, the morbidity risk increases dramatically when one parent also has the illness. However, no significant increase occurs in the Stenstedt study. The reason for the discrepancy is not clear.

Table 7-4

**Morbidity Expectancy in Sibs of a Manic-depressive
Proband, in Relation to Presence or Absence of
Manic-depressive Psychosis in a Parent**

Study	One Parent Manic-depressive		Neither Parent Manic-depressive	
	n*	%	n*	%
Rüdin, 1923	231	23.8	1,525	7.4
Luxenburger, 1942		16.1†		3.4
Stenstedt, 1952	76	6.58	503	5.96

* n's are corrected.
† Some parents were classified as "cycloid," rather than manic-depressive.

Luxenburger reports another puzzling finding. When one parent was not manic-depressive but was *otherwise* abnormal, the risk for manic-depressive psychosis among the children of the couple increased to 7.6 percent, more than double the rate he found when neither parent had any psychiatric illness. The finding suggests that: (1) the genetic factor in manic-depressive psychosis may be nonspecific, heterogeneous, or multifactorial; (2) some of the parents called abnormal may have had *formes frustes* of manic-depressive psychosis; (3) rearing by abnormal parents may increase the possibility of manic-depressive psychosis in their children.

When both parents had manic-depressive psychosis, the morbidity risk for this illness in their children ranged between 20 and 40 percent in a study by Schulz (1940). The rate depended on whether or not the parental illnesses were atypical or exogenously influenced. Elsässer (1952) selected four couples in Schulz's series in which he thought the diagnosis was certain, and estimated the morbidity risk among their children to be 34.5 percent. These findings again suggest that diagnostic considerations influence appreciably the rates reported.

TWIN STUDIES

Some investigators prefer to use the broader designation, *affective psychosis,* rather than the more narrowly defined manic-depressive psychosis. In the affective psychoses, the affected individual must show psychotic symptoms in which affective or emotional disturbances are prominent.

Investigators using this diagnostic term often subsume manic-depressive psychosis under it. Table 7-5 presents a summary of the major twin studies of manic-depressive and affective psychoses.

Twin studies can be helpful in understanding how sampling methods can influence the estimated contribution of genetic factors to a behavioral disorder. In this regard, we can make the following points.

1 The number of manic-depressive twin index cases reported is much smaller than the number of schizophrenic probands, as shown in Table 7-2. What makes this finding puzzling is that the median morbidity rate for schizophrenia in the general population, as shown in Table 6-3, is 0.8 percent, whereas the comparable rate for manic-depressive psychosis, based on the studies in Table 7-1, is 0.7 percent. If the incidence of the two disorders is truly of about the same magnitude, we should expect approximately the same number of manic-depressive as schizophrenic twins. Where have all the manic-depressive twins gone?

One possible explanation is that the median population expectancy rate for manic-depressive psychosis is inflated. In the United States at least, the incidence of diagnosed schizophrenia is much higher than the rate of manic-depressive psychosis, and we saw earlier that the ratio of schizophrenia to manic-depressive psychosis has increased over the years.

A second possible explanation has to do with sampling. If one samples primarily from a resident hospital population, one is bound to

Table 7-5

Concordance Rates for Manic-depressive and Affective Psychosis in MZ and DZ Twins

Study	MZ Twins			DZ Twins		
	Total Pairs	Concordant Pairs	Concordance Rate	Total Pairs	Concordant Pairs	Concordance Rate
Luxenburger, 1930b	4	3	75.0	13	0	0.0
Rosanoff et al., 1934	23	16	69.6	67	11	16.4
Kallmann, 1952c	27	25	92.6; 100.0*	55	13	23.6
Slater, 1953:						
Only manic-depressive psychosis	7	4	57.1; 80.0*	17	4	23.5
Other affective disorders	1	0	0.0	13	3	18.8
Da Fonseca, 1959: affective disorders	21	15	71.4	39	15	38.5
Harvald and Hauge, 1965†	10	5	50.0	39	1	2.6

* Corrected concordance rate.
† According to Zerbin-Rüdin, 1967.

accumulate a large number of schizophrenics, who have a poor prognosis and tend to become chronically ill, and to miss a large number of manic-depressive psychotics, who have a good prognosis and are likely to be discharged back into the community. This could account in part for the high schizophrenic–manic-depressive ratios in the Slater and Kallmann studies, but not in the Essen-Möller study, where sampling was by consecutive admissions. Harvald and Hauge (1965) obtained their sample of twins from records of twin births in Denmark. The names of the twins were matched to a psychiatric register, and they found 71 schizophrenic twin pairs as against 55 manic-depressive twin pairs. These figures are more in keeping with population incidence figures in Denmark.

2 The concordance rates for MZ twins in Table 7-5 are uniformly high, varying from 50 to 100 percent, and considerably higher than the rates for DZ twins. Such findings afford strong support for a genetic etiology in manic-depressive psychosis. But a few cautions are in order. The number of MZ pairs in all studies is small, but especially so in those of Luxenburger (4 pairs) and Slater (7 pairs). Studies that obtained most of their cases from resident hospital populations, such as Kallmann and Slater, probably had an excess of cases with more severe forms of the illness while missing the more benign—and perhaps more common—types of cases. It is possible, perhaps likely, that one might find an appreciably higher frequency of *dis*cordant pairs among the more benign types. Thus the concordance rates for both the MZ and DZ pairs are possibly higher than they should be. Peculiarities that may result from such sampling are reflected in the fact that all eight of the MZ pairs in Slater's study were females; not one was male.

3 The MZ-DZ concordance ratios are not always consistent. We find a high of 19.2:1 in the study by Harvald and Hauge and a low of 2.4:1 in the study by Slater. The ratios in the Kallmann and Rosanoff et al. studies are closer to 4:1. A strict dominance theory which assumes full and equal penetrance for both types of twins would predict a 2:1 ratio. Thus the twin studies do not help us decide between dominance or recessiveness as the probable mode of inheritance.

4 The rates for the affective disorders appear to be consistent with those for manic-depressive psychosis, but they could be considered similar to those for schizophrenia as well. Moreover, they encompass several clinical entities. Slater includes 11 index twins with involutional depressions and 3 with reactive depressions. DaFonseca also includes probands with depressive or hypomanic personalities, and cotwins with such personalities are said to be concordant for affective disorder. Thus, the definition is broad, providing a large umbrella under which to gather many clinical types. Perhaps this accounts for the high DZ concordance

rate of 38.5 percent in his study. That psychological factors may be contributing to these rates is attested to by the fact that DaFonseca finds a concordance rate for sibs of 18.9 percent, which is half the rate for DZ twins.

5 As in the schizophrenia studies, no investigator has attempted to assess the reliability of diagnoses with respect to his own study, and characteristically, diagnoses of the cotwin were made with prior knowledge of the diagnosis in the index twin. For these reasons, we are unable to estimate the margin of error in the diagnostic process. Moreover, failures to take such methodological precautions serve to reinforce the skepticism of those behavioral scientists who ignore or disbelieve in the importance of genetic factors in the behavioral disorders.

BIOLOGICAL UNITY OF
MANIC-DEPRESSIVE PSYCHOSIS

According to Kraepelin (1896):

> Manic-depressive insanity includes on the one hand the entire province of so-called periodic and circular insanity, and on the other hand, the simple manias, the largest part of the clinical pictures designated as melancholias, and also a not inconsiderable number of cases with amentia. Finally, we count as well certain mild and very mild, partly periodic, partly enduring morbid pictures with similar coloring, which may start out as grave disturbances, but which alternatively may pass over without clearly defined boundaries into the realm of deviant personality organization [1]

Thus, Kraepelin believed that a number of milder, somewhat different but related clinical conditions belonged generically and genetically with manic-depressive psychosis. Under the problem of biological unity, one is primarily concerned here with the so-called affective disorders. These include the simple manias and their milder forms, depressive conditions of varying degree, involutional psychosis, and cycloid, circular, or cyclothymic personalities who show periodic mood swings without any ostensible environmental provocation.

Quite early, some investigators wondered whether cases that showed only manic episodes or only depressive episodes (*monopolar*) were genetically the same as cases who fluctuated between manic and depressive episodes (*bipolar*). Some pointed out that no MZ twin pair had been found in which one twin was a monopolar manic and the other a mono-

---

[1] Author's translation.

polar depressive. Leonhard (1959) claimed that the bipolar forms of
manic-depressive psychosis had a greater genetic loading than the monopolar forms. Angst (1966) investigated the relatives of 151 manic-depressive psychotics (of whom 105 were pure depressives and 46 were
circular cases), 104 patients with involutional melancholia, and 73 with
mixed psychoses. Based on differences in "hereditary loading" in families as indicated by the frequency and type of secondary cases, age at
onset, duration of attacks, and intervals between attacks, he concluded
that the pure depressions comprised a disorder which was separate
from the circular forms of manic-depressive psychosis, but which on
the other hand showed a certain similarity to the involutional melan-
cholias. He found the morbidity risk for manic-depressive psychosis, including "uncertain" cases, to be 12.6 and 15.6 percent for the parents and
sibs, respectively, of circular cases, 8.6 and 8.3 percent for the parents
and sibs of pure depressives, and 1.7 and 3.2 percent for the parents and
sibs of cases with involutional melancholia. The morbidity risk for reactive depressions was 3.8 and 8.7 percent, 8.6 and 10.1 percent, and 6.1
and 2.6 percent for the parents and sibs of the circular, pure depressive,
and involutional cases, respectively, suggesting that the greatest genetic
association is between the pure depressive psychoses and the reactive
depressions.

Stenstedt (1952), however, found no difference in hereditary loading among monopolar manics and monopolar depressives, or among cases
with repeated attacks and those with a single attack. Taschev (1965)
found that the circular forms had an earlier onset, on the average, than
the pure depressive forms, and a greater number of attacks. Clayton,
Pitts, and Winokur (1965) found that monopolar manics tended more
often to be male than did monopolar depressives and were hospitalized
at an earlier age. However, the two groups did not differ with respect
to clinical family histories.

Do manic-depressive cases with a late onset have less of a genetic
loading—as might be the case in polygenic theory—than do cases with
earlier onset? Stenstedt found the morbidity risk for manic-depressive
psychosis among sibs of probands whose first attack occurred after age
fifty to be 16.3 percent, as compared with 13.3 percent for sibs of cases
with earlier onset. But Schulz (1951) found the morbidity expectancy
to be 9.3 and 15.7 percent for the parents of late- versus early-onset
cases, respectively.

Hopkinson (1964) began his study with 100 cases of affective psychosis, all over age fifty. Among them 39 had had earlier attacks, 61
had not. He found the morbidity risk for parents, children, and sibs
to be lower (8.3 percent) among the late-onset cases than among those
with earlier attacks (20.1 percent). Angst, grouping age of onset by

decades, found a correlation between age of onset and degree of genetic loading, the greatest loading occurring among cases whose first attack occurred between age twenty and forty. However, Woodruff, Pitts, and Winokur (1964) compared 68 patients who had a family history of affective disorder with 98 who did not. All were age fifty or more and had a diagnosis of endogenous depression. There was no difference between the groups with respect to late or early onset, or number of admissions for affective episodes. The authors concluded that the two groups comprised a single, homogeneous population.

Winokur and Pitts (1964) compared the family histories of 212 cases of manic-depressive disease with those of 75 patients hospitalized with a diagnosis of reactive depression. Although there was a significantly higher rate of affective or possible affective illness among the sibs of the manic-depressive probands, no such difference was found for fathers or mothers, and in other clinical respects the families were quite similar. The authors maintained that the term *reactive* was not warranted and that the two groups were basically alike. The same authors (1965) compared the family histories of cases with a diagnosis of psychotic depression and cases called manic-depressive psychosis. They concluded that no significant differences in frequency of affective disorder occurred between fathers, mothers, or sibs in the two groups and that in this respect the groups comprised a homogeneous population.

Asano (1967) divided his 162 manic-depressive probands in several ways. Of the probands, 30 were classified as *typical*, and 132 as *atypical*, that is, those with *mixed type*, such as agitated depression, clouding of consciousness, severe autonomic symptoms, or "depression plus neurotic symptoms such as depersonalization or compulsive phenomena." The morbidity risk for manic-depressive psychosis was 10.1 and 9.4 percent for sibs of the typical and atypical probands, respectively, but 16.8 and 5.0 percent for parents of the respective groups, the latter difference reaching significance at the 0.01 level. It is not clear why the significant difference occurs for parents but not for sibs. He also classified his probands into three groups: monopolar manic, monopolar depressive, and combined manic and depressive symptoms. The morbidity risk for manic-depressive psychosis for the three groups respectively was 3.1, 8.6, and 11.4 percent for sibs, and 0.0, 6.3, and 9.4 percent for parents. Although the trend seems to be consistent for both sibs and parents, with monopolar manics having the lowest genetic loading and circular forms the highest, in neither case do the differences reach statistical significance.

Thus, on the basis of the findings cited, we find fairly consistent evidence that the various clinical forms of affective disorders are genetically related. When associations are found, as between circular manic-depressive psychosis and monopolar forms, or between severe depressive psychotic reactions and the milder reactive depressions, we do not have any knowledge about the possible role of environmental factors. With respect to late-onset cases, in whom some investigators have reported a reduced genetic association, we cannot be certain that some of these cases are not misdiagnosed in that they may reflect various presenile or senile organic conditions, or that some are not reactions of despair that may occur in individuals with shattered lives whose approaching end looms ominously for them.

Winokur and Clayton (1967), however, come to a different conclusion. Based on a brief review of the literature and on their own research, they inferred that two types of primary affective disorder could be differentiated clinically and genetically. Their conclusions were based on the following findings:

1 The morbidity risk for affective disorder in sibs of affected probands was 43, 26, and 12 percent when both parents were affected, one parent was affected, and neither parent was affected, respectively.

2 The morbidity risk for female sibs was higher than that for male sibs.

3 When family histories were divided into those with a clear two-generation history of affective disorder (the FH+ group) and those who had no family history at all of affective disorder (the FH- group), they found a significantly higher number of manics among the FH+ probands: 16 of 112 versus 4 of 129, $p < 0.003$.

The authors concluded that the FH+ group involves manic-depressive disease with a dominant mode of genetic transmission, and is sometimes clinically manic, whereas the FH- group shows no mania but only depressions similar to other manic-depressive depressions. The authors offer no opinion regarding the latter's mode of genetic transmission, but hold that it differs from the manic-depressive group both clinically and genetically.

The findings by Winokur and Clayton deserve further study and replication. Even if they should recur in additional studies, the interpretations of them could vary appreciably. However, the finding of an increased risk among female as compared with male sibs may simply reflect the common observation that females are more liable to affective disorders than males. The finding of more manics in the FH+ group is consistent with data by some other investigators that the cyclical forms of the illness have a higher heritability than the monopolar forms.

In addition, the authors excluded (justifiably) a third and largest group of probands from their analysis: 185 patients whose family histories were indeterminate with respect to dominant transmission. About 30 percent of these had a history of affective disorder in other than first-degree relatives. Will it be necessary to postulate still another mode of inheritance for the latter group? The authors and Pitts (1965) had previously pointed out themselves that there were no significant differences in the family histories of manics and depressives. Parsimony suggests that we be wary of multiplying hypothesized genotypes too freely, and that alternative explanations involving fewer major "causes" of these disorders may serve as well or better. To complete their view of the affective disorders, the authors postulate two additional entities: (1) *secondary affective disorder,* which occurs in the course of another medical or psychiatric illness and (2) *reactive depression,* which is a short-lived response to psychological factors such as grief or defeat and rarely requires hospitalization. Thus, the authors postulate four distinct groups of affective disorder, and leave some implication regarding the possibility of a fifth.

SPECIFICITY OF THE MANIC-DEPRESSIVE GENOTYPE

Manic-depressive psychosis and schizophrenia

In Chapter 6 we reviewed a good part of the literature regarding manic-depressive psychosis and schizophrenia and concluded that in their prototypical manifestations they were genetically distinct and different disorders. We had omitted studies by Kant (1942), Pollock and Malzberg (1940), and a few others that came to an opposite conclusion. These studies are in the minority, and the question of diagnostic error is perhaps even more at issue in these studies than in most of the others. Nevertheless, they do raise doubt about the genetic heterogeneity of the two disorders.

In the studies summarized in Table 7-3, many of the authors reported the morbidity risk for schizophrenia among the first-degree relatives of manic-depressive probands. Without specifying the particular studies, the risks reported were as follows: for parents: 0.0, 0.0, 0.5, 0.6, 0.6, and 0.8; for sibs: 0.0, 0.4, 0.4, 0.7, 0.8, 0.8, 0.8, 1.6, and 1.6; for children: 0.8, 2.0, 2.5, 3.1, and 3.1. The figures for parents and sibs tend to be approximately the same as the rates of schizophrenia in the general population, but the rates for children tend to be elevated appreciably, if not greatly. Three of the highest rates among children were obtained in studies carried out in Germany, and were about four to five times greater than the median expectancy rate reported for the German population. This finding of an elevated rate for schizophrenia among the children, but not the parents or sibs of manic-depressive probands, has puzzled investigators since Rüdin. It appears to be the only relationship in which this association between the disorders occurs. Some investigators have proposed a complex genetic mechanism to account for it. The possibility of misdiagnosis among the manic-depressive parent probands is not consistent with the findings of nonelevated rates of schizophrenia in the parents and sibs of these same probands. A third possibility is that rearing by a manic-depressive parent can sometimes lead to schizophrenia in his or her children. An even more striking finding indicating a possible genetic overlap between the two psychoses was reported by Schulz (1940). Among the offspring of parents who both had manic-depressive psychosis, the risk for affective psychoses was 28 percent, but for schizophrenia it was actually 12 percent, which is a very high figure. Unless some of the parents were misdiagnosed, this finding poses a serious challenge to specificity theory. Elsässer believed that the schizophrenic children came from parents whose manic-depressive psychosis was atypical. Thus the problems of diagnosis continue to raise difficulties in interpreting such data.

Manic-depressive psychosis and involutional psychosis

The diagnostic category *involutional melancholia,* or *involutional psychosis,* has aroused considerable discussion with respect to whether it is a separate disease entity or not. Kraepelin initially classified the disorder with the manic-depressive psychoses, but he later changed his mind. Many investigators believe that it comprises a motley assortment of clinical pictures whose onset happens to occur at that time of life when menopausal changes take place. However, the diagnosis has been made for men as well as women. By and large, authors who have investigated the genetics of this disorder have also estimated relatives' morbidity risk for other affective psychoses and for schizophrenia as well. We will not go into detail here, but the general picture is that the morbidity risk for other affective psychoses among both first- and second-degree relatives of involutional probands tends to be about as high, and sometimes considerably higher, than the morbidity risk for involutional melancholia. Among parents and sibs in the studies considered here, the morbidity-risk estimates for involutional melancholia range between 1.5 and 9.5 percent, with an approximate median rate of 3.0 percent, whereas the estimates for other affective psychoses range between 1.5 and 16.3 percent, with an approximate median rate of 5.2 percent, and the estimates for schizophrenia from 0.2 to 2.3 percent,

with an approximate median rate of 1.0 percent.   Thus there does seem
to be a genetic association between involutional melancholia and other
affective psychoses, whereas the heritability of involutional melancholia
itself appears to be of a relatively low order.   When the expectancy
rates for both involutional and affective psychoses among relatives are
combined, they are comparable to the rates reported for affective psychoses among the relatives of affective psychotic probands.   On the
other hand, there seems to be no genetic association between schizophrenia and involutional psychosis.

Manic-depressive psychosis and alcoholism

Winokur and Pitts (1965) reported that among the parents of 366
patients hospitalized for affective disorder they found a prevalence of
alcoholism in 1.1 percent of the mothers and 9.5 percent of the fathers.
Among the parents of 180 controls, the prevalence of alcoholism was
0.0 for mothers and 1.7 percent for fathers.   The difference with respect
to fathers is considerable and significant.   However, the authors point
out that the percentage of fathers with alcoholism was 11 percent for
101 schizophrenic probands, 8.6 percent for 82 psychoneurotic probands,
and 7.6 percent for 53 cases with personality disorder.   Thus, alcoholism
appears to be a nonspecific syndrome that is associated in some way
with a variety of disorders.

Manic-depressive psychosis and suicide

Several investigators have reported rather high rates of suicide
among patients diagnosed manic-depressive psychosis.   The rates range
from about 2.8 to 12.0 percent, with an approximate median of 6.25
percent.   Suicide accounted for approximately 15 percent of all deaths
among manic-depressive probands.   An elevated rate of suicide was
also found among the relatives of manic-depressive probands.   The
median rate among first-degree relatives was about 2.5 percent in two
studies, and somewhat less for relatives further removed.   Whether
suicide is itself a heritable trait is rather improbable.   The fact that
suicide should occur so commonly in severely depressed individuals
should occasion no surprise, and in fact, an elevated rate is likely to be
common to all psychological disorders.

THE PREMORBID PERSONALITY
OF MANIC-DEPRESSIVES

It appears that all information available about the premorbid personality
of persons who develop manic-depressive or affective psychosis has been

obtained retrospectively. We have not been able to locate any studies of the predictive or postdictive type. Almost all accounts have been given by German investigators or others following the German tradition. The latter in turn have been strongly influenced by the typological system of Kretschmer, in which personality or temperament is linked closely to body build. Investigators have reported that manic-depressive psychotics tend to be of the *pyknic* type, which is characterized by roundness of contour, amplitude of body cavities, and a plentiful endowment of fat. The face is broad and fleshy, the neck is short and thick, the trunk is thickset and barrel-shaped, the limbs massive, the hands square or broad, and the skin warm and moist with an ample layer of fat beneath it. The associated temperament is *cyclothymic,* and has three subdivisions:

1 *Healthy.* A gay chatterbox; quiet humorist; silent good-tempered person; happy enjoyer of life; energetic practical man

2 *Cycloid.* Cheery, hypomanic; quiet, contented; melancholic

3 *Manic-depressive*

Both the body build and the temperament are thought to be strongly influenced by heredity.

Kretschmer counterposed to the pyknic the *asthenic* type, which is characterized by a long, narrow, and flat chest; long, thin limbs with lean muscles; hips wider than the chest in males; pale, dry, cold skin; and scanty fat. The associated temperament is *schizothymic,* and also has three subdivisions:

1 *Healthy.* Polite; sensitive; world-hostile idealists; cold-hearted egoists

2 *Schizoid.* Hyperesthetic; cold and aristocratic; pathetic idealists; insensitive, despotic, or passionate types; and unsteady loafers

3 *Schizophrenic*

With respect to schizophrenia, the premorbid personalities as depicted by the prediction studies often did not correspond very closely to the traits classified as schizothymic, nor do we know the reliability of assessing the presence, absence, or degree of such traits. With respect to manic-depressive psychotics, most investigators describe their premorbid personality as cyclothymic, but we have little knowledge regarding the reliability of assessing such traits in young, unaffected individuals. Until we have good prediction studies, the attribution of a cyclothymic temperament to the premorbid personality of manic-depressive patients should be held in reservation.   Hopefully, such studies will be carried out in the future.   With respect to the heritability of these types and temperaments in the two major psychoses, Elsässer (1952) found that the frequency of the cycloid and schizoid temperaments in the premorbid personality of manic-depressive and schizophrenic patients, respectively, was less striking than generally supposed, and that among the children of his dual mating probands, he found it impossible to classify no less than 54 percent according to the Kretschmerian typology.

FERTILITY AND MORTALITY

Two investigators, Essen-Möller (1935) and Hopkinson (1963), found that the frequency of marriage and the number of children produced by manic-depressive individuals were approximately like that found in the comparable general population.   However, several others have found reduced rates of marriage and children in their probands. Stenstedt (1952) found the rate of marriage in his manic-depressive male and female probands to be 65.8 and 62.5 percent, respectively, as compared with the population rates of 78.3 and 76.0 percent for men and women, respectively.   Landis and Page (1938) and Norris (1956) reported similar findings.   Kallmann (1952c) compared the marriage rates of manic-depressive probands over age forty-five with those of their healthy sibs as well as controls, and the respective rates for the three groups were 72.5, 92.5, and 87.5 percent.   Moreover, the manic-depressive probands were more often childless and had fewer children: 1.6 versus 2.5 for the combined comparison groups.   Ödegaard (1961) found that among cases with affective psychosis the marriage rate was reduced 10 percent and fertility 20 to 25 percent.   Lewis (1959) also found both rates reduced and associated the reduction to factors such as birth control, severity of illness, social class, and so on.

With respect to mortality, three investigations agree in that after the onset of manic-depressive psychosis, the death rate is increased about $1\frac{1}{2}$-fold and life expectancy is decreased about 15 percent as compared with the average population of the same age.

Thus, the same problem arises in manic-depressive psychosis as in schizophrenia.   If mortality is higher and fertility is reduced, we might expect the incidence of the disorder to decline more or less gradually and slowly, depending on the mode of inheritance.   Moreover, we need to ask why the incidence has become so high.   We have no clear evidence of a decline in the frequency of this disorder.   Some people assume that changed diagnostic practices that have occurred in countries like the United States yield statistics which make it appear that there is a lower incidence of this disorder than there was 40 years ago. Some clinicians currently claim, on the other hand, that they in fact see very few typical cases of manic-depressive psychosis. However, investigators who pay special attention to this disorder and the affective psychoses generally, for example, Winokur and his colleagues, find no dearth of the disorder. Unless clear evidence is produced to the contrary, we cannot assume that an actual decline in the incidence of the disorder has occurred. One might speculate that the genotype that makes for the jolly, warm, friendly, and likeable personality of many manic-depressive probands might in unaffected individuals lead to increased rates of marriage and fertility. In Kallmann's study, the sibs of the manic-depressive probands had a slightly *higher* marriage rate than a control group. Speculations of this kind need to be tested further before we can take them seriously.

MODE OF INHERITANCE

Based on the complexities involved in the collection and diagnosis of the probands and relatives reviewed in this section, and on the considerable deviation of the data from any simple Mendelian distribution, one might assume that investigators would hold varied interpretations regarding the mode of inheritance of manic-depressive psychosis. This is indeed the case. However, no investigator has proposed a simple recessivity theory, although several have favored a theory of simple dominance with considerably reduced penetrance. Dominance is favored when the illness tends to be passed on in a direct line of descent through several generations, and when the morbidity risk tends to be approximately of the same magnitude for parents, sibs, and children of manic-depressive probands. In Table 7-3, we noted considerable variation in the rates across studies for such relatives. The median expectancy rates for the three groups of relatives was 7.6, 8.8, and 11.2 percent, respectively. These appear to be of the same order of magnitude, but they are a far cry from the expected rate of 50 percent which dominance theory predicts. Moreover, there does seem to be a modestly increased rate for children as compared with parents and sibs, and we also noted an increased rate of schizophrenia among children of manic-depressive probands, but not among parents and sibs. One could plausibly claim that such findings can readily be attributed to psychological factors involved in rearing by manic-depressive parents. Another possibility is that manic-depressive probands tend to marry individuals who carry genes that favor the development of manic-depressive psychosis or schizophrenia in their children.

Other investigators have proposed rather complex theories regarding the hereditary transmission of manic-depressive psychosis. Rüdin (1923) considered the probability that three separate genotypes were involved —two recessive and one dominant. Rosanoff, Handy, and Plesset (1934b) postulated an autosomal factor for cyclothymia and an X-chromosomal activating factor to account for the increased cases found among women. Hoffmann also favored a three-factor theory, but he thought that they were all dominant and he attributed different weights to each. Luxenburger (1942) favored a multiple-factor theory, with some being dominant and some recessive. Winokur and Clayton (1967) concluded that there were two genetically different types of primary affective disorder and that the mania group was probably transmitted by a single dominant X-linked gene with diminished penetrance, or two dominant genes, one of which is sex-linked. One could argue that the continual gradation of manic and depressive characteristics in the general population—from mild, normal, and sometimes desirable manifestations through various degrees of intensity to severe manic-depressive psychosis—favors a simple polygenic theory. The latter would, however, have to be modified to account for the generally found higher incidence of affective disorder in women than men, unless one assumes that the rearing, life patterns, or hormonal makeup of women generally favors their developing affective disorders as compared with men.

Despite the strong evidence in favor of considering manic-depressive psychosis to be genetically influenced in good part, we are unable to come to any conclusions regarding its mode of inheritance. Nor have we intended here to evaluate the possible contribution of environmental factors to the clinical conditions included in the affective disorders. With respect to etiological theories, we can classify them as monogenic-biochemical, diathesis-stress, and life-experience theories in much the same way as with schizophrenia. However, research with respect to manic-depressive psychosis and the affective psychoses generally has not been as thorough or as sophisticated as research on schizophrenia. Good prediction and adoption studies have not been tried, and we are badly in need of them. Generally, however, the genetic studies of the two major psychoses done thus far are consistent with the Kraepelinian view that these are two separate illnesses.

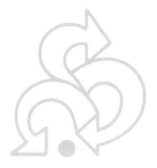

Chapter Eight

Genetic Studies of Psychopathy and Criminality

DEFINITION OF THE DISORDER

In its 1952 classification of mental disorders, the American Psychiatric Association included one major category of disorder which it called *sociopathic personality disturbance.* Subsumed under it were five subtypes: *antisocial reaction, dyssocial reaction, sexual deviation, alcoholism* (*addiction*), and *drug addiction.* The World Health Organization (1957) had four major categories that were clearly related to the sociopathy group:

1 *Antisocial personality.* Subtypes: antisocial personality, constitutional psychopathic state, and psychopathic personality with antisocial trend

2 *Asocial personality.* Subtypes: asocial personality, moral deficiency, pathological liar, psychopathic personality with amoral trend

3 *Sexual deviation.* Subtypes: exhibitionism, fetishism, homosexuality, pathologic sexuality, sadism, sexual deviation

4 *Other* and *unspecified.* Subtype: pathological personality

The German classification system used widely in the 1930s, as recommended by the *Deutscher Verein für Psychiatrie*, included one major group of relevance to this chapter—*nonpsychotic personality disorders.* Relevant subtypes were predominantly endogenous (psychopathic), predominantly exogenous (pseudopsychopathic), and habitual nonpsychotic personality variations, which included inter alia many traits that might be called psychopathic—explosive, callous, unstable, infantile, emotionally labile, homosexual, and other perversions. One separate major category was simply called *criminals.*

One may estimate the likelihood that the sociopathic personality is a simple diagnostic entity or unit character from the American Psychiatric Association definition of it. "Sociopathic reactions are very often symptomatic of severe underlying personality disorder, neurosis, or psychosis, or occur as the result of organic brain injury or disease." Affected individuals "are ill primarily in terms of society and of conformity with the prevailing cultural milieu."

Individuals with antisocial reaction "are always in trouble, profiting neither from experience nor punishment, and maintaining no real loyalties to any person, group, or code. They are frequently callous and hedonistic, showing marked emotional immaturity, with lack of sense of responsibility, lack of judgment, and an ability to rationalize their behavior so that it appears warranted, reasonable, and justified. . . . The term includes cases previously classified as 'constitutional psychopathic state' and 'psychopathic personality.' "

Individuals with dyssocial reaction "manifest disregard for the usual social codes, and often come into conflict with them . . . (and) typically do not show significant personality deviations other than those implied by adherence to the values of their own predatory, criminal, or other social group."

Although there is a strong association between psychopathy and criminality, not all psychopaths are criminals and not all criminals are psychopaths. In a study of 10,000 men incarcerated in Sing Sing prison in New York, 66 percent were classified as antisocial or dyssocial types of sociopathic personality, whereas the remaining 34 percent were diagnosed as neurotics, psychotics, mental defectives, or alcoholics.

INCIDENCE AND DISTRIBUTION

Table 8-1 presents some census studies of populations in which the investigators reported rates for psychopathic personality disorder or some approximately comparable diagnostic term. The rates vary from 0.05

to 15.0 percent, the higher rate being 300 times as large as the lower one. Various factors, however, influence the rates. The first, and perhaps the most important, involves differences in diagnostic preferences among investigators. Ekblad's finding of 15.0 percent of naval conscriptees with psychopathic personality seems extremely high. These were average Swedish youths who were drafted for military service. They did not include professional sailors, who might be suspected of having an elevated rate of psychopathic personality. In fact, Ekblad assigned this diagnosis to 33 percent of the sailors! Another factor influencing the rates in Table 8-1 involves sampling and types of rates calculated. The figure reported by Lemkau et al. represents a one-year prevalence rate. Sjögren's cases had all been found through institutional records. The Nielsen et al. cases were patients seen at a psychiatric clinic. Hagnell surveyed the entire population, interviewed probands, and obtained information about individuals from both official and personal sources. Differences of such kinds are bound to produce variation in the rates obtained.

Surprisingly, the only city district—and a relatively lower-class one at that—in Table 8-1 occurs in the Lemkau et al. study and provides the *lowest* rate shown. At least with respect to crime and delinquency, the highest rates are typically found in the poorer sections of large cities. One might infer that Lemkau et al. used a very restricted definition of psychopathic personality, whereas that of Ekblad was unusually broad. Table 8-1 also suggests two additional points of importance.

Table 8-1

Reported Frequency of Psychopathic Personality Disorder in Different Populations

Study	Location	Diagnosis	Rate Reported, %
Lemkau et al., 1941–1943	Baltimore	Psychopathic personality	0.05
Mayer-Gross, 1948	Rural Scotland area	Neurotics and psychopaths	1.9
Sjögren, 1948	Swedish island	Psychopaths	0.1
Ekblad, 1948	Swedish conscripts	Psychopaths	15.0
Nielsen et al., 1965:	Samsö, Denmark	Character disorders	0.76
Males			0.81
Females			0.71
Hagnell, 1966:	Two parishes, Sweden	Psychopathic personality	
Males			
Continuous residence			3.0
Moved			7.5
Newcomer			10.2
Females			
Continuous residence			1.2
Moved			3.3
Newcomer			3.3

1 The incidence of psychopathic personality disorder appears to be higher among males than females. If this disorder is inherited, the Y chromosome may be providing a contributory factor.

2 There is a clear association between residential instability and psychopathy.

Robins (1966) documents this last point abundantly in her follow-up study of children who had been referred to a psychiatric clinic for antisocial behavior.

Robins, like other investigators, also found that most of her 524 antisocial child probands came from disrupted homes. Only 36 percent had both parents at home; 32 percent had lived in institutions or foster homes for at least six months before referral. In 60 percent of the cases, one or both parents had died, the parents were divorced or separated, or the mother was unmarried. Fathers showed: excessive drinking (32 percent), nonsupport or neglect of the home (26 percent), deserted (21 percent), cruel or physically abusive (20 percent), erratic worker (20 percent), illicit sexual behavior (18 percent), arrests and illegal occupations (11 percent), gambling, extravagance, incompetent work, coldness, and no affection (23 percent). Both mothers (48 percent) and fathers (23 percent) were severely nervous, mentally ill, or feebleminded. The most prominent other characteristics of the mothers were nonsupport or neglect of home (20 percent) and illicit sexual behavior (19 percent).

When parents are so severely disturbed and manifest such psychopathic behavior themselves, it is virtually impossible to tell from the usual family studies how much of the antisocial behavior and personality difficulties in the child can be traced to either genetic or psychological transmission. Studies of sibs do not help either. Robins reports that among 387 sibs of her probands, histories showed: arrests (22 percent), sex problems (19 percent), poor work history (13 percent), aggressive behavior (8 percent), poor school record (33 percent), probable psychiatric illness or feeblemindedness (18 percent), and "other antisocial behavior," such as incorrigibility, runaway, thefts, gambling, and so on (25 percent). In 43 percent of the cases, the sibs showed none of these traits.

TWIN STUDIES

Because of the hopeless entanglement of severe rearing abuse and instability on the one hand, and possible genetic factors on the other, we can hope to learn little from familial morbidity-risk studies about the possible contribution of heredity to these disorders. Twin studies afford better prospects, since psychopathic MZ and DZ twins should both be reared in similar pathological environments, and differences in concordance rates may tell us something about heritability of the disorder under such conditions.

The first twin study was the much-publicized one by Lange (1929), the report of which he called *Crime as Destiny*. The title attempts to dramatize Lange's conviction that such behavior was genetically determined. The belief itself, of course, was not new. The term *constitutional psychopathic state* had already been in widespread use for many decades. But Lange's study seemed to provide the evidence needed to confirm the accepted belief.

To obtain his sample, Lange searched for convicted individuals who had a living twin of the same sex. He also looked for twins in the sibships of prisoners. He examined the records of the prisons under the Bavarian Minister of Justice, the "criminal-biological" files of a house of correction, a psychiatric research institute, and his own hospital. He collected 39 same-sexed pairs, of whom 9 had to be dropped. In addition he learned of 10 opposite-sexed pairs by chance. His main findings are shown in Table 8-2.

Lange determined the zygosity of his twins from various somatic measurements, photographs, and fingerprints. In as many cases as possible, he examined personally both the twins who were in or out of prison. The results show a striking difference in concordance between MZ and same-sexed DZ pairs. We can ignore the opposite-sexed pairs, since they were not obtained systematically. With respect to the same-sexed pairs, Lange was diligent in his search for cases, and it is difficult to know what sorts of bias may have crept into his sample. It often seems

---

Table 8-2
Concordance for Criminality in MZ and DZ Twins*

| Zygosity | Total Pairs | Concordant Pairs | | Male | Female |
		n	%		
MZ twins	13	10	77	12	1
DZ twins:					
Same sex	17	2	12	14	3
Opposite sexes	10	1	10		

* Data from Lange, 1929.

Table 8-3

Concordance Rates for Adult Criminality, Juvenile Delinquency, and Childhood Behavior Problems in MZ and DZ Twins*

Zygosity and Sex of Twins	Adult Criminality†	Juvenile Delinquency	Childhood Behavior Problems
Same-sex twins, probably MZ:			
Males, concordant	22 } (66.7%)	25 } (92.6%)	21 } (84.0%)
Males, discordant	11	2	4
Females, concordant	3 } (75%)	14 } (93.3%)	20 } (91.0%)
Females, discordant	1	1	2
Same-sex twins, probably DZ:			
Males, concordant	3 } (13.1%)	11 } (68.8%)	13 } (56.5%)
Males, discordant	20	5	10
Females, concordant	2 } (40.0%)	9 } (100%)	13 } (35.1%)
Females, discordant	3	0	24
Opposite-sex twins (DZ):			
Concordant	1 } (3.1%)	8 } (20.0%)	8 } (27.6%)
Male affected	21	28	18
Female affected	10	4	3
Total	97	107	136

* Data from Rosanoff et al., 1934*b*.
† (%) = pairwise concordance rate.

to happen in research that pioneering investigations turn up dramatic results that later turn out to be less exciting or that cannot be replicated. This is true—in part—of the Lange study. The next study to follow his (Legras, 1932) found four of four MZ pairs and one of five DZ pairs concordant for criminality, thus seeming to provide confirmation of Lange's findings and conclusions. One point that needs to be made in Lange's study is that the sex differences he obtained reflect sex differences regarding imprisonment rather than psychopathy per se. Lange's sample includes 6.5 male pairs for every female pair. In Table 8-1 we saw that in at least two well-done studies, males are diagnosed psychopathic personality more often than females, but not nearly 6.5 times as often. The study by Rosanoff et al. (1934*b*) throws some light on this problem. The essential data are shown in Table 8-3.

Unfortunately, Rosanoff et al. do not go into details of their sampling procedure, but they solicited information about admitted twins from hospitals, clinics, penal and correctional institutions, and other facilities dealing with mental illness or behavioral disorder. Thus, their sampling was neither systematic nor controlled. Under such circumstances, one might anticipate an excess of concordant MZ pairs. Nor do the authors say how they determined zygosity or how many subjects they saw personally, if any. Usually, when zygosity is guessed from appearance, some MZ cases tend to be classified DZ. Thus, procedurally, the study leaves much to be desired, but the data are of interest because of their size and their breakdown by sex and age-related disruptive or antisocial behavior.

The authors' criteria regarding the three clinical groups are:

1 *Criminal adult.* Any person, eighteen years of age or over, convicted and sentenced by a criminal court

2 *Juvenile delinquent.* Any boy or girl brought to the juvenile court authorities for some offense and placed on probation or committed to a correctional institution

3 *Child with behavior difficulties.* Cases sent to children's, child guidance, school, or neurological clinics because of behavioral difficulties, and to special classes for problem children in public schools, but who have not come into conflict with the law or to a juvenile court

We see in Table 8-3 a preponderance of males as compared with females in the adult and juvenile groups, but not in the children with behavioral difficulties; the male-female ratio for the three groups in the order listed is approximately 4:1, 2:1, and 1:1. If the three groups are diagnostically related, why should such a progression in the male-female ratio occur with age? One must question whether the uncontrolled sampling is implicated in such ratios, but it is difficult to see why possible selective bias would move in this direction with such regularity. An explanation based on acculturation effects has more to recommend it. The number of males seems to be approximately the same from one age group to another, but the number of females declines steadily from childhood to adulthood, except in the case of opposite-sexed twins, where the number is fairly constant. One might infer from such data that courts or legal agencies are much more reluctant to indict and sentence females for antisocial behavior as they grow to adulthood, or that females learn to control their antisocial tendencies sufficiently as they grow older to avoid coming into contact with criminal authorities.

If the latter point is correct, we might assume that if genetic factors are playing a role in such disorders, females who do have difficulties with the law at later ages must be more severely affected by their genetic makeup than males, who, if genes contribute to their antisocial behavior, behave antisocially at all ages with little adjusting to cultural norms or learning from experience as they grow up. On the basis of such reasoning, we would predict fewer female cases with maturation, but higher concordance for female twin pairs in adulthood. For MZ twins, we find little difference between the sexes regarding concordance rates at all ages, the female rate being slightly higher. For same-sexed DZ twins, the rate for females is higher than that for males at both the juvenile and adult ages, but lower in childhood. Thus, the hypothesis of a genetic predisposition of varying degree plus a factor of acculturation in women finds support in the data on same-sexed DZ twins, but not in MZ twins.

With respect to the possible role of heredity in Table 8-3, we can make the following points.

1 Concordance rates are consistently higher for MZ than DZ twins. This finding is consistent with a genetic hypothesis, but we should maintain some reservations because of the method of sampling. The latter may have contributed an excess of concordant MZ pairs, and may have classified a few MZ pairs as DZ. Such errors, if they occurred, tend to exaggerate differences in concordance rates between MZ and DZ twins.

2 The differences between MZ and DZ rates are not as great as in the Lange and Legras studies. In the juvenile and adult groups, the rates for females are not very different in the MZ and same-sexed DZ groups. With respect to juvenile delinquency, the rate for male DZ pairs is almost 70 percent, and for females it is 100 percent, indicating the probably strong role of environmental factors in this regard.

3 The rates for same-sexed DZ twins are consistently higher than for opposite-sexed twins, the differences being greater at the later ages than in childhood. This finding again implies that environmental factors may play a strong role in such disorders.

4 We may use the Weinberg differential method to see if that helps us to estimate the degree of possible bias in the sample. It will be recalled that this method is based on the principle that the number of opposite-sexed and same-sexed twins should be about the same, and the remainder should be MZ. With respect to adult criminality, there are 32 opposite-sexed pairs, 28 same-sexed DZ, and 37 MZ pairs. The difference between same- and opposite-sexed DZ pairs is close to expectancy, but the slightly fewer number of same-sexed pairs suggests that there may in fact be a few MZ pairs too many and a few same-sexed DZ pairs too few. Perhaps a few pairs classified MZ were really DZ. This is the direction of error that we would predict based solely on knowledge of the types of bias that occur when sampling is not strictly controlled. With respect to juvenile delinquency, the pairs number 40, 25, and 42 for the opposite-sexed DZ, same-sexed DZ, and MZ pairs,

respectively. Again we see the same direction of possible error, but to a somewhat more serious extent. Thus, for both clinical groups, the difference in concordance rates between MZ and DZ twins may be somewhat exaggerated. With respect to childhood behavioral difficulties, we find 29 opposite-sexed DZ, 60 same-sexed DZ, and 47 MZ pairs. In this group, there is a clear shortage of opposite-sexed pairs. Sometimes such a bias occurs in that opposite-sexed pairs may be more likely to be overlooked or not reported.

The next two studies to be done were published in the same year and made special efforts to minimize the possibility of bias in their samples. The one by Stumpfl (1936) is summarized in Table 8-4, and the one by Kranz (1936) in Table 8-5.

Stumpfl obtained 550 twin pairs from among an uninterrupted series of admissions to several German provincial prisons and from the files of inmates at a Bavarian institution for "biological criminals," based on a number of selected "sample days." From among the total, he selected for study 65 twin pairs because of their availability. Unfortunately, availability is a criterion that could introduce bias. Stumpfl's study group consisted of 18 MZ, 19 same-sexed DZ, and 28 opposite-sexed pairs. He personally investigated at least one member of each pair and also contacted relatives and official sources. To determine zygosity, he used photographs, and except for a few cases, obtained measurements of the skull, face, hair, and eyes of same-sexed pairs and noted similarities regarding other constitutional traits. He obtained information about the probands from personal interviews, parents, sibs, official sources, and conviction lists.

Stumpfl's major contribution was that he tried to grade concordance

Table 8-4
Levels of Concordance for Criminality in MZ and DZ Twins*

Zygosity and Sex	Pairs	Number Concordant, by Levels				
		(1)	(2)	(3)	(4)	(5)
MZ twins:						
Male	15	9	8	8	13	15
Female	3	2	2	2	2	3
DZ twins:						
Male	17	7	4	3	0	0
Female	2	0	0	0	0	0
Opposite	28	2				

* Data from Stumpfl, 1936.

according to the severity of the crimes or of subjects' antisocial orientation. He defined five levels:

1 Overall concordance or concordance of the first degree.
2 Both twins are concordant for a single offense or for repeated offenses.
3 Both twins committed similar crimes.
4 Both evidence similar day-to-day social orientation.
5 Both have identical deep traits of character or essential personality traits.

Stumpfl's levels do not seem to comprise a unidimensional type of scale and may not be a scale at all. Levels 4 and 5 are personality assessments. There is little question but that MZ twins are more alike in most personality traits than DZ twins, and these levels tell us little more than that. Moreover, the author was not blind with respect to the assessment of the cotwin, and we do not therefore know either the reliability of the assessments or what they would be if made by independent or "blind" raters. The male-female ratio is like that usually obtained for criminality, not psychopathic personality. He has too few same-sexed pairs. And despite his care and effort, some small degree of error in zygosity typing is possible with the similarity method alone.

With these reservations in mind, we may note that for level 1, which is most similar to that of other investigators, the concordance rates for males were 60.0 and 41.2 percent for MZ and DZ pairs, respectively. The number of female pairs is too small to be meaningful. The concordance rate for opposite-sexed pairs is about 7 percent. These findings are not too different from those of Rosanoff et al. (1934b). It is interesting to note that for level 5, the concordance rate is 100 percent for MZ pairs and zero percent for same-sexed DZ pairs! Such a finding makes as little sense genetically as environmentally, unless a clear chromosomal abnormality underlies such personality phenotypes, which is most unlikely. Thus the most that we can conclude from Stumpfl's study is that the role of heredity in criminality as such is not as great as Lange believed, but that it might be very important in shaping the kind of personality that might increase the likelihood of one's coming into conflict with the law.

Methodologically, the study of Kranz (1936) had several advantages over the others. He obtained his sample from:

1 All inmates in Prussian prisons on a given day, each of whom was questioned as to whether or not he was a twin

2 All prisons in four districts, with two sample days for two districts and two different sample days for the other two districts

3 All newly admitted convicts in six institutions in a small region over a one-year period

4 Two concordant pairs (one MZ and one DZ) reported as cases of sentenced twins

The last two, of course, should have been excluded. To determine zygosity, he used the similarity method and blood grouping, including ABO, MN, and others. Of the pairs, 16 were examined together and 13 were examined apart by the author, and 5 pairs were examined by another person. One member of 21 pairs was personally examined. Additional aids such as photographs, descriptions of the pair, and so on, were also used.

In this way, Kranz obtained 552 reported twins. But of these, 127 turned out not to be twins (even the ascertainment of twinship from among such populations can be a precarious enterprise!), one twin had died in 202 pairs, and in 97 pairs the twins were of uncertain zygosity or concordance. The final sample included 32 MZ, 43 same-sexed DZ, and the first 50 opposite-sexed pairs reported. The lower number of MZ and DZ pairs reflects the large number of same-sexed pairs that were excluded because of uncertain zygosity or concordance. This latter factor can have a biasing effect. The main findings regarding concordance are shown in Table 8-5.

We see in Table 8-5 that the concordance rates for MZ and same-sexed DZ pairs are of the same order of magnitude. The difference between them is not statistically significant, but the rate is slightly higher

Table 8-5

Concordance Regarding the Presence of Criminal Records in MZ and DZ Twins*

Zygosity	Total Pairs	Concordant Pairs		Discordant Pairs	
		n	*%*	*n*	*%*
MZ twins	32 (all male)	21	66	11	34
DZ twins:					
Same sex	43 (two female)	23	54	20	46
Opposite sexes	50	7	14	43	86

* Data from Kranz, 1936.

for MZ twins.   There occurs again the marked difference in concordance between same-sexed and opposite-sexed pairs.   These findings support strongly the likelihood that environmental factors are of overriding importance with respect to the legal criterion of whether or not one obtains a criminal record.   It does not by any means exclude the possibility that individuals with a certain type of personality are more likely to commit a crime and to be arrested and sentenced for it, and that heredity can contribute significantly to the formation of that personality.   Kranz reevaluated his same-sexed pairs with such considerations in mind and, with respect to what he called "criminality," the concordance rate for MZ pairs remained the same, whereas the rate for DZ pairs dropped to 44 percent.   Thus, the differences in "tendency" are greater than the differences regarding a criminal record per se.

Kranz also examined his sample to see whether certain aspects of the crime pattern are more heritable than others.   He took all concordant pairs and rated with regard to three degrees of similarity such factors as frequency, severity or type of crime, age at first conviction, and a combination of all of these.   His findings are shown in Table 8-6. With respect to the frequency of crimes, the intrapair similarity is about the same for both MZ and DZ pairs.   With respect to severity and type of crime and age at first conviction, the intrapair similarity is somewhat—but not strikingly—greater for MZ twins.   With respect to a global view of similarity in all four indices of crime pattern, Kranz judges the intrapair similarity to be much greater for MZ than DZ twins. Unfortunately, we do not know the reliability of making such global judgments, but we do know that Kranz was not blind with regard to type of twinship, and such knowledge could have influenced his classifications.   Even if the judgments are objectively veridical, we still could not say how much of the greater similarity in MZ twins stems from psychological rather than genetic factors.

It would be misleading to think that a given type of personality commits a certain type of crime, or that there is a simple relationship between a specific genotype and a particular type of crime pattern.   Let us take a "severe" crime like murder.   Who murders?   Hrebicek et al. examined 70 cases of murder and attempted murder committed by 73 offenders.   They found that 85 percent suffered from a psychiatric disorder.   Of these, 22 percent were judged psychotic, 35.6 percent psychopathic.   The remaining 42.4 percent had some other disorder, and 15 percent had none at all, in the authors' opinion.   Pathological motives were found in 26 percent of the offenders, and contributing or provoking factors included jealousy (21.9 percent), anger (17.8 percent), and alcohol (15.7 percent).   In fact, the trend in criminal law today is to weigh the severity of the crime less and to place greater emphasis on

Table 8-6

Similarity in Concordant MZ and DZ Twins with Respect to Different Aspects of Crime Pattern*

Zygosity	Pairs	Very Similar		Somewhat Similar		Scarcely Similar	
		n	%	n	%	n	%
Frequency							
MZ twins	21	9	43	8	38	4	19
DZ twins:							
Same sex	23	9	39	4	17	10	44
Opposite sexes	7	0		2	28	5	72
Severity							
MZ twins	21	7	33	4	19	10	48
DZ twins:							
Same sex	23	4	17	2	9	17	74
Opposite sexes	7	0		1	14	6	86
Type							
MZ twins	21	9	43	7	33	5	24
DZ twins:							
Same sex	23	6	26	7	30	10	44
Opposite sexes	7	1	14	3	43	3	43
Age at First Conviction							
MZ twins	21	15	71	4	19	2	10
DZ twins:							
Same sex	23	12	52	9	39	2	9
Opposite sexes	7	3	43	3	43	1	14
Global Crime Pattern							
MZ twins	21	11	52	6	29	4	19
DZ twins:							
Same sex	23	5	22	10	44	8	34
Opposite sexes	7	0		3	43	4	57

* Data from Kranz, 1936.

the personality of the offender (including mental illness) in deciding on the disposition of the case. There is a great need today to generate a proper understanding and classification of personality types that evidence proneness to crime, and to evaluate the hereditary—as well as environmental—factors that are associated with such types. Kranz (1937), in a second study, made an attempt along such lines.

The article describing the research was given as a preliminary report at a professional meeting and Kranz stated that he hoped later to present much larger and "unobjectionable" material to his colleagues. Thus, Kranz was himself not satisfied with his reported sample. It is of interest nevertheless. He again conducted a search for twins, this time in Silesian institutions which are somewhat like our "training schools" for youths who are repeatedly in difficulty in the home or community, and who commit crimes. His sample included 14 MZ pairs (8 male, 6 female) obtained in his search, plus 2 MZ pairs who had not been sent to one of the "trustee education institutions," but who had been reported by the Breslau Juvenile Court; 8 same-sexed DZ pairs (6 male, 2 female); and 14 opposite-sexed pairs. His youngest proband was four years old, the oldest thirty-eight. Among the 16 MZ pairs, 11 were concordant and 5 discordant with respect to institutionalization for crime. Among the 22 DZ pairs, 13 were concordant and 9 discordant. The difference is not statistically significant.

However, what makes this article interesting is that Kranz tried with considerable caution and reservation to evaluate the "causes" of the probands' difficulties and criminality as either predominantly "endogenous" or "exogenous." In the endogenous group he included personality inadequacies of the most varied sort: mental retardation, neuropathy, psychopathy, impulsivity, instability, or having a "blameless home environment." In the exogenous group, he included cases who had been grossly neglected at home and in their rearing. Kranz knew that the two categories often occurred hand in hand in real life, but he made the best judgment he could. His main findings are summarized in Table 8-7. Perhaps the most surprising finding in this table is that, if we sum pairs without regard to zygosity, we find among the "endogenous" group 9 concordant and 13 discordant pairs. Among the "exogenous" group, we find 15 pairs concordant and 1 pair discordant. The difference is clearly one of high statistical significance. Also significant is the fact that the twins classified exogenous are first sent to a trustee education institution at a much lower age than those classified endogenous. Kranz attributes this fact to the terribly noxious milieu to which the exogenous children were subjected. Thus, the pernicious environment seems to contribute more to the delinquent behavior than does the presumed inherited personality factor in this series of cases.

Table 8-7

Endogenous and Exogenous Causes of Juvenile Delinquency in Relation to Age at First Institutionalization and Concordance*

Zygosity and Pairs	Total	*Predominantly Endogenous*		*Predominantly Exogenous*		*Psychic Structure*	
		n	*Age at Admission*	*n*	*Age at Admission*	*Concordant*	*Discordant*
16 MZ:							
Concordant	11	7	14, 16, 17, 17, 18, 18, 18	4	4, 6, 7, 14	11	0
Discordant	5	4	8, 15, 16, 16	1	17	3	2
8 DZ (same sex):							
Concordant	5	0		5	3, 3, 3, 10, 15	2	3
Discordant	3	3	12, 14, 15	0		0	3
14 DZ (opposite sexes):							
Concordant	8	2	12, 15	6	1, 3, 4, 7, 8, 8	5	3
Discordant	6	6	13, 14, 15, 15, 16, 17	0		0	6

* Data from Kranz, 1937.

Whether the same pattern continues toward adult criminality, Kranz could not say, but most recidivistic criminals do begin their antisocial careers at tender ages.

WHAT IS INHERITED?

So many studies have reported a relationship between cultural, socio-economic, home environment, and psychological factors and crime rate that it is pointless to recount these here. The importance of environmental causes is beyond question. But hereditary factors are also significant, although these must be diverse and they must operate in different ways. We will indicate four that are clearly involved, although they are probably not major factors in the high crime rate.

1 A considerable number of studies have been reported that indicate a higher incidence of EEG abnormalities and borderline abnormalities in juvenile delinquents and adult criminals than in the general population. In some prison samples, the rate of abnormality hovers at about 75 percent. Although not all EEG abnormalities are inherited, we know that heredity contributes significantly to the EEG pattern and to a number of abnormalities. Thus, such abnormalities comprise one type of diathesis. How does it contribute to criminality? Possibly because it is associated with poor impulse control and bad judgment.

2 A large number of criminals have low IQs. Heredity contributes significantly to intellectual level, but educational and cultural deprivation also produces low IQ test scores in individuals who may otherwise be normally gifted. Also, poor prenatal, paranatal, and postnatal care may lead to organic brain impairment that is reflected in low IQ scores among some criminals who come from severely disadvantaged areas. Mentally retarded individuals in crime-prone areas are generally fair game for the smarter boys and are often led into crimes by them. In at least some of these cases, heredity leads to the low IQ that permits the individual to be lured or tricked into criminality. Sometimes such individuals are simply bewildered, have no skills, and do not know how to make their way in the world, and they may strike out at it through crime, and may be grateful for the simple, ordered life in prison, which they can comprehend and where they have a feeling of belonging.

3 The term *constitutional psychopathic state* has long been a favorite term applied to criminals. However, with respect to Sheldon's somatotypes, criminals seem to be predominantly mesomorphic. The mesomorph is well-muscled, athletic, strong, tough, and durable. Temperamentally, he is aggressive and less fearful than others. He does not brook restraint or opposition easily, and goes after what he wants. Glueck and Glueck (1956) found that about 60 percent of 496 delinquents were mesomorphs. This rate was twice as high as that of a nondelinquent control group. Thus, the concept of constitutional inferiority that is implicit in the older nomenclature not only seems to err in this sense (although not in others), but the reverse seems to be true. In body build, most criminals tend to approach the masculine ideal. It is easy to see why such people, when subjected to an oppressive or frustrating environment, will strike back, sometimes in ways that bring them into conflict with the law. Since the somatotypes are inherited in good part, in this sense too heredity contributes to sociopathy and criminality.

4 We saw in Chapter 5 that some individuals with Klinefelter's syndrome became criminals. Since 1965, a number of cases have been reported of another kind of aneuploidy in criminals. In contrast to Klinefelter's cases, who are XXY, these more recently reported cases are XYY. They have one Y chromosome too many, and in this respect may be thought of as supermale. Such men tend to be of above average height, usually over 6 feet tall, but they seem not to have any major physical abnormalities. Early reports indicated that they frequently had facial acne in adolescence, were usually mentally dull, with IQs in the 80 to 95 range, that their EEG tended to be abnormal, and that they tended to have an elevated incidence of epileptic and epileptiform conditions. Some investigators reported teeth disorders, including

discoloration, malocclusion, and arrested development. They called this disorder the XYY syndrome, but currently only tallness seems to be a consistent aspect of the "syndrome." In 10 studies totaling 3,345 criminals or delinquents, 52, or 1.55 percent, were found to be XYY. This rate is probably higher than the frequency of XYY in the general population, but the latter has not yet been reliably determined. The rates vary appreciably in the studies obtained thus far, although current consensus estimates that about 1 in every 500 to 550 males is XYY. Affected individuals are often thought to be predisposed to aggressive behavior, and in some, their crimes tend to be violent, often including murder.

Thus, we are able to point to at least four disparate groups whose heredity may have "predisposed" them to crime, but in whom the genetic factors are as disparate as the groups themselves. Clearly, if an MZ twin has one of the four diatheses, his cotwin will also have it and both will have an equally elevated risk for criminality. DZ twins are at least as likely to be discordant for the diathesis as concordant. Such factors could make for the MZ-DZ differences found in the twin studies cited. But even in such cases, environmental factors are usually critical in determining whether the affected individual will or will not commit a crime. Now three points should be clear:

1 There is no single genotype that is implicated in criminality. To the extent that heredity is involved at all, it involves biological or genetic heterogeneity.

2 The four types of diatheses indicated to illustrate the first point account for only a part of the genetically "predisposed" criminals, and they may be considered as secondary causes. The major primary group includes the ones who are simply classified as psychopathic or sociopathic personality. We know all too little about the heritability of this personality type. Its study has been limited by the constant confounding of hereditary and environmental variables. A good adoption study is sorely needed to explicate this point, and fortunately, at the present writing, one is already under way. One previous report by Zur Nieden (1951) indicates that criminals' children reared in good homes behave well.

3 In all likelihood, many, if not most, crimes are committed by individuals in whom the role of heredity is minor, nonspecific, or perhaps irrelevant. The latter statement is contingent on the definition of crime, which is a legal one that varies from place to place and time to time, and is not a sensible criterion for a genetic trait. In the Soviet Union, it is a crime to criticize the Communist Party or its government!

In the United States the crime rate has been increasing steadily and sharply for a long time. From a genetic point of view, one might assume that criminal psychopaths have a high fertility rate which contributes an accelerated frequency of the pathological genes into the general population. However, there is no good evidence of such an elevated fertility, and in fact, there is good reason to believe that their fertility rate is *below* that of the general population. If true, the low fertility rate and the increasing crime rate provide additional testimony to the overriding importance of environmental factors in crime

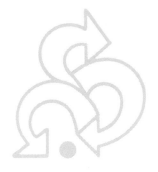

Chapter Nine

Genetic Studies of Psychoneurosis, Homosexuality, and Alcoholism

PSYCHONEUROSIS

Definition of the disorder

According to the 1952 diagnostic manual of the American Psychiatric Association, a major diagnostic group is *psychoneurotic disorders*. The group includes these seven subtypes, called *reactions*: anxious, dissociative, conversion, phobic, obsessive-compulsive, depressive, and "other." Their chief characteristic is anxiety, either expressed or unconscious and controlled by defense mechanisms. Unlike psychoses, psychoneurosis involves no falsification of external reality. Psychoneurotic patients usually present evidence of periodic or constant maladjustment of varying degree from early life. Stresses produce acute symptomatic expression. Anxiety is a danger signal of intrapersonal threat associated with repressed emotions or impulses. The subtypes reflect the ways in which the affected person handles the anxiety.

The 1957 diagnostic manual of the World Health Organization also refers to this group as psychoneurotic disorders and also calls its subtypes reactions. Five reaction types overlap with those in the American classification. These are: anxiety reaction without mention of somatic

240

symptoms, hysterical reaction without mention of anxiety reaction, phobic, obsessive-compulsive, and neurotic-depressive reactions. The two classifications differ in that the WHO scheme also includes subtypes called "psychoneurosis with somatic symptoms," or somatization reactions, which are coded according to the bodily system affected, namely, circulatory, digestive, and "other," the last-named including "psychogenic" reactions of the respiratory, genitourinary, cutaneous, and musculoskeletal systems, and parts of the body not classifiable under these systems. In addition, another subtype is called "other, mixed," and one is called "of other and unspecified types." The American scheme does not group these somatization reactions under psychoneurotic disorders but calls them "psychophysiologic autonomic and visceral disorders," and includes 10 subtypes paralleling those of WHO, but adding a hemic and lymphatic reaction, endocrine reaction, nervous-system reaction, and reaction of organs of special sense.

We present this recital of nosological categories not only to acquaint the reader with them but also to point up the vast breadth of the disorders classified as psychoneurotic. Who has not known anxiety or defended himself against it? How many individuals have not known periods of depression? Should the diagnosis be based on the intensity of such reactions, their duration, their special character? How reliably can this be done? Can anyone be entirely free of neurotic traits? Should the diagnosis be based on the degree of subjective distress of the patient or his reduced social effectiveness? Can one accurately make the diagnosis when one interviews subjects who are not currently having a "reaction," or can one diagnose relatives on the basis of information provided by probands or other secondhand nonprofessional sources? These are basic questions confronting the investigator who wants to learn something about the genetics of such disturbances. In previous chapters, we have already seen that the problem of defining the *unit character* was ever-present and a probable source of error. But in no other disorder does the unit character or diagnostic issue present such great obstacles and difficulties as in the psychoneuroses.

Incidence and distribution

Psychoneurotic reactions occur in all populations. Meaningful figures are hard to obtain. Landis and Page (1938) reported that 1.5 males and 2.0 females per 100,000 population were admitted to state mental hospitals in the United States for psychoneurosis in the year 1933. Such a figure means primarily that psychoneurotics are seldom sufficiently incapacitated to warrant placement in a state mental hospital. By contrast, Rosenthal and Frank (1958) found that among 3,413 first admissions to the Henry Phipps Psychiatric Clinic, Outpatient Department, 1,474, or 43.2 percent, were diagnosed as psychoneurotic. Most of the patients in treatment with psychiatrists, psychologists, counselors, and so on, are neurotics. Bille and Juel-Nielsen (1963) studied the incidence of neurosis in the Danish county of Aarhus in Jutland. They defined incidence as the number of persons in the population who required contact with a public medical or psychiatric service over a 12-month period and received a diagnosis of neurosis. In the population of 161,805 persons aged fifteen or over, 1,173, or about 7 per 1,000, were diagnosed neurotics. Of these, 873 were female and 300 were male. The 3:1 sex ratio is striking, and was even higher in the depressive, anxiety, asthenic, and hysteriform subtypes. For females, the peak incidence occurred in early adulthood (about thirty), but for males, in the forty to fifty year age group.

Nielsen, Wilsnack, and Strömgren (1965) reported all first referrals over a five year period to an easily accessible psychiatric outpatient clinic in the Danish island of Samsø. Diagnosed neurosis occurred at a rate of 2.63 per 100 population. However, the rate was only 1.09 for males as compared with 4.22 for females. Thus, in this study the female-male ratio is about 4:1. Of the 472 referrals, 128, or 27 percent, were diagnosed neurotic as compared with 43.2 percent at the Phipps Clinic in Baltimore. Differences between the two regions may occur with respect to the distribution of psychiatric disorders within each, the referral pattern, that is, which diagnostic groups are more likely to be referred, or diagnostic practices. The differences between the two clinics with respect to sex is much less. Of *all* first referrals, females accounted for 57.2 and 60.6 percent of the Phipps and the Samsø clinics, respectively. Hagnell (1966), in a study of 2,400 persons in southern Sweden who were personally examined psychiatrically over a 10-year period, reported that the lifetime prevalence of psychoneurosis for persons aged ten or over was between 7.8 and 10.0 percent for males, and between 16.5 and 20.4 percent for females. Thus, he finds that about 1 of every 10 men and 1 of every 5 women have psychoneurosis in their lifetime. These figures may be regarded as lowest estimates of the true incidence.

Such reports indicate that psychoneurosis is a very common disorder, that the reported rates vary with the methodology used, and that the disorder is more common in women than men. Studies of the genetics of the neuroses must take such factors into account.

Familial morbidity risk

One might expect that for a disorder as common as psychoneurosis there would be many good studies regarding familial incidence. In fact, the reverse appears to be true. Perhaps because the trait is very common and its diagnosis variably interpreted, its genetic study has been discouraged. Brown (1942) sorted cases of psychoneurosis into three groups: anxiety state (63), hysteria (21), and obsessional state (20). They were selected "at random" from outpatients at three hospitals. The author was psychotherapist of most of the patients. He personally interviewed 500 of their 2,288 relatives. Family histories were obtained from the patient and at least one relative. "Needless to say, a full account was not always available." Interestingly, his index cases numbered 54 males and 50 females, a figure that departs from the more usually reported higher prevalence among females. In evaluating the relatives, he seems to have divided all cases of psychoneurosis among them into three types: anxiety state, hysteria, and obsessional state. However, he did have an additional diagnostic category that he called "anxious personality," its traits including timidity, apprehension, excessive worry, phobias, obsessional personality with *folie de doute,* and depressive personality. Many investigators would undoubtedly have included such cases as psychoneurotic.

Among 573 first-degree relatives (parents and siblings), Brown found 94, or 16.4 percent, to have psychoneurosis. However, he also found 96, or 16.8 percent, to have anxious personality. Therefore, we judge the rate (not age-corrected) among these relatives to be between 16.4 and 33.2 percent. Again, these are minimum rates. Among the 189 first-degree relatives of a control group, Brown found 2 or, 1.1 percent, neurotics and 19 or, 10.1 percent, anxious personalities. Among 1,247 second-degree relatives, he found 35 cases of psychoneurosis, or 2.8 percent, but 153 cases of anxious personality, or 12.3 percent, or a combined total of about 15 percent. Thus if Brown had combined the two diagnostic groups, the rate for second-degree relatives would have been about half that for first-degree relatives, which is what some types of genetic theory would predict.

Oki (1967) collected a sample of 52 children aged four to six who were seen at outpatient clinics and a child psychiatry department and diagnosed "early childhood neurosis." He obtained a control group matched with the probands for sex, age, IQ, parental occupation, and physical state. In evaluating relatives, he called one diagnostic category neurosis and another nervousness. The others were psychosis, psychopathy, and mental deficiency. With respect to parents of probands, 22.05 percent had neurosis and 23.52 percent had nervousness, or 45.47 percent combined. For parents of controls, the corresponding figures were 2.08, 2.08, and 4.16 percent. With respect to sibs of probands, the rate for neurosis was 6.60 percent, for nervousness 26.40 percent, and 33.0 percent for both combined. No sibs of controls had either neurosis or nervousness! For second-degree relatives of probands (grandparents, aunts, and uncles), the rates were 1.58 to 5.17 percent for neurosis and 11.05 to 12.49 percent for nervousness. Again, neither neurosis nor nervousness was found in a single second-degree relative of the controls. As in the Brown study, a correlation occurs between degree of consanguinity and prevalence of neurotic types of disorder.

With respect to the heritability of subtypes of psychoneurosis, we may mention several illustrative studies. Stenstedt (1966) collected a series of probands whom he diagnosed as having neurotic depression. There were 54 males and 122 females. Almost all had been hospitalized. The author interviewed at least 1 member in 143 families personally, in 10 families by telephone and 3 families by questionnaire. The 176 probands had 1,242 first-degree relatives (parents and siblings). Stenstedt found that the expectancy of mental disease and abnormality other than affective disorders among the relatives did not differ appreciably from the rate in the corresponding general population. The expectancy of affective disorders was 2.0 and 7.5 percent for male and female relatives, respectively, and 4.8 percent for all relatives combined. The author believes that this rate is higher than that in the general population. He also believes that neurotic depression is related genetically not to psychoneurosis as such but to the affective disorders, and that the neurotic type of depression is the form with the lowest genetic loading. However, he also shows that a number of nongenetic factors are important in the etiology of the disorder.

Guze (1967) examined the relatives of female probands who had been diagnosed "hysteria" clinically and on the basis of a detailed symptom check list. Of 35 female relatives, 14 percent had hysteria, another 10 percent possible hysteria. In a comparison group of 167 women at a maternity hospital for full-term pregnancies and deliveries, 1.8 percent were diagnosed hysteria. He concluded that if hysteria is carefully defined, its heritability can be demonstrated.

Sakai (1967) obtained a sample of 65 probands (51 male and 14 female) with obsessive-compulsive neurosis. Among the 65 families, in 26 families (40.0 percent) at least one member carried a diagnosis of neurosis. However, 14 families (21.5 percent) also had a member diagnosed as chronic, recovered, or uncertain schizophrenia; 26 families (40.0 percent) had one member diagnosed as psychopathic; 7 families (10.8 percent) had one member with a diagnosis of depression; 8 (12.3 percent) contained epilepsy; 16 (24.6 percent) contained unidentified psychosis; and 11 (16.9 percent) contained mental deficiency. It is difficult to compare this study, and others of Mitsuda and his students, with the usual genetic studies because the calculations are in terms of families rather than individuals. Nevertheless, they do indicate the range of disorders that can occur in families harboring a member with obsessive-compulsive neurosis. Tsuda (1967) reports findings similar to Sakai's when the probands (46 male and 23 female) are diagnosed *depersonalization neurosis*. The rates among families are 37.5 percent for neurosis, 28.6 percent for psychopathy, and 21.4 percent for schizophrenia, but only 3.7 percent for depression.

An earlier study of obsessional neurosis by Rüdin (1953) involved 55 men and 75 women, most of them past age fifty. There was no marked increase of mental disorders among their relatives, except for compulsive neurosis. But even the rates for the latter were low: 4.6 percent for parents, 2.3 percent for sibs, and 1.3 percent for children. Previous studies by other investigators had reported higher rates among relatives.

In the study cited above by Brown, the author compared the diagnosis of relatives with that of his probands. The main results are shown in Table 9-1. Among the subtypes of psychoneurosis, anxiety state accounts for about 70 percent of all cases, whereas obsessional state accounts for about 7 percent. About 59 percent of all parents and sibs were considered to be normal. Among first-degree relatives, Brown

Table 9-1

Relationship between Psychoneurosis Subtypes in Probands and in First- and Second-degree Relatives *

| | Proband Diagnosis | | | | | |
| | Anxiety State | | Hysteria | | Obsessional State | |
Diagnosis of Relatives	n	%	n	%	n	%
First-degree relatives (573):						
Anxiety state	55	15.1	7	6.5	3	3.0
Hysteria	8	2.2	12	11.2	0	0.0
Obsessional state	2	0.5	0	0.0	7	6.9
Anxious personality	61	16.7	10	9.3	25	24.8
Normal	208	57.0	69	64.5	60	59.4
Other conditions	31	8.5	9	8.5	6	5.9
Second-degree relatives (1,247):						
Anxiety state	20	2.7	5	1.9	1	0.4
Hysteria	3	0.4	4	1.5	2	0.8
Obsessional state	0	0.0	0	0.0	2	0.8
Anxious personality	87	11.8	24	9.2	42	16.8

* Data from Brown, 1942.

finds a significant association between their subtype diagnosis and that of the probands. The trend exists in second-degree relatives as well, but is not as pronounced. The concordance rates between probands and their first- and second-degree relatives are 15.1:2.7, 11.2:1.5, and 6.9:0.8 percent for the anxiety, hysterical, and obsessional subtypes, respectively. Thus the degree of familial association drops dramatically from first- to second-degree relationships. The diagnosis of anxious personality occurs mostly among the families of obsessional- and anxiety-state probands, and the rate drops less between first- and second-degree relatives than does the rate for psychoneurosis. But the subtypes seem to be genetically independent, especially hysteria and obsessional state.

Of course, we must have reservations about the findings. Most relatives (1,788) were not personally examined. Brown relied on histories provided by the patient and another relative, and such testimony is hardly ideal for making diagnoses. He knew the subtype diagnosis of the index case when he was diagnosing the relatives and could have been unwittingly influenced by this knowledge. He divided all psychoneuroses into three types, whereas almost all classifications include more than that. He employed a wastebasket category, called anxious personality, which included traits of the three types and which may have blurred the segregation of subtypes had they been included as psychoneuroses. Subtype diagnoses often have low reliability; diagnostic "error" alone should have yielded more of an overlap between subtypes than that found in Table 9-1.

A number of studies have been done in which the association between relatives was based not on the clinical picture but on personality inventories which the subjects fill out themselves. Such studies usually find a modest familial association with respect to self-reported traits that may or may not be related to clinical psychoneurosis.

Twin studies

Kent (1949) obtained a series of childhood twins in which at least one in each pair had been examined at a child guidance institute. Zygosity determination was based on parents' statements about the twins. Diagnoses were based on psychiatric and casework summaries, and consisted primarily of psychoneurosis and a category called *"primary behavior disorder."* Of 6 pairs judged to be MZ, all were concordant for neurosis or nervous symptoms, if we include the primary behavior disorders in the neurosis group. Among the 9 DZ pairs, only 2 were discordant in the sense that the second twin was called healthy. The difference between MZ and DZ pairs is not statistically significant, but the study has obvious methodological difficulties.

Stumpfl (1937) obtained a series of index twins who had what he called an *hysterical reaction*. Of 9 MZ pairs, 3 were concordant for a similar or analogous abnormal reaction, and 4 were discordant. Two pairs were doubtful. Of 9 same-sexed DZ pairs, all were discordant.

Slater (1953) combined a series of twins with diagnoses of neurosis and psychopathy. Of 8 MZ pairs, 2 were concordant. Of 29 same-sexed DZ pairs, 4 were concordant. Of 14 opposite-sexed pairs, only one pair was concordant.

Parker's (1966) twin series included 9 MZ pairs, of whom 6 were concordant for neurosis, 3 discordant; and 11 same-sexed DZ pairs, of whom 4 were concordant and 7 discordant. Parker states that in a second twin series, Slater found 5 of 12 MZ pairs concordant and 4 of 12 DZ pairs concordant for neurosis. Ihda (1961) found that among 20 MZ pairs, 10 were concordant for neurosis, as compared with 2 of 5 DZ pairs. He concluded that hereditary factors in neurosis could be ignored. Tienari (1963) found 12 of 21 MZ pairs concordant for neurosis.

Shields (1954) obtained a sample of normal twins aged twelve to fifteen among schoolchildren in south London. Included in the study were 36 MZ pairs (13 male and 23 female) and 26 same-sexed DZ pairs (14 male and 12 female). Zygosity determination included full blood groupings. Shields divided all subjects according to four degrees of severity of psychiatric maladjustment:

1 *Moderately severe.* Referred to a social agency, $n = 42$

2 *Mild.* Suffered a milder or more transitory but definite psychiatric or behavioral disorder, $n = 25$

Groups 1 and 2 were regarded as neurotic.

3 *Neurotic traits.* Neurotic traits within normal limits, $n = 35$

4 *Well-adjusted.* "No neurotic traits of significance," $n = 22$

Thus, in the entire sample, which is a normative one, only 18 percent have no neurotic traits of significance. Shields believed that the twins did not differ from single-born children in this respect. His main findings are shown in Table 9-2.

Shields divided concordance into four types:

1 *Complete.* Both twins strikingly alike in their outstanding psychiatric characteristics and all other important details

2 *Essential.* Pairs alike in their most distinctive symptoms and in most personality traits, but differ in details

3 *Partial.* Chief symptoms differ, but both have some important characteristic in common

4 *Discordant.* Symptoms and personalities differ in all essential respects

It can be seen in Table 9-2 that among all pairs the MZ twins are consistently more concordant with respect to the complete and essential degrees. Only 6 MZ pairs are said to be discordant. No single DZ pair is completely concordant, and only 8 are essentially or partially concordant. Similar findings occur when the severity of the neurotic symptoms are the basis for classification. Thus, Shields' findings suggest that neurotic traits are almost universal among children aged twelve to fifteen, that such traits are heritable with respect to both type and degree, and that they are continuously distributed and probably polygenically conditioned. The more severely disturbed twin tended to be less intelligent. Shields' study is the best available and the most thoughtful in plan and execution. However, no study of the reliability of assessing severity or concordance type was carried out, and Shields alone made all judgments of these factors in both MZ and DZ twins. A replication of his study with blind raters would be reassuring. Shields points out that environmental factors influenced the occurrence of neurotic traits in the children, but he thought that they were insufficient to explain all the findings.

Eysenck and Prell (1951) attempted to use experimental and factor analytic techniques to study the heritability of core aspects of psychoneurosis. They classified the core syndrome as "neuroticism." Their subjects included 25 MZ and 25 DZ twin pairs, all of them schoolchildren

Table 9-2
Concordance for Severity of Neurotic Traits in Normative Twin Schoolchildren*

Type of Concordance	All Pairs				Both Twins in Group 1 or 2				Both Twins in Same Severity Group			
	MZ	%	DZ	%	MZ	%	DZ	%	MZ	%	DZ	%
Complete	13	36	0	0	6	35	0	0	12	48	0	0
Essential	12	33	3	12	8	47	1	11	10	40	1	13
Partial	5	14	5	19	3	18	3	33	3	12	2	25
Discordant	6	17	18	69	0	0	5	56	0	0	5	63
Total	36		26		17		9		25		8	

* Data from Shields, 1954.

who were located through birth records, and 21 neurotic children matched to the twins for age. All subjects were given a battery of psychological tests which were intercorrelated for all twins. Factor analysis yielded three factors, one of which the authors called neuroticism. Unexpectedly, the MZ and DZ twins differed significantly on a neurotic inventory and a lie scale, the MZ twins scoring higher on the lie scale and containing more pairs who were extremely stable or extremely unstable than the DZ twins!

"Neuroticism" scores were calculated for each twin. The intraclass correlations were .851 and .217 for the MZ and DZ twins, respectively. Heritability (h^2) was .81. The authors took this finding as evidence that "neuroticism . . . constitutes a biological unit which is inherited as a whole."

According to Shields (1954), Blewett tried to repeat the experiment of Eysenck and Prell on Shields' twin series. However, Blewett's tests did not intercorrelate with one another in the expected directions, and he could not identify any of the factors in his analysis as neuroticism. One factor that was defined by tests like body sway (which loaded high on Eysenck and Prell's neuroticism factor) and self-ratings regarding neuroticism gave no evidence of hereditary determination. Thus, the Eysenck and Prell study, which has been widely cited, could not be replicated by the only study that attempted to do so. However, the introduction of experimental psychological sophistication into the study of the inheritance of the behavioral disorders represents an approach that warrants emulation and expansion.

Gottesman (1960) studied 34 MZ and 34 same-sexed DZ twin pairs, all high school adolescents, with the MMPI. Interesting sex differences in heritability occurred with respect to neurotic subtypes: hypochondriasis: 0.29 females, 0.00 males; depression: 0.18 females, 0.66 males; hysteria: 0.00 females, 0.37 males; psychasthenia: 0.45 females, 0.17 males; psychoneuroticism: 0.46 females, 0.20 males; general neuroticism: 0.25 females, 0.00 males. The meaning of these findings is not clear.

By and large, we are limited in our conclusions about the heredity issue in neurosis because of the sparseness of studies, their relative lack of variety, their failure to take various diagnostic precautions, and the difficulty involved in assessing the role of environmental factors. However, the overall evidence points to the likelihood that heredity plays a role in the development of psychoneurotic symptoms, but we can say very little about the genetics involved, except that various polygenic systems may be involved in a more or less low-keyed way. If we sum the concordant and discordant pairs in the twin studies of clinical neurosis (which excludes Shields' study of normative twins) we find a 53 percent concordance rate for MZ pairs and a 40 percent rate for DZ pairs. Thus, the difference is not great and leaves little doubt about the importance of environmental factors in the development of clinical neurosis. But Shields' study suggests with equal strength that an inherited diathesis contributes significantly to the likelihood that clinical neurosis of more or less degree will occur. Future studies with increased methodological sophistication may help us to understand more clearly the diathesis-stress interactions and their relation to subtype syndromes.

HOMOSEXUALITY

Krafft-Ebing (1939), that illustrious, pioneering student of sexual pathology, suggested the possibility that male homosexuality might have an hereditary basis. An equally famous but later scholar (Kinsey et al., 1948) considered genetic factors to be a potential source of variation in sexual responsiveness, factors that were possibly related to personality formation. Some clinicians have claimed to find a number of homosexual males who had the horizontal pubic-hair pattern characteristic of women. Others have noted that many have feminine behavioral traits and special artistic ability. However, at least till now, in the great majority of male homosexuals, no hormonal, chromosomal, or other physical abnormalities have been found. Almost all research on homosexuality has been limited to males, and our knowledge of female homosexuality is meager indeed.

Familial morbidity risk

It is of course obvious that homosexuals are less likely than normals to marry and to have children. This fact limits the study of familial morbidity risk considerably. Moreover, since their parents had to be at least partly heterosexual, we cannot expect to find thoroughgoing homosexuality among them. To make such research even more difficult, a great social stigma is attached to homosexuality, and many subjects might refuse to acknowledge it. Many practicing homosexuals are denizens of the darker corners of our society, and many are treated as criminals and can be found only in prison. Unfortunately, most prisons in Western society permit no conjugal visits and therefore homosexual activities become common practice there, with the younger, weaker, more passive men usually assuming the female role, sometimes willingly or at least with complicity, at other times under coercion and even rape.

Lang (1941) provides what may well be a characteristic family picture of homosexual males. He visited the homes and personally interviewed families of 33 homosexual male probands who were found through a search of prisons in the Munich area. All probands but one were more than 20 years old, 7 were between 21 and 30. The rest ranged in age to the seventh decade of life, with the median age being about 37. Of these, 27 had never married, and 4 were married, 1 widowed, and 1 divorced. Between them, they produced 13 children, among whom only 2 were over 20. Of the 7 male children, 1 had an incestuous relationship with his own father, although Lang says he was primarily heterosexual, and 2 were predominantly homosexual.

Among the probands' mothers, 2 were called psychopaths, one of whom was a criminal, 2 were questionable psychopaths, 1 was alcoholic, 1 was a mental defective who was questionably schizoid, and another was a psychopath who committed suicide. Among the fathers, 3 were psychopathic, 1 of whom was schizoid, a second committed suicide, and the third had questionable endogenous depression; 2 were alcoholic; and 1 had cerebral sclerosis. Among probands' sibs, 35 were below twenty-one, and 85 were twenty-one or older; 6 were diagnosed schizophrenic, including paranoid, catatonic, and hebephrenic subtypes, 5 were psychopaths, usually with criminal records, 1 was called a case of endogenous depressive psychosis with catatonic signs, 1 was unstable, 1 questionably epileptic, and 3 were mental defectives (one an imbecile, one an idiot). Thus, in these 33 families one finds almost every known form of mental disorder.

This familial panorama of psychopathology may reflect the fact that male homosexuality is not a diagnostic entity by itself but is rather a secondary behavioral expression (or symptom) of other disorders. For example, among 40 pairs of homosexual male MZ twins (Kallmann, 1952a,b), 6 pairs were concordant for schizophrenia and 1 of these pairs was also concordant for suicide. At least 22 index cases were definitely schizoid, unstable with obsessive-compulsive features, or excessively alcoholic. Of the index cases, 7 cases evidenced transvestism (a compulsion to wear clothes of the opposite sex). Only 10 of the 80 MZ twins and 18 of the entire twin sample (170 individuals) were thought to be "sufficiently adjusted" emotionally and socially. Of course, the possibility exists that in the homosexual twins the homosexuality is the primary disorder and that the other psychopathology that they harbor is secondary and reactive to it. This could be so in some cases, but it would not account for the wide-ranging and at least partly hereditary psychopathology in Lang's families, most of whom by far were not homosexuals. Such families conjure up too a picture of turbulent interpersonal relationships, and such factors could presumably evoke or precipitate some of the observed behavioral disorders, perhaps most of them.

Twin studies

Since familial-risk studies of this disorder are few and heuristically limited, the main type of data regarding the heritability of homosexuality comes from twin studies. Table 9-3 presents a summary of the main studies reported to date. Lange and Habel obtained their series from imprisoned criminal populations. Kallmann's sample consisted of hard-core homosexuals reported to him by psychiatric, correctional, and charitable agencies and by contacts in the homosexual world. Heston and Shields' sample was obtained from a hospital twins' register. The Sanders study was reported in Dutch, abstracted by Slater, and summarized briefly by Heston and Shields. The fact that it includes six MZ pairs and only one DZ pair suggests that it may not be a representative sample.

Kallmann's 100 percent concordance rate for his MZ pairs also suggests that his method of obtaining probands led to a sample that missed discordant pairs. He himself recognized and emphasized the difficulties involved in obtaining a sample of homosexual twins, and later reported an MZ twin pair in which one twin was both schizophrenic and homosexual and the cotwin was neither. Other investigators were prompted by his findings to report isolated cases of MZ twins discordant for homosexuality. These are not included in the table since they were not part of a systematic sample. Of Kallmann's 11 DZ cotwins classified as homosexual, 7 had a rating of 1 on the Kinsey scale, which means they were "predominantly" heterosexual. One MZ cotwin in the Heston and Shields study showed sexual deviation (that is, he had delusions of

---

Table 9-3
Concordance for Homosexuality in Male Twins

	MZ Twins		DZ Twins	
Study	*Total Pairs*	*Concordant Pairs*	*Total Pairs*	*Concordant Pairs*
Lange, 1931	2	1		
Sanders, 1934	6	5	1	0
Habel, 1950	5	3	5	0
Kallmann, 1952*a,b*	37*	37	26*	4 (+7?)
Heston and Shields, 1968	5	2 (+1?)	7	1

* Three MZ cotwins and nineteen DZ cotwins could not be classified with regard to homosexuality, according to the author.

sex change and exposed himself); both he and his index twin were schizophrenic.

If we exclude the Sanders and Kallmann studies on the grounds that they were probably not representative, we find 6 of 12 MZ pairs concordant for homosexuality, or 50 percent, as compared with 1 of 12 DZ pairs, or 8.3 percent. Thus a clear difference occurs between the two types of twins. The rate for DZ twins, however, may be lower than expected. Kinsey et al. (1948) reported that 37 percent of males had had overt homosexual experiences—to the point of orgasm—and that 4 percent were exclusively homosexual, 8 percent had been exclusively homosexual during a 3-year period, and 18 percent were more homosexual than heterosexual. Kinsey's sampling and findings have been roundly criticized, but it is probably still the best study we have of the prevalence of homosexual behavior among males. Even if Kinsey's rates are too high, they do raise some question about the meaning of an 8.3 percent rate among DZ cotwins of homosexuals, which may well be lower than the population incidence.

Heston and Shields present interesting case summaries of their twins. Of their 5 MZ index cases, 1 was schizophrenic and a second had attacks of anxiety and depression, once with delusions. Their cotwins had clinical pictures similar to their own. The depressive pair was concordant for homosexuality. Of the 3 remaining MZ probands, 2 had no psychiatric abnormality apart from the homosexuality and 1 had a depression that was secondary to the sexual problem. The latter's cotwin showed a similar pattern. The other 2 were heterosexual, 1 of whom was married and had two children. Of their 7 DZ index cases, 1 had severe anxiety attacks, another finally succeeded in suicide at age twenty-two after 11 attempts, a third was *psychopathic,* and a fourth *sociopathic.*

From the environmental side, the authors recount the following events in their subjects' lives:

1 A priest interfered with twin's private parts when he was age ten.

2 Subject treated as a girl by his mother.

3 Mother died; twins, age four, brought up by grandmother, got on indifferently with father.

4 Unhappy home, much parental quarreling, father drinker, mother shrill-voiced and overpowering, sister epileptic.

5 Neglected by mother, parents divorced, unstable background.

6 Father rejecting, mother has disseminated sclerosis.

7 Father eccentric, paranoid.

8 Overpossessive mother.

Heston and Shields also report a remarkable family in their series. The family of 14 children included 3 sets of MZ male twins, of which 2 pairs were concordant for homosexuality, whereas the third pair was free of any sexual or other psychiatric abnormality. Of the heterosexual children, 4 had been enuretic till adolescence and 1 had recurrent depressions and suicidal thoughts. None of the single-born children was homosexual. The father was a heavy drinker who had brutalized the mother and children, threatened to kill them, beat them severely, tied them to a bed, and so on. The mother tried to control the father by threatening suicide.

It is difficult to evaluate this spotty literature. The twin studies suggest that heredity plays an important role with respect to whether males become homosexuals, but even here, we have only a few small samples that at least suggest that they may not be biased, and of these, two were obtained from prison populations, which may in itself be a biasing factor. The study by Heston and Shields provides the least-compromised sample, but here too the index cases were hospital admissions—either inpatients or outpatients. It may be that discordant MZ twins are less likely to seek hospital treatment and that such cases often go unreported. Moreover, a wide range of psychopathology seems to abound in the families of most male homosexuals, and one may not always be able to tell whether the homosexual behavior is secondary to such psychopathology or whether the psychopathology is secondary to the homosexuality. From the hereditary side, it is difficult to see what the genetic association between the homosexuality and all these other disorders might be. From the environmentalist side, a wide variety of pathological behaviors occurs in these families, and though they appear to be pathogenic, their diversity poses as much of a problem for a theory of psychological etiology as for a genetic theory. Perhaps a broad spectrum of diatheses and stresses is involved. Clearly, the biggest impediment to research on these matters has been the social ostracism of homosexuals. However, in the current climate of the United States and some other Western countries, the opprobrium that has attached to homosexuality has been reduced, and many homosexuals have been much more open about their personal lives. It may be that future attempts to study these issues will be less hampered.

From an evolutionary viewpoint, we are confronted with the problem of why, if homosexuality is transmitted genetically, the disorder has come to be so prevalent at all. Moreover, the fertility of homosexuals is probably far lower than that of persons with any of the other behavioral disorders.

Some students of homosexuality claim that the choice of a sex object has to be learned, and that whether an individual chooses a male or female object is a matter solely of the circumstances surrounding his psychosexual development and the way they shape his learning and his preferences. Such a theory ignores evolutionary considerations in that preference for the opposite sex as a sex object is strongly built into the biopsychological apparatus. It is one of the most fundamental mammalian and probably human impulsions. Without it, the species could hardly have survived. One does not need to have cultural dicta prescribe that postadolescent boys must like girls, and girls must like boys. These heterosexual responses occur naturally and spontaneously in all cultures.

It is true that the sex drive is normally strong, and that when the preferred sex object is not available, a displaced object choice to satisfy the drive can and perhaps will occur. It is also true that cultural differences occur regarding the tolerance of homosexuality. Sometimes, psychological events can surely influence an individual's concept of his masculinity or his lack of appeal to the opposite sex, and this may influence his own object choice. People who are chromosomal intersexes learn to accept a "gender role" and identify psychologically with one sex or the other. Overprotective mothers and brutalizing fathers could instill passivity and submissiveness in prone individuals. But these illustrations point only to the fact that some learning regarding our sexual behavior does occur, and that such learning can divert our normal, evolutionarily selected but plastic sexual impulsions regarding object choice. But persistent, exclusive homosexuality is not merely a variation of normal sexual behavior. It is a serious abnormality that probably arises from a combination of unfortunate genetic propensities and a warped psychosexual rearing environment.

ALCOHOLISM

According to the 1952 diagnostic manual of the American Psychiatric Association, habitual alcoholism is considered to be an addiction and a sociopathic personality disturbance. Diagnosis of the addiction to alcohol must be "well established . . . without recognizable underlying disorder." It does not include simple drunkenness. The manual also includes a category called "acute brain syndrome, alcohol intoxication," in which acute recoverable psychotic manifestations occur, such as delirium tremens and acute alcoholic hallucinosis, and a category called "chronic brain syndrome associated with intoxication," which includes "chronic delirium," or Korsakoff's psychosis.

It is worth noting at the outset that this disorder is defined in terms of an environmental agent, since without alcohol an individual clearly cannot suffer from alcoholism. How then can we consider the possibility that alcoholism might have a genetic basis? First, let us recognize that a number of investigators have shown that different strains of rats and mice show clear preferences for alcohol as compared with other strains that avoid it. The pioneer investigator of these studies, R. J. Williams, has referred to alcoholism as a genetotrophic disease in which the genetic pattern calls for an increased supply of a particular nutrient for which there develops a nutritional deficiency. Such a disease would result from a partial genetic block which does not involve a complete inability to carry out a specific enzymatic transformation, but rather a diminished potential for producing the biochemical change. This diminution in turn would make for the increased nutrient demand.

Distribution of the disorder

Descriptions of drunkenness can be found in the ancient literature of most older civilizations. A taste or craving for alcohol is neither new nor confined to particular regions or groups. However, the incidence of alcoholism varies considerably in different national or racial groups. Two groups especially have been known to have very low rates of alcoholism: Jews and Chinese. At a New York psychiatric clinic in which Jews abounded in the surrounding population, this group contained high numbers who sought admission for a variety of psychopathologic disorders, but the clinic, which embarked on a study of alcoholism, could turn up only one Jewish alcoholic. In New York's Chinatown, a search also turned up a low rate of alcoholism. On the other hand, the prevalence of alcoholism among the Irish has been reported to be quite high. Reports of elevated rates among the American Indian, however, were thought to be not justified. According to a "world poll" conducted by the New York Herald Tribune in 1958, in only 2 of 12 countries did more than half the population abstain completely from alcohol. In Austria and France, 4 of every 5 persons drank alcoholic beverages. People described as "frequent users" of alcohol ranged from 1 percent in Mexico to 30 percent in France. The prevalence of chronic alcoholics in the United States has been estimated to be 4.5 to 5 million, the incidence of chronic alcoholism of all degrees being about 4,390 per 100,000 population.

In Canada, first admissions for alcoholism to mental institutions increased in each succeeding year between 1943 and 1956, from 1.6

to 21.4 per 100,000 population aged 20 or more. This represents about a fourteenfold increase over a 14-year period. In Canada, too, people who lived in maritime regions were more frequently abstainers than people living in the prairies and in British Columbia. Males were more often users of alcohol than were females; people in the age range 30 to 49 were more often users than people 21 to 29 and people 50 or more. Catholics and Protestants did not differ appreciably in this respect, but there was an association between alcohol use and education, economic status, and community size. People with a high school education or higher were more frequent users than the less educated; the more prosperous people were more frequent users than the poorer people; and those who lived in more populated communities were the more frequent users. Thus, there appears to be a clear correlation between sex, age, and socioenvironmental factors and alcohol use.

Familial morbidity risk

Table 9-4 shows the prevalence of chronic alcoholism in the parents and sibs of alcoholic probands and of comparison groups who were free of alcoholism. In all samples, the rates are higher for males than females. With respect to the alcoholic probands, rates ranged from 11.4 to 32.6 percent for fathers, 12.2 to 27.7 percent for brothers, 0.4 to 8.2 percent for mothers, and 2.8 to 10.3 percent for sisters. The rates for parents in the Lemere et al. study are appreciably lower than the others. We already noted an association between alcohol use and various nongenetic factors, and on this ground alone we should expect considerable variation across samples. Perhaps more surprising is Bleuler's finding of a lower prevalence among the relatives of schizophrenics than of nonalcoholic surgical patients. As a matter of fact, the rates for the relatives of the surgical patients were higher than those for the relatives of alcoholics in the Lemere et al. study. Thus the fluctuation of rates is great enough that the morbidity risk for a control population may be higher than that of an index sample. This finding does not necessarily constitute grounds for dismissing the genetic hypothesis, but does emphasize the importance of environmental factors and the inadvisability of comparing control and index samples from different populations.

Jellinek (1945) reviewed the reports of different earlier investigators, combined their data, and found that of the 4,372 alcoholics in these reports, 2,799, or 52 percent, "had either an inebriate father or mother." This rate is much higher than the rates in Table 9-4 and suggests again that the early studies of the behavioral disorders often involved biased samples.

Table 9-4

Chronic Alcoholism in the Parents and Siblings of Alcoholic and Nonalcoholic Probands

Study	Fathers		Mothers		Brothers*		Sisters*	
	n	%	n	%	n	%	n	%
Alcoholic probands:								
Brugger, 1934	70	24.3	72	5.5	83	27.7	107	2.8
Lemere et al., 1943	500	11.4	500	0.4		14.0%		
Åmark, 1951	186	26.0	200	2.0	349	21.0	365	†
Bleuler, 1955, United States	50	22.0	50	6.0	27	22.3	29	10.3
Bleuler, 1955b, Switzerland	49	32.6	49	8.2	49	12.2	61	3.3
Nagao, 1967		13.1%				8.8%		
Nonalcoholic probands:‡								
100 schizophrenics	100	3.0	100	1.0	54	3.7	59	1.7
200 surgical patients	200	13.0	200	3.0	192	13.0	185	3.3

* The brothers and sisters are all over forty years of age, except in the study by Åmark and in the one by Lemere et al., where the ages and n's for sibs are not stated and where the 14.0 percent figure refers to *families* with an affected sib.
† About the same as the general population. Only three sisters of age twenty and over were alcoholic.
‡ As reported by Bleuler, 1964.

Adoption study

We are fortunate to have a well-carried-out adoption study of alcoholism. Roe (1945) obtained her subjects from among children referred to the State Charities Aid Association of New York City. The children came from all over the state and from private and public agencies. Roe and her colleagues reviewed the records of the child-placing department and selected as subjects those who were white, non-Jewish, age twenty-one or more at the time of the study, placed originally before they were ten years old, and about whose parents adequate data were available. Those who met these criteria but who could not be located or who lived too far away were excluded.

Of the 61 subjects obtained in this way, 25 had both parents normal; that is, neither parent was alcoholic, psychotic, epileptic, criminal, feeble-minded, a sex deviant, inadequate, or guilty of mistreatment or neglect of the child. Each parent showed adequate adjustment with respect to family, job, and community and manifested no grossly inadequate behavior in the immediate situation leading to the child's becoming a public charge. These children were either illegitimate or had lost one or both parents and had no relatives to care for them.

The 36 index children had a father classified as "heavy drinker with syndrome"; that is, he was overaggressive, disorganized, had repeated loss of jobs, and manifested disorderly conduct, neglect, or mistreatment of the wife or children. Among the fathers, 25 percent were criminal or possibly criminal, and 3 were sex deviants. Of the mothers, only 4 were considered normal; 5 drank heavily. Over half were sex deviants; 44 percent mistreated or neglected the children. Psychotic, epileptic, and feeble-minded parents were excluded.

Information about the child was obtained by carefully trained field workers who interviewed at length the child, the foster parent, or both, using a prepared schedule. The main findings relevant to this section are shown in Table 9-5.

Roe points out that when children are first placed in foster homes, they are likely to experience difficulties, no matter how nice the child or how good the home. Enuresis, temper tantrums, stealing from the foster parents, and other problems are very common, but they are usually only temporary. In Roe's series, however, several children had serious difficulties in late adolescence. Of these, 10 were index cases; 5 were girls who were all sex delinquents, and of the 5 boys, 2 got into trouble for drinking too much, 2 for stealing, and 1 for forgery. Of the control

Table 9-5
Foster-home-reared Children of Alcoholic and Control Parents*

Major Characteristics	*Index Group*	*Control Group*
Males	21	11
Females	15	14
Mean age when placed (years)	5.56	2.60†
Placed in rural or small towns	67%	28%†
Mean age at study (years)	32	28
Married	83%	64%
Children	67%	50%
Use of alcohol:		
Total abstinence	30%	36%
Occasional	63%	55%
Regular, not necessarily heavy	7%	9%

* Data from Roe, 1945.
† Indicates a statistically significant difference between the groups.

boys, 2 had serious difficulties: 1 for drinking and 1 for truancy. The higher frequency of such problems in the index group could reflect the fact that they were placed at later ages, spent their early childhood with seriously disturbed biological parents, or had poorer foster homes. Roe points out that no child reared in a foster home rated *satisfactory* became delinquent.

Most important here is the low rate of alcoholism in the index group. In their adulthood, not a single one of the index children was an excessive drinker. There is no significant difference in the drinking habits of the two groups despite the fact that the index group is older and included relatively more males as compared with the control group. Thus, whatever role heredity may play with respect to the development of chronic alcoholism, this study suggests that the contribution of environmental factors is of overriding importance with respect to whether addiction does or does not occur.

Twin studies

In the study of possible genetic factors in alcoholism, we are fortunate in having two major twin studies, both well conceived and analyzed. Kaij (1960) obtained his sample of probands from a twins' register in Sweden. The names on this register were compared with names and other identifying data in registers maintained by temperance boards. The method produces minimal sampling bias. In the final study sample, there were 174 pairs of male twins, or 348 individuals of whom the author examined 292 personally. Zygosity was determined by the similarity method, and when possible, by blood grouping. Kaij classified drinking habits into five classes as follows:

0 Abstainers or almost total abstainers

1 A drink now and then; never or seldom drunk; buy spirits regularly; successful in concealing alcohol abuse

2 Weekend drinkers and above-average consumers

3 Heavy abusers who have none or one of the cardinal symptoms

4 Chronic alcoholics with two or three cardinal symptoms, including (*a*) a pathological desire for alcohol after ingestion of small quantities or "trigger dose," (*b*) regular blackouts during intoxication with alcohol, (*c*) a physical dependence on alcohol after withdrawal following a drinking bout

In evaluating concordance, Kaij counted as concordant any pair in which both members had the same class rating with respect to drink-

Table 9-6

Concordance and Discordance with Respect to Similarity of Drinking Habits of MZ and DZ Male Twins*

Grades of Concordance†	MZ Twins		DZ Twins		Total	
	n	%	n	%	n	%
C	31	53.5	39	28.3	70	35.6
D_1	18	31.0	53	38.4	71	36.2
D_2	8	13.8	26	18.8	34	17.3
D_3	1	1.7	15	10.9	16	8.3
D_4			5	3.6	5	2.6
Total	58		138		196‡	

* Data from Kaij, 1960.
† For explanations of code designations, see text.
‡ The number exceeds the actual 174 pairs because in some pairs, both members were probands.

ing habits. These were designated C. Those only one-scale-point apart were called D_1, and those who were two, three, or four scale points apart were designated D_2, D_3, and D_4, respectively. The major findings are summarized in Table 9-6. Kaij, in the analysis of his data, does not treat concordance with respect to alcoholism as a yes or no matter. Rather, he takes recognition of alcohol consumption as a graded, quantitative character and correspondingly examines concordance with respect to the *degree* to which it occurs. Although he chooses to say that when the two twins in a pair both have the same scale-point rating, they are concordant, and that when they do not, they are manifesting different degrees of discordance, the code designations in Table 9-6 could as well have been represented as C_1, C_2, C_3, C_4, and C_5 to emphasize the continuum of degrees of concordance. We should recognize too that the scale is ordinal; that is, it does not assume that the differences between scale points are equidistant. If one pair has a 3 and a 4 rating, the twins may in some sense be more concordant than a pair that has a 1 and 2 rating, or vice versa. Kaij knew the zygosity of the pairs when making his ratings, and recognized that this could introduce bias, but he checked his own reliability against ratings by five experienced psychiatrists who reviewed the written records of 32 MZ pairs. Interrater correlations ranged from .54 to .92.

The difference between MZ and DZ pairs with respect to the frequency of identical ratings within pairs is significant at the 0.001 level. Among the 3 MZ cotwins who had a 0 rating, their twin probands had ratings of 1 or 2. Regardless of how the data are analyzed, the intrapair similarity is greater for MZ than DZ twins. However, the degree of similarity is also high for DZ pairs. The two highest degrees of concordance, $C + D_1$, account for 84.5 and 64.7 percent of all MZ and DZ pairs, respectively. The concordance rates of the MZ pairs increased with increasing degree of alcohol abuse of the probands, but no corresponding increase occurred in the DZ pairs.

Kaij interpreted his findings to mean that the development of alcohol abuse and chronic alcoholism was greatly influenced by genetic factors. Although his findings are strongly suggestive that genetic factors are implicated, the probable role of environmental influences in interaction with the inferred genetic factors cannot be estimated from this study.

The second study was carried out by Partanen et al. (1966) in Finland. The twins were obtained through a twins' register, and the analysis of the material was highly sophisticated. We will not review the study in detail here. The authors factor-analyzed 13 drinking variables and generated 3 drinking factors: "density," "amount," and "lack of control." Of these, density and amount were thought to show significant heritability, whereas lack of control, and another factor called "social complications," seemed to be "predominantly environmentally determined." Thus, some aspects of drinking behavior may be heritable and others may not be.

Is alcoholism a disease?

In the nineteenth century, a great controversy arose around the issue of whether chronic alcoholism should or should not be considered a disease, and the issue has still not been resolved. Many hold that it is a psychological or emotional disorder secondary to underlying psychoneurotic conflicts or personality problems. Others regard it as a disease, some considering it to be an allergy, others as resulting from biochemical or physiological imbalances, and others as due to brain pathology, nutritional deficiencies, or endocrinological dysfunctioning.

Whichever is correct, it should be clear that these different proposals regarding the nature of the disorder arise from the heterogeneity of characteristics of alcoholics. For example, in a study of alcoholics admitted to the Payne Whitney Clinic in New York, Sherfey (1955) found that 8.7 percent had schizophrenia (mostly paranoid), 6.8 percent had manic-depressive psychosis, 6.8 percent had poorly organized, asocial psychopathic personalities, 9.3 percent had poorly organized, psychoneurotic psychopathic personalities, 4.3 percent had epilepsy and epileptoid reactions, 3 percent had brain damage, 13.6 percent were males with obsessive-compulsive personalities, 10 percent were females with rigidly organized neurotic personalities with paranoid features, 18.6 percent were males with poorly organized, inadequate psychoneurotic personalities, 7.4 percent were females with dependent psychoneurotic personalities with depression and tension, and 6.8 percent had depressions of middle and late life.   Other studies have consistently revealed a wide variety of disorders among alcoholics.   Kaij has questioned whether a number of neurological disorders thought to be the consequences of alcoholism may not indeed have antedated and perhaps even precipitated the alcoholism.   We must indeed assume multiple motivations and etiologies in the persistent resort to alcohol of many individuals, and among them perhaps an inherited factor which may be simple or heterogeneous, primary or secondary.   It has in fact been suggested that alcoholism is associated with a sex-linked recessive gene, but Winokur (1967) reviewed the evidence on which the hypothesis was based and correctly concluded that the support for it was lacking.

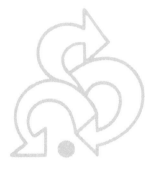

Chapter Ten

Some Methodological and Theoretical Considerations for Future Studies

We have tried to present a balanced review of the major evidence that implicates genetic factors in the most serious "functional" behavioral disorders. These disorders have two primary characteristics in common.

1 Their distribution does not follow a Mendelian pattern.
2 No evidence of a specific metabolic, biochemical dysfunction that is etiological with respect to the disorder has been found in any of them.

We have not discussed other serious disorders that are clearly genetic or that have demonstrable organic pathology and devastating effects on behavior, or are lethal. This group includes such disorders as epilepsy, a variety of disorders with more or less severe mental defect, brain or generalized CNS diseases, diseases of old age, and others.

In the preparation of such a review, it is necessary to be sufficiently critical that sources of error or possible error are exposed and examined.

All scientific data must at some time be treated in this fashion. We have not intended that such a critique should be equated with outright rejection of the studies cited.   Those who did the pioneering work could not have anticipated all issues and problems, methodological or substantive, nor did they always have the wherewithal to carry out the studies in the way they would have liked.   The early investigators did conceive many basic questions and techniques with which to study them.   Many exercised great ingenuity in designing their experiments.   Each moved the field under review forward—some more, some less.   This is the way every science and every body of knowledge grows.   At the beginning there always tends to be faltering, but gradually the steps become steadier and better integrated into the overall movement.   We seem now to have reached this stage of development with respect to the role of genetics in abnormal behavior.

If there is a lesson to be learned from such a review, it is that the contributions of heredity to abnormal behavior ought not, indeed, cannot, be ignored, and that the opportunities for research that will enlarge our understanding of this important matter constitute a golden field waiting to be harvested.   Those who see the potential and have the will and imagination required for such research will reap many rewards.   Future investigators will of course want to build on the work of their predecessors and avoid some of the pitfalls that beset such research.   We have dealt with them in the previous chapters but we wish to emphasize and expand upon them here.

SAMPLING

Even when early investigators approached their method of sampling with great sophistication, difficulties frequently arose with respect to the avoidance of bias in the ascertainment of probands.   We now have a better understanding of these difficulties and can use this knowledge to reduce such bias and to estimate the degree to which unavoidable bias may influence one's findings.   Unavoidable bias includes such factors as loss of legitimate probands or relatives through death, migration, insufficient information, or refusal to cooperate.   The subjects who are missed for these reasons are always the most worrisome.   The mere fact that they differ from the remaining subjects in these respects suggests that they might also differ with regard to others, for example, the kinds of psychopathology that concern the investigator.   One can only try to get as much information as possible about these individuals and evaluate it as best he can.

DIAGNOSIS

Although knowledge about sampling has progressed, problems of diagnosis and the ascertainment of unit characters constitute as much of a problem today as in the days of Rüdin. For various reasons, this problem has been the most neglected by previous investigators. One has the impression that each investigator approached this aspect of his study with the certain belief that he could recognize a case of hebephrenia or affective disorder when he saw one. By and large, especially with regard to the selection of index cases, his self-confidence may have been warranted. With regard to the diagnosis of relatives, however, the margin of error that could occur might be well beyond what is permissible.

For example, Schmidt and Fonda (1956) had pairs of psychiatrists diagnose independently 426 state hospital patients. Classification of the diagnoses into three major categories—organic, psychotic, and characterological—showed that both psychiatrists agreed about 80 percent of the time. One could argue that a 20 percent margin of error for such gross classification is already considerable. However, reliability of the diagnosis of schizophrenia varied between .73 and .95, depending on the range of discrimination required. Such margins of error are tolerable. However, agreement with respect to the specific subtype of disorder was only about 50 percent, and was almost absent in cases involving personality pattern-and-trait disorders and psychoneuroses.

Wallinga (1956) found that patients seen at more than one psychiatrically staffed medical facility were likely to have a change of diagnosis, and that such changes involved psychoses and character disorders more than neuroses. Diagnostic disagreement was related to the training, experience, administrative demands, and emotional characteristics of the diagnosticians.

Ash (1949) evaluated the reliability of diagnosis at a clinic whose function it was to screen out psychotic and mentally defective individuals. They used five major diagnostic categories: mental deficiency, psychosis, psychopathic personality, neurosis, and predominant personality characteristic. Three psychiatrists achieved a consensus on the major category in only 45.7 percent of the cases, and a consensus on subcategory diagnoses in only 20 percent of the cases.

A recent study, not yet published, compares equally experienced American and British psychiatrists, both groups of whom viewed films of hospitalized American patients. The Americans reported twice as many symptoms as did the British psychiatrists. The latter, however, saw more elation, excitement, and grandiosity than did the Americans, who saw more underactivity, dependency, or indecisiveness. Previous studies had reported that social class was a factor in diagnosis: the poor and uneducated were more likely to be labeled schizophrenic by middle-class psychiatrists. In another study, 9 percent of 344 patients initially diagnosed schizophrenic were later given a different diagnosis, while 5 percent of cases with a different initial diagnosis were later called schizophrenic. Kendell (1968) showed that psychiatrists were biased in their ratings of depressive and neurotic symptoms by their opinions about the relationship between different types of depression, the bias occurring in such a way as to confirm those opinions.

These studies and others indicate that the presumed self-confidence of investigators studying the genetics of behavioral disorders is not warranted. Kendell's study suggests that many of the past studies may have been nothing more than self-fulfilling prophecies. All future research in this field, if it is to achieve acceptance, must be carried out in such a way that the diagnosis of the index cases is confirmed independently by at least two investigators, the diagnosis of relatives is also made by at least two people, and the diagnosticians should not know whether the subject under evaluation is a relative of an index or control case. Even better, they should not know which diagnostic entity is under study.

One possible way to reduce the amount of bias is to use a standardized questionnaire which the investigator follows precisely with respect to every subject interviewed. This method, however, has its limitations in that it cannot anticipate all manner of symptoms or behaviors in all subjects, and may inhibit spontaneity and full communication on the part of the respondent. Sometimes, too, the interviewer believes he does not get as much of a "feel" about the subject as he would like. If he wishes to rate observed behavior in addition to the verbal report of the respondent, the latter's range of behavior is likely to be restricted by a formal-questionnaire method of interviewing.

The relatively low reliability of diagnoses obtained in the studies just cited suggests that the standard diagnostic categories may not be the unit characters that we are looking for. However, the genetic studies—with their sundry faults—provide strong evidence for the view that schizophrenia and manic-depressive psychosis are valid, distinctive, genetic disorders and that unless future studies provide evidence to the contrary, it would be foolhardy to dismiss them out of hand. However, the diagnostic categories might possibly be refined through the use of factor-analytic techniques. Several studies have been carried out in which hospitalized populations were rated for presence or absence of various symptoms, the ratings intercorrelated, and various factors abstracted. Although the factors vary somewhat from study to study, by and large they provide support for the schizophrenic–manic-depressive distinction, although mania and depressive psychosis may turn up as different factors.   Whether factors so obtained would be useful in evaluating relatives would remain to be seen.   No such study has been attempted as yet.   The factors obtained from assessments of hospitalized patients could apply to only a small fraction of all relatives.   However, if such a study revealed factorial similarities between probands and relatives, this finding would both justify the use of factor-analytic methods as possible indicators of unit characters and support the view that such unit characters are genetically based.

Another advance in methodology that is only beginning to be exploited involves the use of psychological tests along with other measures of psychophysiological and biological functioning.   With such methods, the subjective impressions of the investigators become less critical and the possibility of defining clearly and quantifying the unit characters increases considerably.

TWIN STUDIES

Since twin studies have such saliency and often provide the best evidence we have regarding the heritability of a disorder, it is worth reiterating a few precautions regarding the interpretation of findings obtained from twins.   The validity of comparisons between MZ and DZ twins depends on the assumptions that the two types of twins are not essentially different from the single-born population or from one another, and that intrapair environmental differences are the same for the two types of twins.   There is a growing body of evidence that these assumptions may not be entirely correct.   Some studies show that twins learn to talk later than single borns, and some suggest that a population of twins has a somewhat reduced IQ as compared with a population of singletons.   Psychologists and psychiatrists, especially psychoanalysts, who have studied both types of twins intensively, have reported psychological mechanisms and traits that differ in the two types of twins. In the previous chapter, we cited the findings of Eysenck and Prell, who came up with the surprising finding that MZ twins had higher scores on a lie scale than did DZ twins, and that the MZ group had greater numbers of pairs who were more extremely stable and more extremely unstable than the DZ pairs, whereas the mean scores did not discriminate the two groups at all.   Such findings support the clinical impressions of important differences between the two types of twins.

Additional words of caution come from R. C. Nichols (1966), who collected abundant data from large numbers of twins of high school age.   Nichols was interested in the heritability of a wide variety of behaviors and personality traits, as well as intelligence.   He reported:

"Identical twins were more similar than were fraternal twins on almost all the measures used, but three troublesome findings prevent us from interpreting this to mean that heredity is necessarily an important factor for most dimensions of personality and interest." The three findings were:

1 "The failure to find agreement between the results for boys and those for girls."

2 "The sheer size of the differences in similarity between the two kinds of twins. The many values of HR (the ratio of the hereditary variance to the hereditary plus the common environmental variance) *greater* than 1.0 could not have been produced by the simple additive effects of hereditary factors alone."

3 "The lack of agreement with results obtained by others."

Correlations of h^2 values for 18 personality traits as assessed by self-rating scales were actually somewhat *negative* when Nichols compared his results with those of another investigator. He thought most of the variance in his data was error that in turn was associated with random events that were probably more common for both members of MZ than DZ pairs.

Now, there are studies that provide strong evidence for the heritability of some personality characteristics, most notably those of Freedman (1967), but we must be wary about jumping to conclusions from evidence obtained in the usual kind of twin study alone. Some of the same factors that made for the interpretational difficulties in Nichols' study could possibly also apply to studies of the behavioral disorders.

Another study that should give us pause was reported by Wilde (1964). He found that DZ twins living apart more than five years were more alike with respect to neurotic instability and test-taking attitude than DZ twins living together. Correlations for DZ twins living apart were .64 and .49 respectively, $P < 0.01$, but on five different personality measures, DZ twins reared together did not correlate at a level significantly above zero. In the past, it has always been assumed that rearing apart means rearing in environments that differ more, so that if the rearing environment plays any etiological role at all, twins who are reared apart should differ more than twins who are reared together. From a psychological point of view, this is a most inadequate way to conceptualize the environment. Wilde's study suggests that, at least with DZ twins, their common association during their growing-up years may be a more relevant variable with respect to their similarity or dissimilarity than is the household in which they live. It also suggests that DZ twins might tend to polarize themselves psychologically so that natural differences between them tend to be increased.

On the other hand, a common rearing of MZ twins could possibly increase their similarity rather than their dissimilarity. Wilde found that MZ twins living together correlated .58 regarding extraversion, $P < 0.01$, whereas MZ twins living apart for 5+ years correlated .19, which was not significantly above zero. The possibility exists that a common rearing could influence MZ and DZ twins in opposite directions with respect to a number of variables, and on this ground alone we should exercise caution in evaluating intrapair differences in MZ and DZ twins. One of the most important contributions that future research can make is to define in the best traditions of psychology the environmental variables that are relevant and influential with respect to the possible development of behavioral disorder in differently vulnerable individuals. The determination of such variables will require special research designs and studies.

In this regard, let us take one more look at the logic of the classical twin-study research design. We select MZ and DZ twins because heredity is the independent variable that we wish to study. In the case of the MZ twins, heredity is the same for both. With respect to DZ twins, heredity of the effective, relevant genetic factor varies between members of a pair to the extent that it involves aneuploidy or a dominant, recessive, or polygenic mode of transmission. Thus, we design the experiment so as to achieve greater intrapair genetic variation in one type of twin as compared with the other. However, with respect to the potentially effective, relevant environmental variable, whatever it might be, we make no effort to increase its variation in one of the two types of twins relative to the other. That is, we do not treat it as a systematically varied and controlled independent variable, but rather we permit it to be randomly distributed across both groups. Such a design virtually assures that heredity will account for more of the variance regarding a particular phenotype than any particular environmental variable. Thus, heredity may appear to be "more important" than environment regarding the phenotype in question.

In the opposite vein, if we study only discordant MZ twins, we do not permit heredity to vary at all, so that all the known variation within pairs regarding any phenotype must be due to variation of nongenetic factors. Thus, even the uncontrolled or randomly distributed environmental factors may seem to be "more important" than hereditary factors. Ideally, at least with respect to the behavioral disorders, we should like to have studies in which both the genetic and relevant environmental variables are systematically varied with regard to one another to evaluate their relative and interactional contributions to the phenotype in question. Perhaps the best illustration of this point is to be found in the section on alcoholism. There we had two excellent studies that seemed to lead to opposite conclusions. The classical twin study by Kaij yielded findings that led him to conclude that alcoholism was greatly influenced by genetic factors. The classical adoption study by Roe led her to conclude that rearing factors were critical with respect to the development of alcoholism. Kaij controlled the genetic variables and let the environmental factors vary "randomly" across both twin groups. Roe controlled for environmental variables—especially with respect to ratings of the quality of household and foster rearing—as well as the genetic variable and concluded that environmental factors predominated with respect to whether alcoholism did or did not occur. The counterposed methods of study and conclusions provide pointed evidence for the philosophical dictum that there is no true separation of means and ends, in science as in life.

SEX DIFFERENCES

With respect to schizophrenia, both sexes appear to be affected equally, although males tend to be admitted to hospitals at earlier ages. In manic-depressive psychosis, females tend to be admitted earlier. Moreover, females have manic-depressive psychosis, affective disorder, and psychoneurosis more frequently than males, whereas there is a preponderance of males with psychopathy and criminality, homosexuality, and alcoholism. With respect to suicide, women attempt suicide more often than men, but men actually commit suicide more often than women, are older than female suicides, use more violent methods, and are less often diagnosed as depressed (Davis, 1968). Do these sex differences betoken different but specific genetic mechanisms in the various disorders? Do they reflect hormonal differences deriving from an XX as compared to an XY constitution? Or do they reflect cultural influences that prescribe different behavioral patterns for the two sexes?

To hypothesize a specific sex-linked genetic mechanism for each disorder invites not only multiple hypotheses, but these would have to be modified, each in turn, to account for secondary aspects of the disorder such as age at "onset" or first admission. Such theorizing becomes unparsimonious. The hormonal and cultural theories could account nicely for the various sex findings considered together. Males are biologically more aggressive than females, and the culture reinforces this aggressive-passive distinction between the sexes. The heredity-environment interaction here appears to be that of augmentation. Females beset by psychological stresses or disturbing conflicts should be more prone to inhibit aggressive responses, which could in turn lead to increased depressions or psychoneurotic manifestations and less violent suicidal attempts, whereas afflicted males might experience increased disinhibition of aggressive, rebellious behavior and resort to more antisocial and violent acts.

With respect to schizophrenia, the picture is less clear. Many investigators have considered schizophrenia to be primarily a postpubescent disorder that is linked somehow to the hormonal changes that occur with adulthood. Some indirect evidence for this viewpoint was provided by Rosenbaum (1968), as shown in Figure 10-1.

Rosenbaum noted a remarkable similarity between age-at-first-admission curves for schizophrenia and age-orgasm frequency curves regarding the two sexes. The curves are plotted together to show the striking parallels. Orgasms before age ten were considered to be zero,

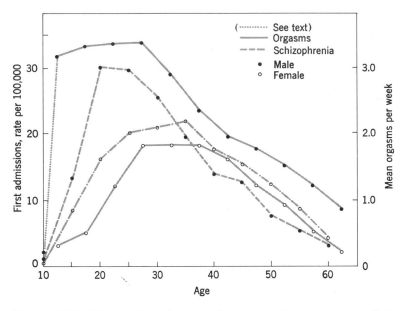

Figure 10-1. The relation between frequency of orgasms and first admissions for schizophrenia in males and females, according to age. (From C. P. Rosenbaum, Metabolic, physiological, anatomic and genetic studies in the schizophrenias: A review and analysis, *J. Nervous Mental Disease*, 1968, **146**. Reprinted with permission of C. P. Rosenbaum, M.D., and The Williams & Wilkins Company, Baltimore.)

and the part of the orgasm curve between ages ten and fifteen is drawn as a straight line to reflect this warranted assumption. The orgasm curves are based on the reports of Kinsey et al. (1948, 1953). The first-admission curves for schizophrenia are based on the previously cited data of Landis and Page. Rosenbaum drew the inference that the parallel curves represented a probable interaction of factors—hormonal, psychological, and environmental—and that these "can lead to behavior which varies from being predominantly sexual to predominantly schizophrenic." Research to date has failed to turn up any primary disturbance of sex-hormone metabolism in schizophrenics. Since the factor probably underlying the parallel curves is one that must be common to both schizophrenia and sexual behavior, we can infer that it may concern something akin to "sex drive," which in turn could have an hormonal basis.

MATING PATTERNS

Much of the genetic analysis and theorizing regarding behavioral disorders has assumed that random mating occurs with respect to them. Even a casual look at married couples would suggest that the assumption does not hold with respect to a variety of traits, such as intelligence, social class, height, and so on. The same is probably true for personality factors and mental disorders. Kreitman (1968) found 74 married couples who had been inpatients in mental hospitals at some time during their lives. Among them, 42 percent had the same diagnosis. Concordance rates were 45.7 percent for manic-depressive illness, 30.8 percent for personality disorder, 17.4 percent for schizophrenia, and 23.1 percent for neurosis. Among the 43 couples who became ill after marriage, 44 percent had the same diagnosis. Thus, the concordances could reflect true assortative mating as well as the effects of a common association. In fact, future studies of behavioral disorders should make it a point to examine both marital partners carefully to ascertain their common behavioral and personality characteristics as well as their diagnoses to see what bearing such concordances might have with respect to the characteristics of their children. For example, most schizophrenics do not have a parent who has been hospitalized for schizophrenia, but intensive examination often reveals mild to severe behavioral and personality disturbances in both parents. Investigators who attempt to calculate frequencies of the assumed pathological genes in different populations will have to take into account that assortative mating with re-

spect to the disorder under study is probably occurring in more or
less degree.

BIOLOGICAL FITNESS

We have seen that in at least four major types of disorder—schizophrenia, manic-depressive psychosis, psychopathy, and homosexuality, biological fitness or fertility is reduced, but no evidence exists to indicate
that the incidence of these disorders has declined.   Each disorder seems
to involve a genetic component, but in each we may well be dealing
with polygenic systems or with genetic heterogeneity.   A small fraction
of the cases involves aneuploidies that may occur at a constant rate,
but these alone could not explain the probable lack of a declining incidence.   Genetic mutations at multiple loci could occur at rates that
would not be unusually high yet would be sufficient to maintain the
incidence of the disorder, but the likelihood is that one would probably
have to assume a large number of loci for such a common disorder.   Possibly, too, the implicated environmental stresses in these disorders may
be increasing sufficiently to produce clinical cases in sufficient numbers
to compensate for the gene loss due to reduced fitness.   According to
the latter view, the contribution of genetic factors to such disorders
would be decreasing, whereas that of environmental factors would be
increasing.   We have no clear evidence of such a changing balance,
especially since genetic selection would be so slow.
    Let us consider another possibility.   Let us begin with the hypothe-
sis that in man, as in many other species, a group of individuals tends
to organize itself in a dominance hierachy.   The dominance may be
physical, perhaps involving strength or attractiveness, sexual or social,
explicit or implicit.   Let us assume too that such organization fulfills
a selective function with respect to evolution in that dominance is correlated with fitness.   Those who are dominant are more likely to survive
and reproduce than those who are not.   Individuals at the bottom rungs
of the dominance ladder have the lowest fitness and are subject to the
most obnoxious, rejecting, and derogating behavior by themselves or
by other members of the group.   Although age factors play a role in
this process, it is peer relationships with which we are essentially concerned.   There is a general need to fit somewhere in the peer hierarchy
and we assume that individuals are always trying to find a self-satisfying
rank order in it for themselves.   The lowest rank of all is complete
extrusion from the group.
    Now we make the likely assumption that individuals have geneti-
cally conditioned characteristics which contribute significantly to the

position in the group hierarchy that they are able to attain. We also assume that the ones who either objectively or subjectively find themselves at the lowest rungs of the ladder can react in various ways. They may resignedly accept their fate, withdraw physically, emotionally, or cognitively, become depressed by their failure and lowliness, strike out blindly in rebellion against the oppressive social organization, flout the group mores, or act out their consigned role of submissiveness through passive sexuality, impotence, or other sexual deviancy, or with some combination of such behaviors. The particular kind of response reflects the combination of genetic and experiential factors that is each one's lot. Each generation establishes its own dominance hierarchy, and in each generation it is those at the lowest rungs of the ladder who have the lowest fitness. In this way there occurs a gradual weeding out—up to a point—of those who are least well equipped genetically to exist in a complex socially organized group life, and a gradual improvement of the species with respect to adaptability to group living. For each generation, the proportion of the entire group occupying the lowest rungs of the subjective or objective hierarchy is constant, and so the morbidity rate overall shows no appreciable change.

This fleeting sketch is proposed not so much as a theory, but as an illustration of how we might account for a constant morbidity rate in the face of a presumptive gene loss. Nevertheless, such a model, and others drawn in the same mode, at least possess the scientific virtue that they can probably be subjected to empirical study, and either accepted or found wanting.

MENTAL ILLNESS:
ONE, MANY, OR NONE?

Earlier we pointed out that many workers in the mental health field wish to do away with psychiatric classification schemes or diagnostic categories on the ground that they have no essential meaningfulness or that they merely represent degrees of a single entity, which can be called mental illness. Others go even farther and repudiate the medical model entirely, saying that behavioral disorders do not represent anything that can be called an illness or a disease, but are simply patterns of adjustment or learned reaction to various kinds of life experiences. Nosologists, many clinical psychiatrists, some clinical psychologists, and virtually all workers in the field of psychiatric genetics believe that the different diagnostic groups are different diseases with distinct and separate genetic and metabolic bases. Who is correct?

Based on our summary of the literature, we are led to the view that schizophrenia and manic-depressive psychosis may well be different mental illnesses. Their clinical pictures can be sharply discriminated, even though there are disorders, called schizo-affective, which have some clinical features of each. Each seems to represent the endpoint of a gradation or spectrum of clinical-behavioral manifestations that are genetically linked. In German, the term for such a spectrum is *Erbkreis*, or circle of heredity, a term that describes the concept well. Not only are the clinical features distinctive, but the clinical course and outcome for each is fairly predictable. Moreover, therapeutic measures affect the two groups differently. For example, electroconvulsive shock is virtually a specific for the affective disorders, achieving a high yield of remissions, whereas it seems to have little beneficial effect with schizophrenics. In addition, the two groups respond differently to different drugs. Lithium salts, for example, are reported to have a strikingly ameliorative effect on patients in manic excitement, and also help to keep cyclical cases on a more even keel. This drug, however, has little therapeutic effect with most schizophrenics. Antidepressant drugs are often effective in alleviating depression but tend to make schizophrenics worse. On the other hand, drugs called phenothiazines have been effective in calming schizophrenics, making them more accessible, and permitting many to take up life in the community. The schizophrenic subtypes, in turn, respond somewhat differently to different phenothiazines.

None of these points alone is conclusive, yet when they are considered together, one must be impressed by their combined weight. With respect to the genetic contribution to this general picture, we hope that in future studies diagnosticians will heed the methodological precautions that we have urged at several places in this book. If indeed studies using blind diagnostic procedures support the findings of earlier studies, confidence in the two separate diseases formulation will probably increase sharply. But if they fail to provide support, the basic foundation for the formulation crumbles.

With respect to whether the other behavioral disorders reviewed here should be thought of as separate diseases, the picture is less clear. Some neuroses are probably in the Erbkreis of either schizophrenia or manic-depressive psychosis. For example, some obsessive-compulsive, anxiety, and depersonalization neuroses may be in the schizophrenic spectrum, whereas reactive and neurotic depressions appear to belong genetically in the spectrum of affective disorders. Some psychoneuroses seem not to involve any specific genetic mechanism, although some diathetic types may be more likely to develop some kinds of neurosis rather than others. However, life experiences provide critical factors for such individuals. Nor do we have any reason to assume that psychopathy or homosexuality are distinct diseases. We saw that psychopathic behavior could be associated with several different diatheses, and there are as yet no positive findings of genital or hormonal abnormalities in most homosexuals. For the time being, these disorders are better thought of as behavioral syndromes. A variable number of cases may simply involve learned behavioral patterns.

The disease controversy with regard to alcoholism will undoubtedly continue until such time as a metabolic abnormality or deficiency may be found in affected individuals. The data on the genetics of this disorder indicate that a wide variety of genetic and nongenetic disorders are associated with alcoholism, and this fact reduces one's confidence in finding a specific metabolic abnormality. However, animal studies show strain differences in alcohol preference or tolerance, and if similar differences occur in man, an individual with such preference could readily increase his intake under stress or habit until withdrawal problems occur. At this point, the individual is clearly a medical problem, as in other addictions, and the condition clearly fits the generally accepted definitions of a disease.

Part of the disease-nondisease controversy may arise because of differing conceptualizations regarding the implications of genetic influences on behavior generally, and on abnormal behavior particularly. Some people seem to believe that heredity is synonymous with predetermination, inevitability, and immutability. This is of course not so, especially with regard to behavior. There is many a step—genetic, constitutional, and environmental—between the genotype and the phenotype. Almost everyone can learn, and learning can modify and shape behavior. A severely mentally retarded or autistic child can be taught many things if one uses the appropriate techniques. However, their ability to learn does not signify that the retardation is less or the autism learned. An individual may suffer serious brain damage, and he may later learn or relearn many skills, but he is still brain-damaged.

What heredity seems to do—metabolic considerations aside—is to restrict the range and modulation of responses that an individual evinces under usual living conditions, or to make some responses more probable than others. The degree of genetic determination is associated with the degree of restriction or probability of response. Thus, a child may have a tendency to be shy and avoid people. The probability of such behavior occurring may well be associated with genetic factors. The likelihood of shy behavior occurring is negatively correlated with the likelihood that other types of behavior will occur. But environmental conditions can also be arranged to restrict one's range of responses and to make some responses more probable than others. By appropriate measures, we may help the shy child to expand his range of behaviors and perhaps even make responses other than shyness the more probable ones. We do not in the process change the child's predisposition to shyness, but we do change his behavior. However, we need to know more about what these diatheses are and what kinds of constraints they tend to impose on the individual's behavior, and we may then be able to design better environmental regimens to help him learn to modify undesirable behavior patterns. In the process, we may generate more precise conceptions of how humans behave, and why they behave in ways that we call abnormal.

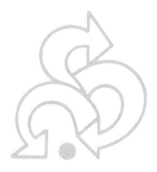

Glossary of Genetic Terms

Adaptation. The adjustment of an organism or a population to an environment.

Alleles, or allelomorphs. Alternative forms of a gene occurring at the same locus on homologous chromosomes.

Anaphase. The stage of cell division when the chromosomes leave the equatorial plate and migrate to opposite poles of the spindle.

Aneuploidy. A condition in which the number of chromosomes is not an exact multiple of the monoploid or basic number; for example, $2n - 1$ or $2n + 1$ chromosomes would be aneuploid.

Assortative mating. Nonrandom mating. High-IQ people marrying high-IQ people is an example of assortative mating.

Autosome. Any chromosome other than a sex chromosome.

Balanced polymorphism. The equal weighting of positive- and negative-selection effects in two or more genotypes.

Chromosomes. The threadlike, deep-staining nucleoprotein bodies which carry the genes.

Concordant. Having the same characteristic or trait.

Crossing over. The exchange of genetic material between homologous chromosomes.

Dihybrid. An individual who is heterozygous with respect to two pairs of alleles.

Diploid. Refers to a cell or organism with two sets of chromosomes, or two genomes.

Discordance. Dissimilarity between two individuals in that one has the trait or characteristic in question and the other does not.

Dizygotic twins. Fraternal twins, produced by the fertilization of two eggs by two different sperms.

DNA. Deoxyribonucleic acid, in which the genetic information is coded.

Dominant trait. A trait that is expressed in individuals who are heterozygous or homozygous for a particular gene.

Dual mating. Mating of two spouses who have the same trait or characteristic.

Epistasis. The suppression of gene action by a gene or genes not alleles of those suppressed.

Expressivity. The degree or severity of expression of a trait controlled by a particular gene.

Fitness, biological. Refers to the number of offspring reaching maturity. Two such offspring constitute a fitness of 100 percent, or unity.

Gamete. A mature germ cell, sperm, or egg.

Gene. A unit particle of DNA, or a unit of heredity with a fixed location on a given chromosome.

Genotype. The genetic constitution, or makeup, of an individual.

Haploid, or monoploid. Refers to a cell or organism containing one set of chromosomes, or one genome, as in a gamete.

Hardy-Weinberg law. The law, shown mathematically by Hardy and Weinberg, that alleles segregating in a population tend to establish an equilibrium with reference to each other.

Heritability. The proportion of the total variation regarding a given characteristic that is accounted for by genetic factors.

Heterozygous. Possessing two different alleles at a particular locus on a pair of homologous chromosomes.

Homologous chromosomes. Chromosomes which pair during meiosis, similar in size and shape, one coming from the male and one from the female parent.

Homozygous. Possessing two identical alleles at a particular locus on a pair of homologous chromosomes.

Index case (also *proband* or *propositus*). One of the starting cases who possesses the trait under study.

Intermediate inheritance. A pattern of inheritance in which the heterozygote's phenotype is distinguishable from those of both homozygotes.

Interphase. The stage in the cell cycle when the cell is not dividing, that is, after telophase of one cell division and before prophase of the next division. In this phase the normal metabolic processes of the cell proceed.

Inversion. A chromosomal abnormality in which one segment of a chromosome is reversed.

Karyotype. The chromosome set of an individual as shown by a photomicrograph of a somatic cell in which the number, size, and shape of the chromosomes are displayed.

Lethal gene. A gene that renders a cell or an organism inviable.

Linkage. Genes whose loci occur in different places on the same chromosome are said to be linked.

Locus. The position or site of a gene on a chromosome.

Meiosis. The type of cell division that results in the formation of gametes in animals.

Metaphase. The stage of mitosis or meiosis during which the chromosomes line up on the equatorial plate and the nuclear membrane disappears.

Mitosis. Somatic cell division which results in the formation of two cells, each having the same complement of chromosomes as the parent or the parent cell.

Modifier, or modifying gene. A gene that affects the expression of a nonallelic gene.

Monohybrid cross. A cross between two parents in which only one trait is being considered.

Monoploid, or haploid. Having a single set of chromosomes, or one genome.

Monosomy. A condition in which one chromosome of a pair is missing; the individual has one less than the diploid number of chromosomes $(2n - 1)$.

Monozygotic twins. Twins derived from a single fertilized ovum, commonly called identical twins.

Mosaicism. A condition in which part of the individual's tissue or cells is genetically or chromosomally different from other parts of his tissue or from other cells.

Multifactorial inheritance (also called *multiple-factor inheritance, quantitative inheritance,* or *polygenic inheritance*). Inheritance controlled by many genes with small additive effects.

Mutation. A sudden change in the genetic material of an organism, usually of a single gene. A gametic mutation is inherited; a mutation in a somatic cell is not inherited.

Mutation rate. The number of mutations at a single locus which occur per gamete per generation.

Nondisjunction. The failure of homologous chromosomes to separate during anaphase so that both pass to the same daughter cell.

Pedigree. A diagrammatic representation of one's ancestral history.

Penetrance. The proportion of individuals with a particular genotype that manifests the corresponding phenotype.

Phenocopy. An environmentally caused trait or characteristic that resembles one which is genetically caused.

Phenotype. The appearance of an individual arising from his genotype in interaction with his environment.

Pleiotropy. Instances in which a single gene influences more than one trait, or has multiple effects.

Polygene. One of a number of genes involved in the quantitative inheritance of a trait or characteristic.

Position effect. A difference in phenotype that is related to the position of a gene or genes relative to other genes.

Proband. See *Index case.*

Prophase. The first visible stage of cell division in which the chromosomes contract and thicken.

Propositus. See *Index case.*

Quantitative inheritance. See *Multifactorial inheritance.*

Recessive. Strictly speaking, refers to a trait; less precisely, refers to a gene. A recessive trait is not expressed in individuals who are heterozygous for a given gene but is expressed in the homozygote.

RNA. Ribonucleic acid, which is a nucleic acid formed upon a DNA template and found mainly in the nucleolus and ribosomes.

Segregation. The separation of paternal and maternal chromosomes or alleles during meiosis; Mendel's first principle of inheritance.

Sex linkage. Inheritance of a trait stemming from genes on the sex chromosomes, especially the X chromosome.

Telophase. The last stage of cell division in mitosis when the chromosomes have completely separated into two groups, each in its own nuclear membrane.

Threshold character. A trait dependent upon the additive effects of multiple genes, but whose characteristics may appear to be discontinuous or quasi-continuous in that the phenotype shows apparent discontinuity.

Translocation. The transfer of genetic material from one chromosome to a nonhomologous chromosome.

Trisomy. A condition in which there is one extra chromosome per cell so that one particular chromosome occurs three times rather than twice.

Zygote. The cell resulting from the union of a maternal and paternal gamete.

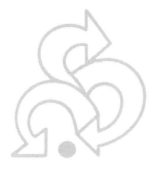

References

GENERAL REFERENCES

Readers who are interested in having a broader introduction to the basic concepts of evolution can find many good books on the subject with little difficulty. Here are a few suggestions:

Darwin, Charles: *The Origin of Species,* Great Books of the Western World, vol. 49, Encyclopaedia Britannica, Inc., Chicago, 1955, pp. 1–252.
——— : *The Descent of Man,* Great Books of the Western World, vol. 49, Encyclopaedia Britannica, Inc., Chicago, 1955, pp. 253–600.
Dobzhansky, T.: *Evolution, Genetics, and Man,* John Wiley & Sons, Inc., New York, 1955, 398 pp.
———: *Mankind Evolving,* Yale University Press, New Haven and London, 1962, 381 pp.
Huxley, J.: *The Living Thoughts of Darwin,* Fawcett World Library, New York, 1963, 176 pp.
Simpson, G. G.: *The Meaning of Evolution: A Study of the History of Life and of Its Significance for Man,* Yale University Press, New Haven, 1949, 364 pp.
———: *The Major Features of Evolution,* Columbia University Press, New York, 1953, 434 pp.
Tax, S. (ed.): *Evolution after Darwin,* University of Chicago Press, Chicago, 1960, 3 vols.:
Vol. 1, *The Evolution of Life: Its Origin, History, and Future,* 629 pp.
Vol. 2, *The Evolution of Man: Man, Culture, and Society,* 473 pp.
Vol. 3, *Issues in Evolution* (edited with C. Callender), 310 pp.

Readers who wish to have a broader introduction to genetics can also find
a wide selection of helpful textbooks. Some suggested references are:

Asimov, I.: *The Genetic Code,* Signet Books, New American Library, Inc.,
New York, 1962, 187 pp.
Ebert, J. D., with F. E. Sampson, Jr.: Gene expression, *Bull. Neurosci. Res.
Progr.,* 1967, **5**(3):223–306.
Falconer, D. S.: *Introduction to Quantitative Genetics,* The Ronald Press
Company, New York, 1960, 365 pp.
Fuller, J. L., and W. R. Thompson: *Behavior Genetics,* John Wiley & Sons, Inc.,
New York, 1960, 396 pp.
Gardner, E. J.: *Principles of Genetics,* John Wiley & Sons, Inc., New York,
1960, 386 pp.
Li, C. C.: *Human Genetics: Principles and Methods,* McGraw-Hill Book
Company, New York, 1961, 218 pp.
Neel, J. V., and W. J. Schull: *Human Heredity,* University of Chicago Press,
Chicago, 1954, 361 pp.
Stern, C.: *Principles of Human Genetics,* W. H. Freeman and Company,
San Francisco, 1960, 753 pp.
Whittingill, M.: *Human Genetics and Its Foundations,* Reinhold Publishing
Corporation, New York, 1965, 431 pp.

Readers who would like to learn more about the history of psychiatry and
psychiatric nosology will find the following references helpful:

Alexander, F. G., and S. T. Selesnick: *The History of Psychiatry,* Harper and
Row, Publishers, Incorporated, New York, 1966.
American Psychiatric Association: *Diagnostic and Statistical Manual of Mental
Disorder,* New York, 1952.
Goshen, D. E. (ed.): *Documentary History of Psychiatry,* Philosophical
Library, Inc., New York, 1967.
Menninger, K., with Martin Mayman and Paul Pruyser: *The Vital Balance,* The
Viking Press, Inc., New York, 1963.
Zilboorg, G.: *A History of Medical Psychology,* W. W. Norton & Company, Inc.,
New York, 1941.

Readers who would like an entree into the literature on the genetics of the
diseases cited in Chapter 5 will do well to consult the following articles:

Phenylketonuria
Jervis, G. A.: The genetics of phenylpyruvic oligophrenia, *J. Mental Sci.,* 1939,
85:719–762.
Lang, K.: Die Phenylpyruvische Oligophrenie, in *Ergebnisse der inneren
Medizin und Kinderheilkunde,* Springer-Verlag OHG, Berlin-Gottingen-
Heidelberg, 1955, vol. 6, pp. 78–99.
Perry, T. L., Bluma Tischler, and J. A. Chapple: The incidence of mental

illnesses in the relatives of individuals suffering from phenylketonuria or mongolism, *J. Psychiat. Res.*, 1966, **4**:51–57.

Stewart, Janet M., and C. G. Ashley: Phenylketonuria: Report of the Oregon detection and evaluation program, *Journal-Lancet*, 1967, **87**:162–166.

Huntington's chorea

Chandler, J. H., T. E. Reed, and R. N. DeJong: Huntington's chorea in Michigan: III.   Clinical observations, *Neurology*, 1960, **10**:148–153.

Goodman, R. M., C. L. Hall, L. Terango, G. A. Perrine, Jr., and Patricia L. Roberts: Huntington's chorea: A multidisciplinary study of affected parents and first generation offspring, *Arch. Neurol.*, 1966, **15**:345–355.

Heathfield, K. W. G.: Huntington's chorea: Investigation into the prevalence of this disease in the area covered by the North East Metropolitan Regional Hospital Board, *Brain*, 1967, **90**:203–232.

Down's syndrome

Allen, G., and G. S. Baroff: Mongoloid twins and their siblings, *Acta Genet.*, 1955, **5**:294–326.

McDonald, A. D.: Mongolism in twins, *J. Med. Genet.*, 1964, **1**:39–41.

Penrose, L. S.: Mongolism, *Brit. Med. Bull.*, 1961, **17**:184–189.

Turner's syndrome

Alexander, D., A. A. Ehrhardt, and J. Money: Defective figure drawing, geometric and human, in Turner's syndrome, *J. Nervous Mental Disease*, 1966, **142**:161–167.

de la Chapelle, A.: Cytogenetical and clinical observations in female gonadal dysgenesis, *Acta Endocrinol., Suppl.* 65, 1962, **40**:1–122.

Kinch, R. A. H., E. R. Plunkett, M. S. Smout, and D. H. Carr: Primary ovarian failure: A clinicopathological and cytogenetic study, *Am. J. Obstet. Gynecol.*, 1965, **91**:630–644.

Klinefelter's syndrome

Barr, M. L., Evelyn L. Shaver, D. H. Carr, and E. R. Plunkett: The chromatin-positive Klinefelter syndrome among patients in mental deficiency hospitals, *J. Mental Deficiency Res.*, 1960, **4**:89–107.

Klinefelter, H. F., Jr., E. C. Reifenstein, Jr., and F. Albright: Syndrome characterized by gynecomastia, aspermatogenesis without aleydigism, and increased excretion of follicle stimulating hormone, *J. Clin. Endocrinol. Metab.*, 1942, **2**:615–627.

Rohde, R. A.: Chromatin-positive Klinefelter's syndrome: Clinical and cytogenetic studies, *J. Chron. Diseases*, 1963, **16**:1139–1149.

Diabetes mellitus

Conn, J. W., and S. S. Fajans: The prediabetic state, *Am. J. Med.*, 1961, **31**:839–850.

Hanhart, E.: Die erbliche Anlage der Zuckerkrankheit, heutiger Stand, *Deut. Z. Verdauungskr.*, 1953, **13**:145–147.

Kubany, A. J., T. S. Danowski, and C. Moses: The personality and intelligence of diabetics, *Diabetes*, 1956, **5**:462–467.

Neel, J. V., S. S. Fajans, J. W. Conn, and Ruth T. Davidson: Diabetes mellitus, in J. V. Neel, Margery W. Shaw, and W. J. Schull (eds.), *Genetics and the Epidemiology of Chronic Diseases*, U.S. Department of Health, Education, and Welfare, PHS, Division of Chronic Diseases, Washington, D.C., 1965, pp. 105–132.

Pincus, G., and Priscilla White: On the inheritance of diabetes mellitus: I. An analysis of 675 family histories, *Am. J. Med. Sci.*, 1933, **186**:1–14.

Rimoin, D. L.: Genetics of diabetes mellitus, *Diabetes*, 1967, **16**:346–351.

TEXT REFERENCES

Alanen, Y. O.: The mothers of schizophrenic patients, *Acta Psychiat. Neurol. Scand.*, Suppl. 124, 1958, **33**.

———, in collaboration with J. K. Rekola, A. Stewen, K. Takala, and M. Tuovinen: The family in the pathogenesis of schizophrenic and neurotic disorders, *Acta Psychiat. Scand.*, Suppl. 189, 1966, **42**.

Allen, G., B. Harvald, and J. Shields: Measures of twin concordance, *Acta Genet.*, 1967, **17**:475–481.

Åmark, C.: A study in alcoholism, *Acta Psychiat. Neurol. Scand.*, Suppl. 70, 1951.

Angst, J.: Zur Ätiologie und Nosologie endogener depressiver Psychosen, *Monograph. Gesamtgeb. Neurol. Psychiat. (Berlin)*, 1966, **112**.

Anthony, E. J.: The developmental precursors of adult schizophrenia, in D. Rosenthal and S. S. Kety (eds.), *The Transmission of Schizophrenia*, Pergamon Press, London, 1968, pp. 293–316.

Asano, N.: Clinico-genetic study of manic-depressive psychoses, in H. Mitsuda (ed.), *Clinical Genetics in Psychiatry*, Igaku Shoin, Tokyo, 1967, pp. 262–275.

Ash, P.: The reliability of psychiatric diagnoses, *J. Abnormal Soc. Psychol.*, 1949, **44**:272–276.

Bakwin, H.: Early infantile autism, *J. Pediat.*, 1954, **45**:492–497.

Banse, J.: Zum Problem der Erbprognosebestimmung, *Z. Ges. Neurol. Psychiat.*, 1929, **119**:576–612.

Bender, Lauretta: Childhood schizophrenia, *Nervous Child*, 1942, **1**:138–141.

———: Childhood schizophrenia, *Psychiat. Quart.*, 1953, **27**:663–681.

———: Twenty years of research of schizophrenic children with special reference to those under six years of age, in G. Caplan (ed.), *Emotional Problems of Early Childhood*, Basic Books, Inc., Publishers, New York, 1955, pp. 503–519.

———: Treatment of juvenile schizophrenia, in *Neurology and Psychiatry in Childhood*, The Williams and Wilkins Company, Baltimore, 1956, pp. 462–477.

———: The concept of pseudopsychopathic schizophrenia in adolescents, *Am. J. Orthopsychiat.*, 1959, **29**:491–512.

———: Childhood schizophrenia and convulsive states, in *Recent Advances in Biological Psychiatry*, 1961, 3:96–103.

———: Mental illness in childhood and heredity, *Eugenics Quart.*, 1963, 10:1–11.

——— and A. M. Freedman: A study of the first three years in the maturation of schizophrenic children, *Quart. J. Child Behavior*, 1952, 1:245–272.

——— and A. E. Grugett: A study of certain epidemiological factors in a group of children with childhood schizophrenia, *Am. J. Orthopsychiat.*, 1956, 26:131–145.

Benedict, P. K., and I. Jacks: Mental illness in primitive societies, *Psychiatry*, 1954, 17:377–390.

Bille, M., and N. Juel-Nielsen: Incidence of neurosis in psychiatric and other medical services in a Danish county, *Danish Med. Bull.*, 1963, 10:172–176.

Bleuler, E.: Primäre und sekundäre Symptome der Schizophrenie, *Z. Ges. Neurol. Psychiat.*, 1930, 124:607–646.

———: *Dementia Praecox or the Group of Schizophrenias*, International Universities Press, Inc., New York, 1950.

Bleuler, M.: *Vererbungsprobleme* bei Schizophrenen, *Z. Ges. Neurol. Psychiat.*, 1930, 127:321–388.

———: Psychotische Belastung von körperlich Kranken, *Z. Ges. Neurol. Psychiat.*, 1932, 142:780–810.

———: Krankheitsverlauf, Persönlichkeit und Verwandtshaft Schizophrener und ihre gegenseitigen Beziehungen, in *Sammlung Psychiatrischer und Neurologischer Einzeldarstellungen*, vol. 16, Georg Thieme Verlag, Leipzig, 1941.

———: Familial and personal background of chronic alcoholics, in O. Diethelm (ed.), *Etiology of Chronic Alcoholism*, Charles C Thomas, Publisher, Springfield, Ill., 1955, pp. 110–166.

———: A comparative study of the constitutions of Swiss and American alcoholic patients, in O. Diethelm (ed.), *Etiology of Chronic Alcoholism*, Charles C Thomas, Publisher, Springfield, Ill., 1955*b*, 167–178.

———: Ursache und Wesen der schizophrenen Geistesstörungen: I. Forschungsergebnisse, *Deutsch. Med. Wschr.*, 1964, 89:1865–1870.

Böök, J. A.: A genetic and neuropsychiatric investigation of a North-Swedish population with special regard to schizophrenia and mental deficiency, *Acta Genet.*, 1953, 4:1–139.

———: Schizophrenia as a gene mutation, *Acta Genet. Statist. Med.*, 1953*b*, 4:133–139.

Brown, F. W.: Heredity in the psychoneuroses, *Proc. Royal Soc. Med.*, 1942, 35:785–790.

Brugger, C.: Die erbbiologische Stellung der Pfropfschizophrenie, *Z. Ges. Neurol. Psychiat.*, 1928, 113:348.

———: Zur Frage einer Belastungsstatistik der Durchschnittbevolkerung, *Z. Ges. Neurol. Psychiat.*, 1929, 118:459–488.

———: Versuch einer Geisteskrankenzählung in Thüringen, *Z. Ges. Neurol. Psychiat.*, 1931, 133:352–390.

———: Psychiatrische Ergebnisse einer medizinischen, anthropologischen, und soziologischen Bevolkerungsuntersuchung, *Z. Ges. Neurol. Psychiat.*, 1933, **146**:489–524.

———: Familienuntersuchungen bei chronischen Alcoholikern, *Z. Ges. Neurol. Psychiat.*, 1934, **151**:103–129.

———: Psychiatrische Bestandsaufnahme in Gebiet eines medizinisch-anthropologischen Zensus in der Nähe von Rosenheim, *Z. Ges. Neurol. Psychiat.*, 1938, **160**:189–207.

Chapman, A. H.: Early infantile autism in identical twins, *Arch. Neurol. Psychiat.*, 1957, **78**:621–623.

Clayton, P. J., F. N. Pitts, Jr., and G. Winokur: Affective disorder: IV. Mania, *Comprehensive Psychiat.*, 1965, **6**:313–322.

Cowie, Valerie: The incidence of neurosis in the children of psychotics, *Acta Psychiat. Neurol. Scand.*, 1961, **37**:37–87.

Craike, W. H., and E. Slater: Folie à deux in uniovular twins reared apart, *Brain*, 1945, **68**:213–221.

Da Fonseca, A. F.: Analise heredo-clinica des perturbacoes affectivas, Ph.d. dissertation, Universidade do Porto, Portugal, 1959.

Davis, F. B.: Sex differences in suicide and attempted suicide, *Diseases Nervous System*, 1968, **29**:193–194.

Edwards, J. H.: The simulation of Mendelism, *Acta Genet. (Basel)*, 1960, **10**:63–70.

Eisenberg, L.: The autistic child in adolescence, *Am. J. Psychiat.*, 1956, **112**:607–612.

———: The fathers of autistic children, *Am. J. Orthopsychiat.*, 1957, **27**:715–724.

———: The course of childhood schizophrenia, *AMA Arch. Neurol. Psychiat.*, 1957b, **78**:69–83.

Ekblad, M.: A psychiatric and sociological study of a series of Swedish naval conscripts, 1948, cited by E. Strömgren (1950).

Elsässer, G.: *Die Nachkommen geisteskranker Elternpaare*, Georg Thieme Verlag, Stuttgart, 1952.

Erlenmeyer-Kimling, L., and W. Paradowski: Selection and schizophrenia, *Am. Naturalist*, 1966, **100**:651–665.

Essen-Möller, E.: Untersuchungen über die Fruchtbarkeit gewisser Gruppen von Geisteskranken, *Acta Psychiat. Neurol.*, Suppl. 8, 1935.

———: *Psychiatrische Untersuchungen an einer Serie von Zwillingen*, Munksgaard, Copenhagen, 1941.

———: Individual traits and morbidity in a Swedish rural population, *Acta Psychiat. Neurol. Scand.*, Suppl. 100, 1956.

———: Twin research and psychiatry, *Acta Psychiat. Neurol. Scand.*, 1963, **39**:65–77.

Eysenck, H. J., and D. B. Prell: The inheritance of neuroticism: An experimental study, *J. Mental Sci.*, 1951, **97**:441–467.

Falconer, D. S.: The inheritance of liability to certain diseases, estimated from the incidence among relatives, *Ann. Human Genet.*, 1965, **29**:51–76.

Falek, A.: Methods to investigate the interaction of environmental and genetic factors in normal and deviant traits, Paper presented at the 75th annual meeting of the American Psychological Association, 1967.

Fischer, Margit: Preliminary report of a Danish twin study on schizophrenia, prepublication copy, 1968.

Fish, Barbara: The detection of schizophrenia in infancy, *J. Nervous Mental Diseases*, 1957, **125**:1–24.

———: Longitudinal observations of biological deviations in a schizophrenic infant, *Am. J. Psychiat.*, 1959, **116**:25–31.

———: The study of motor development in infancy and its relationship to psychological functioning, *Am. J. Psychiat.*, 1961, **117**:1113–1118.

———: The maturation of arousal and attention in the first months of life: A study of variations in ego development, *J. Am. Acad. Child Psychiat.*, 1963, **2**:253–270.

Freedman, D. G.: Personality development in infancy: A biological approach, in Y. Brackbill (ed.), *Infancy and Childhood*, The Free Press, New York, 1967.

Fremming, K. H.: The expectation of mental infirmity in a sample of the Danish population, *English Society Occasional Papers on Eugenics*, no. 7, Cassell & Co., Ltd., London, 1951.

Freud, S.: Analysis terminable and interminable, in *Collected Papers*, vol. 5, The Hogarth Press, Ltd., London, 1937.

Galatschjan, A.: Die Vererbung der Schizophrenie, *Schweiz. Arch. Neurol. Psychiat.*, 1937, **39**:291–319.

Gardner, G. G.: The relationship between childhood neurotic symptomatology and later schizophrenia in males and females, *J. Nervous Mental Diseases*, 1967, **144**:97–100.

Garmezy, N.: Process and reactive schizophrenia: Some conceptions and issues, in *The Role and Methodology of Classification in Psychiatry and Psychopathology*, U.S. Department of Health, Education, & Welfare, Washington, D.C., 1965, pp. 419–466.

Garrone, G.: Étude statistique et genetique de la schizophrenie á Génève de 1901 á 1950, *J. Genet. Humaine*, 1962, **11**:89–219.

Gedda, L.: *Twins in History and Science*, Charles C Thomas, Publisher, Springfield, Ill., 1961, 240 pp.

Gengnagel, E.: Beitrag zum Problem der Erbprognosebestimmung, *Z. Ges. Neurol. Psychiat.*, 1933, **145**:52–61.

Glueck, S., and E. Glueck: *Physique and Delinquency*, Paul B. Hoeber, Inc., New York, 1956.

Goldfarb, W.: The subclassification of psychotic children: Application to a study of longitudinal change, in D. Rosenthal and S. S. Kety (eds.), *The Transmission of Schizophrenia*, Pergamon Press, London, 1968, pp. 333–342.

Gottesman, I. I.: *The Psychogenetics of Personality*, University Microfilms, Ann Arbor, 1960, 147 pp.

———: Heritability of personality: A demonstration, *Psychol. Monographs*, 1963, **77**(9):1–21.

———: Severity/concordance and diagnostic refinement in the Maudsley-Bethlem schizophrenic twin study, in D. Rosenthal and S. S. Kety (eds.), *The Transmission of Schizophrenia*, Pergamon Press, London, 1968, pp. 37–48.

———— and J. Shields: Schizophrenia in twins: 16 years, consecutive admissions to a psychiatric clinic, *Brit. J. Psychiat.*, 1966, **112**(489):809–818.

Guze, S. B.: The diagnosis of hysteria: What are we trying to do? *Am. J. Psychiat.*, 1967, **124**:491–498.

Habel, H.: Zwillingsuntersuchungen an Homosexuellen, *Z. Sex Forsch.*, 1950, **1**:161–180.

Hagnell, O.: *A Prospective Study of the Incidence of Mental Disorder,* Svenska Boknorlaget Norstedts-Bonniers, Stockholm, 1966, pp. 1–175.

Hallgren, B., and T. Sjögren: A clinical and genetico-statistical study of schizophrenia and low-grade mental deficiency in a large Swedish rural population, *Acta Psychiat. Neurol. Scand.,* Suppl. 140, 1959.

Hamburger, E.: The penitentiary and paranoia, *Corrective Psychiat.*, 1967, **13**:225–230.

Hanhart, E.: Die genetischen Probleme der Schizophrenien, *Acta Genet. Med.* (*Rome*), 1965, **14**:13–40.

Harvald, B., and M. Hauge: Hereditary factors elucidated by twin studies, in J. V. Neel, M. W. Shaw, and W. J. Schull (eds.), *Genetics and the Epidemiology of Chronic Diseases,* U.S. Department of Health, Education, & Welfare, Washington, D.C., 1965.

Held, J. M. and R. L. Cromwell: Premorbid adjustment in schizophrenia, *J. Nervous Mental Diseases,* 1968, **146**:264–272.

Helgason, T.: Epidemiology of mental disorders in Iceland, *Acta Psychiat. Neurol. Scand.,* Suppl. 173, 1964.

Heston, L. L.: Psychiatric disorders in foster home reared children of schizophrenic mothers, *Brit. J. Psychiat.*, 1966, **112**(489):819–825.

———— and J. Shields: Homosexuality in twins: A family study and a registry study, *Arch. Gen. Psychiat.*, 1968, **18**:149–160.

Hoch, P.: Clinical and biological interrelationship between schizophrenia and epilepsy, *Am. J. Psychiat.*, 1943, **99**:507–512.

———— and P. Polatin: Pseudoneurotic forms of schizophrenia, *Psychiat. Quart.,* 1949, **23**:248–276.

Hoffer, A., W. Pollin, J. R. Stabenau, M. Allen, and Z. Hrubec: Schizophrenia in the National Research Council's register of 15,909 veteran twin pairs (to be published).

Hoffmann, H.: *Die Nachkommenschaft bei endogenen Psychosen,* Springer-Verlag OHG, Berlin, 1921.

————: *Studien über Vererbung und Entstehung geistiger Störungen,* Springer-Verlag OHG, Berlin, 1921b.

Hollingshead, A. B., and F. C. Redlich: *Social Class and Mental Illness,* John Wiley & Sons, Inc., New York, 1957.

Hopkinson, G.: Celibacy and marital fertility in manic-depressive patients, *Acta Psychiat. Neurol. Scand.,* 1963, **39**:473–476.

————: A genetic study of affective illness in patients over 50, *Brit. J. Psychiat.,* 1964, **110**:244–254.

Hrebicek, S., A. Topiar, V. Mikula, and L. Puszkeiler: Psychiatric problems of murder, *Cesk. Psychiat.,* 1967, **63**:325–329. Abstract in *Crime Delin-*

quency Abst., 1967, **5**(7), National Clearing House for Mental Health Information, Chevy Chase, Md.

Huxley, J., E. Mayr, H. Osmond, and A. Hoffer: Schizophrenia as a genetic morphism, *Nature*, 1964, **204**:220–221.

Ihda, S.: A study of neurosis by twin method, *Psychiat. Neurol. Japan*, 1961, **63**:861–892.

Inouye, E.: Similarity and dissimilarity of schizophrenia in twins, *Proc. III World Congr. Psychiat. Montreal*, 1961, **1**:524–530. Published in book form by University of Toronto Press, Toronto.

Jellinek, E. M.: Heredity of the alcoholic, in *Alcohol, Science, and Society*, published by *Quart. J. Studies Alc.*, 1945, pp. 105–114.

———: *The Disease Concept of Alcoholism*, Hillhouse Press, New Haven, Conn., 1960.

Jensen, A. R.: Estimation of the limits of heritability of traits by comparison of monozygotic and dizygotic twins, *Proc. Natl. Acad. Sci.* 1967, **58**:149–156.

Juda, A.: Zum Problem der empirischen Erbprognosebestimmung, *Z. Ges. Neurol. Psychiat.*, 1928, **113**:487–517.

Juel-Nielsen, N.: *Individual and Environment: A Psychiatric-Psychological Investigation of Monozygotic Twins Reared Apart*, Munksgaard, Copenhagen, 1965, 292 pp.

Kahn, E.: Studien über Vererbung und Enstehung geistiger Störungen: IV, Schizoid und Schizophrenie im Erbung, *Monograph. Ges. Neurol. Psychiat.*, 1923, **36**:1.

Kaij, L.: *Alcoholism in Twins: Studies on the Etiology and Sequels of Abuse of Alcohol*, Almquist and Wiksell, Stockholm, 1960.

Kaila, M.: Über die Durchschnittshäufigkeit der Geisteskrankheiten und des Schwachsinns in Finnland, *Acta Psychiat. Neurol.*, 1942, **17**:47–67.

Kallmann, F. J.: *The Genetics of Schizophrenia*, J. J. Augustin, Publisher, Locust Valley, N.Y., 1938.

———: The genetic theory of schizophrenia, *Am. J. Psychiat.*, 1946, **103**:309–322.

———: The genetics of psychoses: An analysis of 1,232 twin index families, in *Congrès Internationale de Psychiatrie, Rapports VI Psychiatrie Sociale*, Paris, 1950, pp. 1–27.

———: Twin and sibship study of overt male homosexuality, *Am. J. Human Genet.*, 1952, **4**:136–146.

———: Comparative twin study on the genetic aspects of male homosexuality, *J. Nervous Mental Disease*, 1952b, **115**:283–298.

———: Genetic principles in manic-depressive psychoses: Depression, *Proc. 42d Ann. Meeting Am. Psychopathol. Assoc.*, 1952c.

———: *Heredity in Health and Mental Disorder*, W. W. Norton & Company, Inc., New York, 1953.

———: The genetics of mental illness, in S. Arieti (ed.), *American Handbook of Psychiatry*, vol. 1, Basic Books, Inc., Publishers, New York, 1959.

——— and B. Roth: Genetic aspects of preadolescent schizophrenia, *Am. J. Psychiat.*, 1956, **112**:599–606.

Kamp, L. N.: Autistic syndrome in one of a pair of monozygotic twins, *Psychiat. Neurol. Neurochir.*, 1964, **67**:143–147.

Kanner, L.: Autistic disturbances of affective contact, *Nervous Child*, 1943, **2**:217–250.

————: To what extent is early infantile autism determined by constitutional inadequacies?, in *Genetics and the Inheritance of Integrated Neurological and Psychiatric Patterns,* The Williams and Wilkins Company, Baltimore, 1954, pp. 378–385.

Kant, O.: Incidence of psychosis and other mental abnormalities in families of recovered and deteriorated schizophrenic patients, *Psychiat. Quart.*, 1942, **16**:176–186.

Karlsson, J. L.: *The Biologic Basis of Schizophrenia*, Charles C Thomas, Publisher, Springfield, Ill., 1966.

Kaufman, I., H. Durkin, Jr., T. Frank, L. W. Heims, D. B. Jones, Z. Ryter, E. Stone, and J. Zilbach: Delineation of two diagnostic groups among juvenile delinquents: The schizophrenic and the impulse-ridden character disorder, *J. Am. Acad. Child Psychiat.*, 1963, **2**:292–318.

Kendell, R. E.: An important source of bias affecting ratings made by psychiatrists, *J. Psychiat. Res.*, 1968, **6**:135–142.

Kent, E.: A study of maladjusted twins, *Smith Coll. Studies Soc. Work*, 1949, **19**:63–77.

Kety, S. S., D. Rosenthal, P. H. Wender, and F. Schulsinger: The types and prevalence of mental illness in the biological and adoptive families of adopted schizophrenics, in D. Rosenthal and S. S. Kety (eds.), *The Transmission of Schizophrenia*, Pergamon Press, London, 1968, pp. 345–362.

Kinsey, A. C., W. B. Pomeroy, and C. E. Martin: *Sexual Behavior in the Human Male*, W. B. Saunders Company, Philadelphia, 1948.

————, ————, ————, and P. H. Gebhard: *Sexual Behavior in the Human Female*, W. B. Saunders Company, Philadelphia, 1953.

Kishimoto, K.: A study on the population genetics of schizophrenia, *Proc. 2d Intern. Congr. Psychiat.* (*Zurich*), 1957, **2**:20–28.

Klemperer, J.: Zur Belastungstatistik der Durchschnittsbevölkerung, *Z. Ges. Neurol. Psychiat.*, 1933, **146**:277–316.

Kolle, K.: *Die Primäre Verrücktheit*, Georg Thieme Verlag, Leipzig, 1931.

Konstantinu, T.: Zum Problem der Erbprognosetimmung, *Z. Ges. Neurol. Psychiat.*, 1930, **125**:103–133.

Kraepelin, E.: *Psychiatrie*, Johann Ambrosius Barth, Leipzig, 5th ed., 1896.

————: Dementia praecox (Insanity of adolescence), in C. E. Goshen (ed.), *Documentary History of Psychiatry*, Philosophical Library, Inc., New York, 1967, pp. 200–210.

Krafft-Ebing, R. von: *Psychopathia sexualis* (12th ed.), Pioneer Publications, New York, 1939.

Kranz, H.: *Lebenschicksale krimineller Zwillinge*, Springer-Verlag OHG, Berlin, 1936.

————: Untersuchungen an Zwillingen in Fursorgeerziehungsanstalten, *Z. Induktive Abstammungs-Vererbungslehre*, 1937, **73**:508–512.

Kreitman, N.: Married couples admitted to mental hospital, *Brit. J. Psychiat.,* 1968, **114**:699–718.

Kretschmer, E.: *Physique and Character,* Harcourt, Brace and Company, Inc., New York, 1923.

Kringlen, E.: *Schizophrenia in Male Monozygotic Twins,* University Press, Oslo, 1964, and *Acta Psychiat. Scand.,* Suppl. 178, 1964.

———: Hereditary and social factors in schizophrenic twins: An epidemiological-clinical study, in J. Romano (ed.), *The Origins of Schizophrenia,* Excerpta Medica Foundation, New York, 1967, pp. 2–14.

Landis, C., and J. D. Page: *Modern Society and Mental Disease,* Farrar & Rhinehart, Inc., New York, 1938.

Lang, T.: Untersuchungen an männlichen Homosexuellen und deren Sippen-zwischen Homosexualität und Psychose, *Z. Ges. Neurol. Psychiat.,* 1941, **171**:651–679.

Lange, J.: *Verbrechen als Schieksal,* Georg Thieme Verlag, Leipzig, 1929.

———: *Crime as Destiny* (trans. C. Haldane), George Allen & Unwin, Ltd., London, 1931.

———: *Kurzgefasstes Lehrbuch der Psychiatrie,* Georg Thieme Verlag, Leipzig, 1935.

Langfeldt, G.: *The Schizophreniform States,* Munksgaard, Copenhagen, 1939.

Langner, T. S., and S. T. Michael: *Life Stress and Mental Health,* Glencoe Press, The Macmillan Company, New York, 1963.

Legras, A. M.: *Psychose en Criminaliteit bij Tweelingen,* University of Utrecht, 1932, cited by Rosanoff et al., 1934.

Lehrman, E., J. Haber, and S. R. Lesser: The use of reserpine in autistic children, *J. Nervous Mental Disease,* 1957, **125**:351–356.

Leighton, A. H., T. A. Lambo, C. C. Hughes, D. C. Leighton, J. M. Murphy, and D. B. Mackline: Psychiatric disorder in West Africa, *Am. J. Psychiat.,* 1963, **120**:521–525.

Lemere, F., W. L. Voegtlin, W. R. Broz, P. O'Hallaren, and W. E. Tupper: Heredity as an etiologic factor in chronic alcoholism, *Northwest Med.,* 1943, **42**:110–111.

Lemkau, P., C. Tietze, and M. Cooper: Mental hygiene problems in an urban district, *Mental Hygiene,* 1941, **25**:624; 1942, **26**:100, **26**:275; 1943, **27**:279.

Leonhard, K.: *Die Defektschizophrenen Krankheitsbilder,* Georg Thieme Verlag, Leipzig, 1936.

———: *Aufteilung der endogenen Psychosen,* Akademie-Verlag GmbH, Berlin, 1959.

Lewis, A. J.: The offspring of parents both mentally ill, *Acta Genet. (Basel),* 1957, **7**:349–365.

———: Families with manic-depressive psychosis, *Eugenics Quart.,* 1959, **6**:130–137.

Lin, Tsung-Yi.: A study of the incidence of mental disorder in Chinese and other cultures, *Psychiatry,* 1953, **16**:313–336.

Luxenburger, H.: Vorläufiger Bericht über psychiatrische Sereinuntersuchungen an Zwillingen, *Z. Ges. Neurol. Psychiat.,* 1928, **116**:297–347.

————: Demographische und psychiatrische Untersuchungen in der engeren biologischen Familie von Paralytikerehegatten, *Z. Ges. Neurol. Psychiat.*, 1928*b*, **112**:331–492.

————: Heredität und Familientypus der Zwangsneurotiker, *V. Kongr. Psychother.* (Baden-Baden), 1930.

————: Psychiatrisch-neurologische Zwillingspathologie, *Zbl. Ges. Neurol. Psychiat.*, 1930*b*, **56**:145–180.

————: Die Manifestationswahrscheinlichkeit der Schizophrenie im Lichte der Zwillingsforschung, *Z. Psychol. Hyg.*, 1934, **7**:174–184.

————: Untersuchungen an schizophrenen Zwillingen und ihren Geschwistern zur Prüfung der Realität von Manifestationsschwankungen, *Z. Ges. Neurol. Psychiat.*, 1935, **154**:351–394.

————: Zur frage der Erbberatung in den Familien Schizophrener, *Med. Klin.*, 1936, **32**:1136–1138.

————: Das zirkuläre Irresein, in A. Gutt (ed.), *Handbuch der Erbkrankheiten*, Georg Thieme Verlag, Leipzig, vol. 4, 1942.

MacLean, Paul D.: New findings relevant to the evolution of psychosexual functions of the brain, *J. Nervous Mental Disease*, 1962, **135**:289–301.

————: Man and his animal brains, *Modern Med.*, February 3, 1964, 95–106.

————: The brain in relation to empathy and medical education, *J. Nervous Mental Disease*, 1967, **144**:374–382.

MacSorley, K.: An investigation into the fertility rates of mentally ill patients, *Ann. Human Genet.*, 1964, **27**:247–256.

Malzberg, B.: A statistical study of age in relation to mental disease, *Mental Hygiene*, 1935, **19**:449–476.

Mayer-Gross, W.: Mental health survey in a rural area, *Eugenics Rev.*, 1948, **40**:140–148.

Mednick, S. A.: A learning theory approach to research in schizophrenia, *Psychol. Bull.*, 1958, **55**:315–327.

———— and F. Schulsinger: Some premorbid characteristics related to breakdown in children with schizophrenic mothers, in D. Rosenthal and S. S. Kety (eds.), *The Transmission of Schizophrenia*, Pergamon Press, London, 1968, pp. 267–291.

Meduna, J. L.: *Die konvulsive Therapie der Schizophrenie*, Carl Mahrhold, Halle, 1937.

Meehl, P. E.: Schizotaxia, schizotypy, schizophrenia, *Am. Psychol.*, 1962, **17**:827–838.

Merrell, D. J.: Inheritance of manic-depressive psychosis, *AMA Arch. Neurol. Psychiat.*, 1951, **66**:272–279.

Mitsuda, H.: The concept of "atypical psychoses" from the aspect of clinical genetics, *Acta Psychiat. Scand.*, 1965, **41**:372–377.

————: A clinico-genetic study of schizophrenia, in H. Mitsuda (ed.), *Clinical Genetics in Psychiatry*, Igaku Shoin, Tokyo, 1967, pp. 49–90.

————: Genealogical and clinical study on the relationship between schizophrenia and genuine epilepsy, in H. Mitsuda (ed.), *Clinical Genetics in Psychiatry*, Igaku Shoin, Tokyo, 1967*b*, pp. 98–107.

————, T. Sakai, and J. Kobayashi: A clinico-genetic study on the relationship between neurosis and psychosis, in H. Mitsuda (ed.), *Clinical Genetics in Psychiatry*, Igaku Shoin, Tokyo, 1967, pp. 27–35.

Murphy, H. B. M.: Cultural factors in the genesis of schizophrenia, in D. Rosenthal and S. S. Kety (eds.), *The Transmission of Schizophrenia*, Pergamon Press, London, 1968, pp. 137–153.

Nagao, S.: Clinico-genetic study of chronic alcoholism, in H. Mitsuda (ed.), *Clinical Genetics in Psychiatry*, Igaku Shoin, Tokyo, 1967, pp. 288–302.

Nameche, G., M. Waring, and D. Ricks: Early indicators of outcome in schizophrenia, *J. Nervous Mental Disease*, 1964, **139**:232–240.

Newman, H. H., F. N. Freeman, and K. J. Holzinger: *Twins: A Study of Heredity and Environment*, University of Chicago Press, Chicago, 1937.

Nichols, R. C.: The resemblance of twins in personality and interests, *Natl. Merit Scholarship Corp. Res. Rep.*, 1966, **2**(8):1–23.

Nielsen, J., W. Wilsnack, and E. Strömgren: Some aspects of community psychiatry, *Brit. J. Prevent. Social Med.*, 1965, **19**:85–93.

Nixon, W. L. B., and E. Slater: A second investigation into the children of cousins, *Acta Genet.*, 1957, **7**:513–532.

Norris, V.: Mental illness in London: A statistical study of the influence of marriage on the hospital care of the mentally sick, *J. Mental Sci.*, 1956, **102**:467.

Ödegaard, Ö.:The epidemiology of depressive psychosis: Depression, *Acta Psychiat. Neurol. Scand.*, Suppl. 162, 1961, 33–38.

————: The psychiatric disease entities in the light of a genetic investigation, *Acta Psychiat. Neurol. Scand.*, 1963, **39**:94–104.

Oki, T.: A psychological study of early childhood neuroses, in H. Mitsuda (ed.), *Clinical Genetics in Psychiatry*, Igaku Shoin, Tokyo, 1967, pp. 344–359.

Oppler, W.: Zum Problem der Erbprognosebestimmung, *Z. Ges. Neurol. Psychiat.*, 1932, **141**:549–616.

Panse, F.: Beitrag zur Belastungsstatistik einer Durchschnittsbevolkerung, *Z. Ges. Neurol. Psychiat.*, 1936, **154**:194–222.

Parker, N.: Twin relationships and concordance for neurosis. *Proc. 4th World Cong. Psychiat.*, Excerpta Medica International Congress Series, no. 150, New York, 1966, pp. 1112–1115.

Partanen, J., K. Bruun, and T. Markkanen: *Inheritance of Drinking Behavior: A study on intelligence, personality, and use of alcohol of adult twins*, The Finnish Foundation for Alcohol Studies, no. 14, 1966, 159 pp., Almquist and Wiksell, Stockholm.

Penrose, L. S.: Mutations in man, *Acta Genet.*, 1956, **6**:160 182.

Planansky, K., and R. Johnston: The incidence and relationship of homosexual and paranoid features in schizophrenia, *J. Mental Sci.*, 1962, **108**:604–615.

Pollin, W., and J. R. Stabenau: Biological, psychological, and historical differences in a series of monozygotic twins discordant for schizophrenia, in D. Rosenthal and S. S. Kety (eds.), *The Transmission of Schizophrenia*, Pergamon Press, London, 1968, pp. 317–332.

Pollock, H. M., and B. Malzberg: Hereditary and environmental factors in the causation of manic-depressive psychoses and dementia praecox, *Am. J. Psychiat.*, 1940, **96**:1227–1247.

Pugh, T. F., and B. MacMahon: *Epidemiologic Findings in United States Mental Hospital Data*, Little, Brown and Company, Boston, 1962.

Reid, D. D.: *Epidemiological Methods in the Study of Mental Disorders*, World Health Organization, Geneva, 1960, 79 pp.

Rin, H., and T-Y. Lin: Mental illness among Formosan aborigines as compared with the Chinese in Taiwan, *J. Ment. Sci.*, 1962, **108**:134–146.

Robins, Lee N.: *Deviant Children Grown Up*, The Williams and Wilkins Company, Baltimore, 1966.

Roe, Anne: Children of alcoholic parentage raised in foster homes, in *Alcohol, Science, and Society*, published by *Quart. J. Studies Alc.*, 1945, pp. 115–127.

Rohr, K.: Beitrag zur Kenntnis der sogenannten schizophrenen Reaktion, *Arch. Psychiat. Nervenkr.*, 1961, **201**:626–647.

Röll, A., and J. L. Entres: Zum Problem der Erbprognosebestimmung, *Z. Ges. Neurol. Psychiat.*, 1936, **156**:169–202.

Rosanoff, A. J., L. M. Handy, and I. R. Plesset: The etiology of manic-depressive syndromes with special reference to their occurrence in twins, *Am. J. Psychiat.*, 1934, **91**:247–286.

———, ———, and ———: Criminality and delinquency in twins, *J. Crim. Law Criminol.*, 1934b, **24**:923–934.

———, ———, ———, and S. Brush: The etiology of so-called schizophrenic psychoses, *Am. J. Psychiat.*, 1934–1935, **91**:247–286.

Rosenbaum, C. P.: Metabolic, physiological, anatomic and genetic studies in the schizophrenias: A review and analysis, *J. Nervous Mental Disease*, 1968, **146**:103–126.

Rosenthal, D.: Some factors associated with concordance and discordance with respect to schizophrenia in monozygotic twins, *J. Nervous Mental Disease*, 1959, **129**:1–10.

———: Confusion of identity and the frequency of schizophrenia in twins, *Arch. Gen. Psychiat.*, 1960, **3**:297–304.

———: Sex distribution and the severity of illness among samples of schizophrenic twins, *J. Psychiat. Res.*, 1961, **1**:26–36.

———: Problems of sampling and diagnosis in the major twin studies of schizophrenia, *J. Psychiat. Res.*, 1962, **1**:116–134.

———: Familial concordance by sex with respect to schizophrenia, *Psychol. Bull.*, 1962, **59**:401–421.

——— (ed.): *The Genain Quadruplets*, Basic Books, Inc., Publishers, New York, 1963.

———: The offspring of schizophrenic couples, *J. Psychiat. Res.*, 1966, **4**:169–188.

——— and J. D. Frank: The fate of psychiatric clinic outpatients assigned to psychotherapy, *J. Nervous Mental Disease*, 1958, **127**:330–343.

——— and S. S. Kety (eds.): *The Transmission of Schizophrenia*, Pergamon Press, London, 1968.

────── and J. Van Dyke: The use of monozygotic twins discordant as to schizophrenia in the search for an inherited characterological defect, *Acta Psychiat. Scand.*, in press.

──────, P. H. Wender, S. S. Kety, F. Schulsinger, J. Welner, and L. Östergaard: Schizophrenics' offspring reared in adoptive homes, in D. Rosenthal and S. S. Kety (eds.), *The Transmission of Schizophrenia*, Pergamon Press, London, 1968, pp. 377–391.

Rüdin, E.: *Zur Vererbung und Neuentstehung der Dementia praecox*, Springer Verlag OHG, Berlin, 1916.

──────: Über Vererbung geistiger Störungen, *Z. Ges. Neurol. Psychiat.*, 1923, **81**:459–496.

Rüdin, Edith: Ein Beitrag zur Frage der Zwangskrankheit, insbesondere ihre hereditären Beziehungen, *Arch. Psychiat. Nervenkr.*, 1953, **191**:14–54.

Sakai, T.: Clinico-genetic study on obsessive-compulsive neurosis, in H. Mitsuda (ed), *Clinical Genetics in Psychiatry*, Igaku Shoin, Tokyo, 1967, pp. 332–343.

Sanders, J.: Homosexueele tweelingen, *Ned. Tijdschr. Gennesk*, 1934, **78**: 3346–3352.

Schade, H.: Ergebnisse einer Bevolkerungsunterschung in der Schwalm, *Abhandl. Deut. Akad. Wiss. Kl. Math. Allgem. Naturw. Mainz*, 1950, **16**:1–75.

Schaedler, E.: *Eine Untersuchung uber die Nachfahren Manisch-Depressiver*, Ph.D. dissertation, University of Wurzburg, Wurzburg, 1938. Cited by Zerbin-Rüdin, 1967.

Scheinfeld, A.: *Your Heredity and Environment*, J. B. Lippincott Company, Philadelphia, 1965, 830 pp.

──────: *Twins and Supertwins*, J. B. Lippincott Company, Philadelphia, 1967, 292 pp.

Schmidt, H. V., and C. P. Fonda: The reliability of psychiatric diagnoses: A new look, *J. Abnormal Social Psychol.*, 1956, **52**:262–267.

Schmidt-Kehl, L.: Die Erkrankungswahrscheinlichkeit der Enkel für Manisch-Depressiven Irresein, *Allgem. Z. Psychiat.*, 1939, **113**:83–85.

Schulz, B.: Zum Problem der Erbprognosebestimmung, *Z. Ges. Neurol. Psychiat.*, 1926, **102**:1–37.

──────: Zur Belastungsstatistik der Durchschnittsbevolkerung, *Z. Ges. Neurol. Psychiat.*, 1931, **136**:386–411.

──────: Zur Erbpathologie der Schizophrenie, *Z. Ges. Neurol. Psychiat.*, 1932, **143**:175–293.

──────: Kinder manisch-depressiver und anderer affektivpsychotischer Elternpaare, *Z. Ges. Neurol. Psychiat.*, 1940, **169**:311–412.

──────: Kinder schizophrener Elternpaare, *Z. Ges. Neurol. Psychiat.*, 1940*b*, **168**:332–381.

──────: Kinder von Elternpaaren mit einem schizophrenen und einem affektivpsychotischen Partner, *Z. Ges. Neurol. Psychiat.*, 1940*c*, **170**:441–514.

──────: Sterblichkeit endogen Geisteskranker und ihrer Eltern, *Z. Menschl. Vererb.-Konstit.-Lehre*, 1949–1950, **29**:338–367.

──────: Auszählungen in der Verwandtschaft von nach Erkrankungsalter und

Geschlecht gruppierten Manisch-Depressiven, *Arch. Psychiat. Nervenkr.,* 1951, **186**:560–576.

Sherfey, M. J.: Psychopathology and character structure in chronic alcoholism, in O. Diethelm (ed.), *Etiology of Chronic Alcoholism,* Charles C Thomas, Publisher, Springfield, Ill., 1955, pp. 16–42.

Sherwin, A. C.: Reactions to music of autistic (schizophrenic) children, *Am. J. Psychiat.,* 1953, **109**:823–831.

Shields, J.: Personality differences and neurotic traits in normal twin school-children, *Eugenics Rev.,* 1954, **45**:213–246.

———: *Monzygotic Twins: Brought Up Apart and Together,* Oxford University Press, London, 1962, 264 pp.

Sjögren, T.: Investigations of the heredity of psychoses and mental deficiency in two north Swedish parishes, *Ann. Eugenics,* 1935, **6**:253–318.

———: Genetic-statistical and psychiatric investigations of a West Swedish population, *Acta Psychiat. Neurol.,* Suppl. 52, 1948.

Slater, E.: Erbpathologie des manisch-depressiven Irreseins, Die Eltern und Kinder von Manisch-Depressiven, *Z. Ges. Neurol. Psychiat.,* 1938, **163**:1–47.

———: *Psychotic and Neurotic Illnesses in Twins,* Her Majesty's Stationary Office, London, 1953.

———: Genetic investigations in twins, *J. Mental Sci.,* 1953b, **99**:44–52.

———: Clinical aspects of genetic mental disorders, in J. N. Cummings and M. Kremer (eds.), *Biochemical Aspects of Neurological Disorders,* 2d series, Blackwell Scientific Publications, Ltd., Oxford, 1965, pp. 271–285.

———: A review of earlier evidence on genetic factors in schizophrenia, in D. Rosenthal and S. S. Kety (eds.), *The Transmission of Schizophrenia,* Pergamon Press, London, 1968, pp. 15–26.

Smith, J. C.: Dementia-praecox problems, *Z. Ges. Neurol. Psychiat.,* 1936, **156**:361–381.

Sobel, D. E.: Children of schizophrenic patients: Preliminary observations on early development, *Am. J. Psychiat.,* 1961, **118**:512–517.

Stenstedt, A.: A study in manic-depressive psychosis: Clinical, social and genetic investigations, *Acta Psychiat. Neurol. Scand.,* Suppl. 79, 1952.

———: Genetics of neurotic depression, *Acta Psychiat. Scand.,* 1966, **42**:398–409.

Strömgren, E.: *Beiträge zur psychiatrischen Erblehre,* Munksgaard, Copenhagen, 1938.

———: Statistical and genetical population studies within psychiatry: Methods and principal results, in *Congrès International de Psychiatrie, Paris, 1950,* part VI, Hermann & Cie, Paris 1950, pp. 155–188.

Stumpfl, F.: *Die Ursprunge des Verbrechens am Lebenslauf von Zwillingen,* Georg Thieme Verlag, Leipzig, 1936.

———: Untersuchungen an psychopathischen Zwillingen, *Z. Ges. Neurol. Psychiat.,* 1937, **158**:480–482.

Taschev, T.: Statistisches über die Melancholie, *Fortschr. Neurol. Psychiat.,* 1965, **33**:25–36.

Tienari, P.: Psychiatric illness in identical twins, *Acta Psychiat. Neurol. Scand.,* Suppl. 171, 1963.

————: Schizophrenia in monozygotic male twins, in D. Rosenthal and S. S. Kety (eds.), *The Transmission of Schizophrenia*, Pergamon Press, London, 1968, pp. 27–36.

Tsuda, K.: Clinico-genetic study of depersonalization neurosis, in H. Mitsuda (ed.), *Clinical Genetics in Psychiatry*, Igaku Shoin, Tokyo, 1967, pp. 332–343.

Turner, J. J.: A syndrome of infantilism, congenital webbed neck, and cubitus valgus, *Endocrinology*, 1938, **23**:566–574.

Vaillant, G. E.: The prediction of recovery in schizophrenia, *J. Nervous Mental Disease*, 1962, **135**:534–543.

————: Twins discordant for early infantile autism, *Arch. Gen. Psychiat.*, 1963, **9**:163–167.

von Tomasson, H.: Further investigations on manic-depressive psychosis, *Acta Psychiat. Neurol.*, 1938, **13**:517–526.

Walker, H.: Zum Problem der empirische Erbprognosebestimmung, *Z. Ges. Neurol. Psychiat.*, 1929, **120**:100–120.

Wallinga, J. V.: Variability of psychiatric diagnosis, *U.S. Armed Forces Med. J.*, 1956, **7**:1305–1312.

Ward, T. F., and B. A. Hoddinott: Early infantile autism in fraternal twins: A case report, *Can. Psychiat. Assoc. J.*, 1962, **7**:191–195.

Weinberg, I., and J. Lobstein: Beitrag zur Vererbung des manisch-depressiven Irreseins, *Psychiat. Neurol. Bull.* (Amsterdam), 1936, **1a**(1):339–372.

———— and ————: Inheritance in schizophrenia, *Acta Psychiat. Neurol.*, 1943, **18**:93–140.

Welner, J., and E. Strömgren: Clinical and genetic studies on benign schizophreniform psychoses based on a follow-up, *Acta Psychiat. Neurol. Scand.*, 1958, **33**:377–399.

Wender, P. H., D. Rosenthal, and S. S. Kety: A psychiatric assessment of the adoptive parents of schizophrenics, in D. Rosenthal and S. S. Kety (eds.), *The Transmission of Schizophrenia*, Pergamon Press, London, 1968, pp. 235–250.

Wilde, G. J. S.: Inheritance of personality traits: An investigation into the hereditary determination of neurotic instability, extraversion, and other personality traits by means of a questionnaire administered to twins, *Acta Psychol.*, 1964, **22**:37–51.

Winokur, G.: X-borne recessive genes in alcoholism, *Lancet*, 1967, p. 466.

———— and P. Clayton: Family history studies: I. Two types of affective disorders separated according to genetic and clinical factors, in *Recent Advances in Biological Psychiatry*, vol. 9, Plenum Press, Plenum Publishing Corporation, 1967.

———— and F. N. Pitts, Jr.: Affective disorder: I. Is reactive depression an entity? *J. Nervous Mental Disease*, 1964, **138**:541–547.

———— and ————: Affective reaction: V. The diagnostic validity of depressive reaction, *Psychiat. Quart.*, 1965, **39**:1–2.

Wittermans, W., and B. Schulz: Genealogischer Beitrag zur Frage der geheilten Schizophrenien, *Arch. Psychiat. Nervenkr.*, 1950, **185**:211–232.

Woodruff, F. N., Jr., F. N. Pitts, Jr., and G. Winokur: Affective disorder: II. A comparison of patients with and without family history of affective disorder, *J. Nervous Mental Disease*, 1964, **139**:49–52.

World Health Organization: *Manual of the International Statistical Classification of Diseases, Injuries and Causes of Death*, Geneva, 1957.

Zerbin-Rüdin, Edith: Über den Gesundheitszustand von Kindern aus nähen Blutsverwandtenehen, *Z. Menschl. Vererb.-Konstit.-Lehre*, 1960, **35**:233–302.

————: Endogene Psychosen, in P. E. Becker (ed.), *Humangenetik: ein kurzes Handbuch in fünf Bänden*, vol. 2, Georg Thieme Verlag, Stuttgart, 1967, pp. 446–577.

Zolan, H., and N. Bigelow: Family taint and response to treatment in functional disorder, *Psychiat. Quart.*, 1950, **24**:672–676.

zur Nieden, M.: The influence of constitution and environment upon the development of adopted children, *J. Psychol.*, 1951, **31**:91–95.

Name Index

Name Index

Subject Index

Subject Index